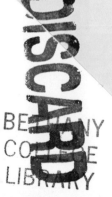

PROSTAGLANDINS IN CLINICAL MEDICINE
Cardiovascular and Thrombotic Disorders

PROSTAGLANDINS IN CLINICAL MEDICINE
CARDIOVASCULAR AND THROMBOTIC DISORDERS

Edited by

KENNETH K. WU, M.D.
Professor and Chief
Coagulation and Thrombosis Unit
Rush Medical College
Chicago, Illinois

ENNIO C. ROSSI, M.D.
Professor and Chief
Section of Hematology
Northwestern University
School of Medicine
Chicago, Illinois

Proceedings of an International Symposium
"Prostaglandins in Cardiovascular and Thrombotic Disorders"
Chicago, Illinois, May 7–9, 1981

YEAR BOOK MEDICAL PUBLISHERS, INC.
Chicago • London

Library of Congress Cataloging in Publication Data
Main entry under title:

Prostaglandins in clinical medicine.

    Includes index.
    1. Cardiovascular system—Diseases—Chemotherapy—
Congresses. 2. Prostaglandins—Therapeutic use—
Congresses. 3. Thrombosis—Chemotherapy—Congresses.
I. Wu, Kenneth K. II. Rossi, Ennio C.
[DNLM: 1. Prostaglandins—Therapeutic use—Congresses.
2. Prostaglandins—Pharmacodynamics—Congresses.
3. Cardiovascular diseases—Drug therapy—Congresses.
4. Thrombosis—Drug therapy—Congresses. 5. Lung
diseases—Drug therapy—Congresses. QU 90 P969 1981]
RC684.P76P76   616.1'061   81-23995
ISBN 0-8151-9609-1   AACR2

Contributors

C. ARÉN, Sahlgrenska Sjukhuset, Göteborg, Sweden

NAJAM A. AWAN, University of California, Davis, School of Medicine; Sacramento (Calif.) Medical Center

R. N. BAIRD, Bristol (England) Royal Infirmary

JAMES M. BEATTIE, University of California, Davis, School of Medicine; Sacramento (Calif.) Medical Center

VITTORIO BERTELE, Mario Negri Institute for Pharmacological Research, Milan, Italy

EUGENE H. BLACKSTONE, University of Alabama, School of Medicine, Birmingham

F. WILLIAM BLAISDELL, University of California, Davis, School of Medicine

M. J. BROEKMAN, New York Veterans Administration Medical Center, New York

W. P. BROWN, Upjohn Company, Kalamazoo, Michigan

WILLIAM B. CAMPBELL, University of Texas Health Science Center, Dallas

CHIARA CERLETTI, Mario Negri Institute for Pharmacological Research, Milan, Italy

DENNIS E. CHENOWETH, Scripps Clinic and Research Foundation, La Jolla, California

P. C. CLIFFORD, Bristol (England) Royal Infirmary

F. COCEANI, Hospital for Sick Children, Toronto, Canada

JOANN L. DATA, Burroughs Wellcome Company, Research Triangle Park, North Carolina

GIOVANNI DE GAETANO, Mario Negri Institute for Pharmacological Research, Milan, Italy

GARRY L. DE GRAAF, Upjohn Company, Kalamazoo, Michigan

MRINAL K. DEWANJEE, Mayo Clinic and Foundation, Rochester, Minnesota

P. A. DIEPPE, Bristol (England) Royal Infirmary

GIOVANNI DI MINNO, Mario Negri Institute for Pharmacological Research, Milan, Italy

DONALD W. DUCHARME, Upjohn Company, Kalamazoo, Michigan ·

v

MICHAEL J. DUNN, Case Western Reserve University; University Hospitals of Cleveland (Ohio)

A. J. DUTKA, Naval Medical Research Institute, Bethesda, Maryland

H. H. G. EASTCOTT, St. Mary's Hospital, London, England

N. EGBERG, Karolinska Sjukhuset, Stockholm, Sweden

ANDERS ERIK EKLUND, Danderyd Hospital, Stockholm, Sweden

BRITA EKLUND, Karolinska Hospital, Stockholm, Sweden

GUNNEL ERIKSSON, Danderyd Hospital, Stockholm, Sweden

MARK K. EVENSON, University of California, Davis, School of Medicine; Sacramento (Calif.) Medical Center

THOMAS F. FERRIS, University of Minnesota Hospitals, Minneapolis

BRIAN G. FIRTH, University of Texas Health Science Center, Dallas

GARRET A. FITZGERALD, Vanderbilt University, Nashville, Tennessee

F. A. FITZPATRICK, Upjohn Company, Kalamazoo, Michigan

HO-LEUNG FUNG, State University of New York, Buffalo

ROBERT R. GORMAN, Upjohn Company, Kalamazoo, Michigan

L. J. GREENBAUM, JR., Naval Medical Research Institute, Bethesda, Maryland

RYSZARD J. GRYGLEWSKI, N. Copernicus Academy of Medicine, Krakow, Poland

J. M. HALLENBECK, Naval Medical Research Institute, Bethesda, Maryland

KATHLEEN E. HARRIS, Northwestern University Medical School, Chicago

MICHAEL A. HEYMANN, University of California, San Francisco, School of Medicine

L. DAVID HILLIS, University of Texas Health Science Center, Dallas

PAUL D. HIRSH, University of Texas Health Science Center, Dallas

JOHN C. HOAK, University of Iowa College of Medicine, Iowa City

JAMES W. HOLCROFT, University of California, Davis, School of Medicine

STEPHEN J. HUMPHREY, M.D., Upjohn Company, Kalamazoo, Michigan

E. A. JAFFE, Cornell University Medical College, New York

TORBJÖRN JORETEG, Karolinska Hospital, Stockholm, Sweden

LENNART KAIJSER, Karolinska Hospital, Stockholm, Sweden

MICHAEL P. KAYE, Mayo Clinic and Foundation, Rochester, Minnesota

JOHN W. KIRKLIN, University of Alabama, School of Medicine, Birmingham

D. R. LEITCH, Naval Medical Research Institute, Bethesda, Maryland

PETER R. LICHTENTHAL, Northwestern University Medical School, Chicago

O. I. LINET, Upjohn Company, Kalamazoo, Michigan

JOHN E. LUND, Upjohn Company, Kalamazoo, Michigan

JOHN C. MC GIFF, New York Medical College, Valhalla

A. J. MARCUS, New York Veterans Administration Medical Center, New York

M. F. R. MARTIN, Bristol (England) Royal Infirmary

DEAN T. MASON, University of California, Davis, School of Medicine; Sacramento (Calif.) Medical Center

LAWRENCE L. MICHAELIS, Northwestern University School of Medicine, Chicago

KATHLEEN E. NEEDHAM, University of California, Davis, School of Medicine; Sacramento (Calif.) Medical Center

PHILIP NEEDLEMAN, Washington University Medical School, St. Louis

MARK NEMEROVSKI, UCLA School of Medicine; Cedars-Sinai Medical Center, Los Angeles

CARL R. NOBACK, Mayo Clinic and Foundation, Rochester, Minnesota

P. M. OLLEY, Hospital for Sick Children, Toronto, Canada

ANDERS G. OLSSON, Karolinska Sjukhuset, Stockholm, Sweden

C. PAPACONSTANTINOU, Karolinska Sjukhuset, Stockholm, Sweden

BRUCE J. PARDY, St. Mary's Hospital, London, England

ROY PATTERSON, Northwestern University Medical School, Chicago

NORBERTO PERICO, Ospedali Riuniti di Bergamo, Bergamo, Italy

KEVIN A. PETERSON, Mayo Clinic and Foundation, Rochester, Minnesota

CH. PUNZENGRUBER, University of Vienna, Vienna, Austria

K. RADEGRAN, University of Göteborg (Sweden)

GIUSEPPE REMUZZI, Ospedali Riuniti de Bergamo, Bergamo, Italy

ENNIO C. ROSSI, Northwestern University School of Medicine, Chicago

L. B. SAFIER, New York Veterans Administration Medical Center, New York

EDWIN W. SALZMAN, Beth Israel Hospital, Boston

WILLIAM E. SHELL, UCLA School of Medicine, Cedars-Sinai Medical Center, Los Angeles

K. SILBERBAUER, University of Vienna, Vienna, Austria

H. SINZINGER, University of Vienna, Vienna, Austria

ERIC G. SPOKAS, New York Medical College, Valhalla

ROBERT W. STEWART, University of Alabama School of Medicine, Birmingham

ANDREW SZCZEKLIK, N. Copernicus Academy of Medicine, Krakow, Poland

K. TACK-GOLDMAN, New York Veterans Administration Medical Center, New York

A. C. TEGER-NILSSON, Sahlgrenska Sjukhuset, Göteborg, Sweden

L. TREGERMAN, Upjohn Company, Kalamazoo, Michigan

H. L. ULLMAN, New York Veterans Administration Medical Center, New York

B. B. WEKSLER, Cornell University Medical College, New York

J. T. WHICHER, Bristol (England) Royal Infirmary

JAMES T. WILLERSON, University of Texas Health Science Center, Dallas

PATRICK Y. K. WONG, New York Medical College, Valhalla

KENNETH K. WU, Rush Medical College, Chicago

M. A. WYNALDA, Upjohn Company, Kalamazoo, Michigan

EDWARD J. ZAMBRASKI, Rutgers University, New Brunswick, New Jersey

Contents

I. Basic Principles of Prostaglandins

II. Physiologic Effects of Prostaglandins

III. Prostaglandins in Peripheral Vascular Disease

VI. Prostaglandins in Thrombosis

VII. Prostaglandins in Cardiopulmonary Bypass Surgery

Preface

Fifty-one years ago, human seminal fluid was shown to produce contraction of smooth muscle. Von Euler found this activity in extracts of the prostate gland and named the active principle "prostaglandin." These early observations, which introduced a new era, did not receive much attention for two decades. Subsequently, however, prostaglandins have been characterized, and their biological actions have been well described. They appear to play an important role in the regulation of many physiologic systems, and the steady flow of new information continually broadens the arena in which prostaglandins appear to act. Important clinical applications seem inevitable.

On the 7th, 8th, and 9th of May, 1981, an international symposium sponsored by Rush Medical College and the Northwestern University School of Medicine, was held in Chicago to explore the clinical applications of prostaglandins in cardiovascular and thrombotic disorders. This volume contains the proceedings of that symposium. The first two sections deal with the basic principles and physiologic effects of prostaglandins. They are followed by sections that describe clinical trials of prostaglandins in peripheral vascular and coronary artery disease; their potential role in asthma, persistent fetal pulmonary circulation, and thrombotic disorders; and the use of prostacyclin in cardiopulmonary bypass surgery.

Frequently, the goal of symposia proceedings is limited to the gathering and organization of previously published information. We believe these proceedings may exceed this limitation. Because of the rapid progress in prostaglandin research, a significant amount of the information presented—especially on clinical trials—is new. We hope the reader will share our view that the clinical data obtained to date confirm the promise of prostaglandin research and foreshadow clinical applications yet to come.

ACKNOWLEDGMENTS

We wish to thank Drs. Udo Axen, Edmond Cole, Francesco del Greco, John Phair, and Max Rafelson for their assistance in organizing the symposium that led to these proceedings. We also express our gratitude to the Upjohn Company, Kalamazoo, Michigan and to the Division of Blood Diseases and Resources of the National Heart, Lung, and Blood Institute for financial support; and to Dr. Harold Paul, Dr. Joseph Vaal, and the staff of Rush-Presbyterian-St. Luke's Medical Center Office of Continuing Education for logistic support. Finally, we wish to express our special appreciation to the investigators who participated in the symposium and provided manuscripts for these proceedings.

KENNETH K. WU
ENNIO C. ROSSI

PART I

BASIC PRINCIPLES OF PROSTAGLANDINS

Lipids, Membranes, and Essential Fatty Acids

A. J. MARCUS, B. B. WEKSLER, E. A. JAFFE,
M. J. BROEKMAN, L. B. SAFIER, H. L. ULLMAN,
K. TACK-GOLDMAN

*Divisions of Hematology/Oncology, Departments of
Medicine, New York Veterans Administration Medical
Center, and Cornell University Medical College,
New York*

Introduction

Lipids can be broadly defined as a chemically heterogeneous group of biomolecules with the common property of insolubility in water but solubility in nonpolar solvents.[1] In this chapter, we will mainly confine our discussion to lipids that are esters of long-chain fatty acids. Three major classes of lipids contain esterified fatty acids: phospholipids, glycolipids, and neutral lipids.[1]

Phospholipids serve as structural components in mammalian cells and tissues. In addition, phospholipids can be conceived as metabolic storage depots for essential fatty acids (EFA). Some phosphoglycerides, such as phosphatidyl-inositol (PI) and phosphatidic acid (PA), turn over rapidly when the cell is stimulated.[2] Tissue fractionation studies have indicated that phospholipids in subcellular compartments usually have similar fatty acid compositions.[3] These similarities may relate to a requirement of phospholipids for normal cell structure and function. Turnover of intact phosphoglyceride molecules is slow. Only the fatty acid moiety is renewed rapidly by intracellular fatty acid transfer. Although arachidonate is the precursor of prostaglandins and hydroxy acids, it may also lend a certain degree of stability to phospholipid components in cell membranes.

Glycolipids contain one or more sugar molecules, and some also have a sialic acid moiety (gangliosides). In human platelets the major

1

glycolipids are gangliosides known as hematosides.[4] Knowledge of the analytic biochemistry of glycolipids has exceeded concepts of their function.[1] They may be involved as receptor components of cell membranes,[4] or in certain aspects of membrane transport.

The neutral lipids, which include cholesteryl esters, triglycerides, free fatty acids, free cholesterol, monoglycerides, and diglycerides, are classified as a group because they are readily soluble in apolar solvents, such as the hydrocarbons. Thus, during chromatographic procedures they migrate with high Rf values and are easier to elute than polar lipids.[1] In contrast to many tissues as well as plasma, platelets contain little esterified cholesterol.[3] Instead, free cholesterol is the major neutral lipid component of platelet membranes (90%). Only 2% of the neutral lipids of platelet membranes is present as free fatty acids, mainly palmitate, stearate, and oleate, with little or no arachidonate.[3] Thus, the arachidonate must be made available in unesterified form for thromboxane and hydroxy acid formation by the action of phospholipases.

Essential fatty acids are polyunsaturated acids, which cannot be synthesized or formed in adequate amounts by animals.[5] The EFA are required nutrients for maintenance of growth and for certain physiologic processes. At present, it is clear that many more functions of EFA remain to be identified. Biosynthesis of unsaturated fatty acids begins with 9-monoenoic acids by insertion of a second double bond into the 12-13 position. In animals, oleic acid (9-octadecenoic acid) cannot be converted into the 9,12 doubly unsaturated acid known as linoleic. The step in desaturation between oleate and linoleate has been lost in the course of metazoan evolution.[5] This occurrence is rather perplexing, since linoleic acid is essential for animal nutrition. Interestingly enough, mechanisms for converting linoleate to arachidonate are present in almost all animal species thus far studied—even though mammals cannot synthesize linoleate de novo. Furthermore, although mammals cannot synthesize arachidonate, an animal fed radiolabeled arachidonate absorbs and retains 90% of the acid.[5] In experimental EFA deficiency, arachidonic acid is initially selectively retained. When animals are fed both linoleate and arachidonate, only the arachidonate is quantitatively inserted into the 2-position of cell phospholipids. Nonessential fatty acids are metabolized more rapidly than EFA. Thus, animals tend to conserve their stores of essential fatty acids.[5]

During experimental essential fatty acid deficiency states, pathologic changes occur that might be related to a lack of prostaglandin production, but there are clearly other defects as well. The changes observed have included low fertility, increased susceptibility to lung infection, low resistance to *Escherichia coli* infections, diminished growth, hair loss, degeneration of reproductive tissues, and depigmentation of the skin. In EFA-deficient animals, concentrations of arachidonate in tissue phospholipids eventually become markedly decreased. The quantity of eicosatrienoic acid is increased at the expense of arachidonate. However, this eicosatrienoic compound is not the essential fatty acid dihomo-gamma-linoleic (derived from linoleate), but 5,8,11-eicosatrienoic acid derived from oleate (Mead acid). The latter is not a precursor of arachidonic acid and cannot perform the normal metabolic functions associated with phospholipids.[5]

Oxygen "Burst" and Aggregation Response in Human Platelets

The early studies of Hamberg and Samuelsson,[6] as well as those of other investigators,[7-11] demonstrated that the oxygen burst in stimulated platelets was a reflection of arachidonic acid oxygenation.[12] In 1979, we developed a new approach to the study of oxygen consumption in stimulated human platelets.[13] A Clark oxygen monitor and a Payton aggregation module were connected to the same recorder, enabling us to obtain simultaneous tracings of oxygen consumption and platelet aggregation. The studies were initially carried out with washed platelet suspensions, but we have recently adapted the system for platelet-rich plasma (PRP).[14] It was already known that following addition of thrombin or arachidonic acid to washed platelets, there was an abrupt, transient increase in oxygen consumption over baseline values.[7-11] We examined the role of collagen in this oxygen consumption system and obtained results that were in agreement with those previously reported by Feinstein and associates.[15]

When collagen was added to washed platelets in the presence of calcium, a burst of O_2 consumption was observed after a lag phase of 25 to 35 seconds. The burst occurred concomitantly with the aggregation response. At the termination of the burst, consumption of oxygen by washed platelets returned to baseline levels. A second burst of O_2 consumption could not be elicited by addition of either collagen or thrombin. In contrast, when sodium arachidonate was added following the initial collagen response, a second burst was indeed elicited. Sequential stimulation with arachidonate elicited additional O_2 bursts of lesser intensity. The latter procedure could be repeated until the oxygen in the chamber was completely consumed. This phenomenon had been demonstrated previously by Pickett and Cohen.[11] The implication of the latter experiment is that platelet cyclo-oxygenase is not inactivated by repeated stimulation with arachidonate. Whereas the oxygen burst elicited by collagen required extracellular calcium, this was not true in the case of thrombin or arachidonate, both of which induced an oxygen burst in the presence or absence of extracellular calcium.[13]

We next studied the oxygen burst as induced by collagen in the presence of scavengers of released adenosine diphosphate (ADP) and in the presence of agents that interfere with arachidonic acid oxygenation. Apyrase, an enzyme that removes released ADP from the medium, had no effect on the magnitude of the burst rate, but did reduce the aggregation response. Extracellular ADP was also removed by another enzyme system, i.e., creatine phosphate/creatine phosphokinase (CP/CPK), and this had the same effect as apyrase. Controls utilizing CP or CPK alone had no effect on aggregation. Eicosatetraynoic acid (ETYA), an inhibitor of both the cyclo-oxygenase and lipoxygenase pathways of arachidonic acid oxygenation, completely blocked the oxygen burst and reduced, but did not totally abolish, the aggregation response (microscopic aggregates were noted by phase microscopy).[13]

In an attempt to "compromise" the entire system, we utilized ETYA and apyrase in combination. Under these circumstances the collagen-induced O_2 burst and aggregation response were completely inhibited. The latter effect was not observed when ETYA or apyrase was used alone. We then substituted indomethacin (8 μM), a cyclo-oxygenase inhibitor, for ETYA. This resulted in abolition of the oxygen burst and marked inhibition of the aggregation response, although microscopic aggregates were observed. The observation with indomethacin suggests that in intact platelets the lipoxygenase pathway may not play a significant role in production of the O_2 burst.[13]

Agents that raise platelet cyclic adenosine monophosphate (cAMP) levels were then tested for their effect on the oxygen burst as induced by collagen. Prostacyclin (PGI_2) or prostaglandin D_2 (PGD_2) produced complete inhibition of the oxygen burst and aggregation response. Pretreatment of the platelets with 2 mM dibutyryl cyclic AMP also abolished the O_2 burst and aggregation response in the presence of collagen.[13]

Antimycin, an inhibitor of oxidative phosphorylation, reduced basal oxygen consumption and slightly inhibited the O_2 burst. However, antimycin had no effect on aggregation. Deoxyglucose, an inhibitor of glycolysis, had no effect on the basal rate or burst rate of O_2 consumption, nor on the aggregation response. In contrast, combining antimycin and deoxyglucose resulted in ablation of the oxygen burst in the presence of a slight aggregation response. In a final experiment we added antimycin, deoxyglucose, plus apyrase to the preincubation mixture. The latter resulted in complete inhibition of the oxygen burst and aggregation response. Antimycin plus apyrase or deoxyglucose plus apyrase could not induce the effects seen when all three agents were combined. These results were comparable to those reported by Mürer, who used thrombin as the stimulus.[10]

The effects of apyrase on the oxygen burst induced by thrombin and

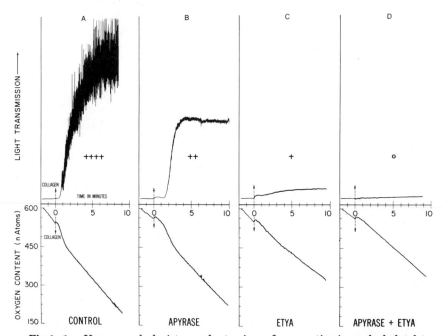

Fig 1–1.—Upper panels depict recorder tracings of aggregation in washed platelets as induced by collagen. Lower panels represent recordings of oxygen consumption, which was measured concomitantly with aggregation. *Arrows* indicate points where 40 µg/ml collagen was added to the aggregometer cuvette. **A,** control. Thirty seconds after collagen addition, and concomitant with initiation of the aggregation response, an abrupt increase in the slope of the line is recorded. This increase represents the burst of O_2 consumption in the stimulated platelets. **B,** effect of preincubation of platelets with apyrase (70 U/ml). An aggregation response is still present, although reduced, due to removal of ADP from the system. **C,** response to collagen after preincubation with ETYA (30 µM). Microscopic aggregates were visible by phase microscopy, although the recorded aggregation response was low. Note that the oxygen burst was completely inhibited. **D,** effects of both blocking arachidonic acid oxygenation and scavenging of free ADP from the incubation mixture. Oxygen burst and aggregation response were totally ablated. Apyrase or ETYA alone did not produce this effect. (Courtesy of Bressler N.M., et al.: *Blood* 53:167–178, 1979.)

arachidonate were also investigated. When thrombin was used as stimulus, apyrase had no effect on the oxygen burst or aggregation response. However, when arachidonate was the stimulus, incubation of apyrase with the platelet suspension resulted in an immediate burst of oxygen consumption, but there was a 2-minute delay in the aggregation response. Increasing the concentration of apyrase was followed by an immediate oxygen burst after arachidonate addition, but aggregation was completely inhibited. Substitution of CP/CPK for apyrase also resulted in an oxygen burst, but no aggregation in response to arachidonate. These results provided evidence that aggregation induced by arachidonic acid was mediated by released ADP. This was in contrast to thrombin, which induced a normal O_2 burst and a normal aggregation response in the presence of apyrase. The results are summarized in Figure 1–1.

The foregoing experiments can be criticized because they were carried out on washed platelet suspensions, which are not as responsive to ADP as are PRP. We postulate that small quantities of ADP released in the microenvironment of the platelet played a role in the results obtained.

It can be concluded that the oxygen burst occurring in stimulated platelets represents oxygenation of arachidonic acid and is the first step leading to the formation of prostaglandin endoperoxides and thromboxane A_2. The oxygen burst as elicited by collagen requires extracellular calcium and is inhibited by agents that elevate intracellular cyclic AMP or by those that completely block energy metabolism.

The oxygen burst in platelets does not appear to be analogous to the burst of oxygen consumption observed in polymorphonuclear leu-

TABLE 1–1.—ARACHIDONIC ACID METABOLITES IN THE SUPERNATE OF STIMULATED, RADIOLABELED PLATELETS*

PRODUCT	IONOPHORE (1μM)		THROMBIN (5 U/ML)		COLLAGEN (30 μG/ML)	
	cpm	%†	cpm	%	cpm	%
PGF$_{2\alpha}$	806	2.4	469	2.2	180	1.4
TXB$_2$	12,471	37.2	9,268	43.1	4,974	39.8
PGE$_2$	998	3.0	467	2.2	210	1.7
PGD$_2$	1,255	3.7	607	2.8	292	2.3
Hydroxy acids	15,551	46.4	9,855	45.8	5,985	47.9
20:4	635	1.9	229	1.1	314	2.5

*Total of 1×10^8 platelets (783,678 cpm) = 200,000/μl. Total volume was 0.5 ml. Ca^{++} (3 mM) included when thrombin or collagen was the stimulus.
†Percentage of recovered counts minus phospholipid and solvent front. Radioactive areas on TLC plates that did not correspond to standards are not included.

kocytes. The leukocyte O_2 burst is mainly associated with production of superoxide radicals and hydrogen peroxide (for further discussion, see reference 16). In stimulated platelets, formation of oxygen radicals does not occur to any significant degree,[17] but arachidonic acid oxygenation is prominent.

Transformation of arachidonate into prostanoids and hydroxy acids, as induced by different stimuli, varies mainly in a quantitative manner. Table 1–1 demonstrates the thin-layer radiochromatographic profile of products observed when radiolabeled platelets are stimulated by ionophore, thrombin, or collagen. It can be seen that the proportions of products are similar, but the stimuli vary in potency with regard to the quantity of radioactivity appearing in different metabolites.

Studies of Prostacyclin Production by Cultured Human Endothelial Cells

The studies to be summarized here represent a collaborative effort involving the laboratories of Drs. Babette B. Weksler and Eric A. Jaffe, as well as our own.

In 1977, we reported that cultured endothelial cells that originated from human umbilical veins and bovine aortas produced a lipid substance that inhibited platelet aggregation. The active principle was further identified by incubating microsomal fractions prepared from the endothelial cells with radiolabeled arachidonate. By means of thin-layer radiochromatography, we identified prostacyclin as a product of the incubation system.[18] These studies were extended with the use of endothelial cell monolayers, which were incubated with ^{14}C arachidonate (20 µM, 0.4 µCi).[19] Following a 20-minute incubation period, prostacyclin was identified as its stable end product, 6-keto-$PGF_{1\alpha}$. It was noted at that time that all the measurable PGI_2 appeared in the supernatant of these monolayers. In addition, small quantities of prostaglandins $F_{2\alpha}$ and E_2 were detected. PGI_2 synthesis could be inhibited by pretreatment of the cells with 100 µM acetylsalicylic acid (ASA) or 15-hydroperoxy arachidonic acid. In these experiments the only cell-associated radioactivity was that identified in the phospholipid fraction and in the unconverted arachidonate.[19]

We next incubated endothelial cell monolayers with radiolabeled PGH_2, which had been biosynthesized in our laboratory.[19] The endothelial cells were pretreated with ASA in order to block endogenous prostaglandin synthesis. They were then treated with ^{14}C PGH_2 (2 µM, 0.06 µCi). By radio-thin-layer chromatography, PGI_2, $PGF_{2\alpha}$,

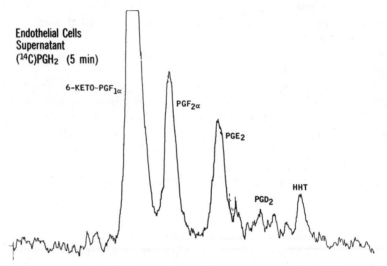

Endothelial Cells
Supernatant
(^{14}C)PGH$_2$ (5 min)

6-KETO-PGF$_{1\alpha}$

PGF$_{2\alpha}$

PGE$_2$

HHT

PGD$_2$

Fig 1–2.—Scan of arachidonic acid metabolites as separated by thin-layer radio-chromatography. Endothelial cells were incubated with (1-^{14}C) PGH$_2$ as synthesized in our laboratory for 5 minutes. The cells were removed by centrifugation, and the supernatant fluid was acidified and extracted.[20] Most of the radioactivity was not associated with the cells themselves. The major product was prostacyclin, as measured by its end product, 6-keto-PGF$_{1\alpha}$. It was concluded from these experiments that prostacyclin was either synthesized intracellularly and released, or generated at the cell surface. Incubation of radiolabeled PGH$_2$ in flasks devoid of endothelial cells resulted in generation of PGF$_{2\alpha}$, PGE$_2$, PGD$_2$, and HHT, but no prostacyclin.[19, 20]

PGE$_2$, PGD$_2$, and 12-L-hydroxy-5,8,10-heptadecatrienoic acid (HHT) were identified. Again, all measurable radioactive products were present in the supernatants, and no counts were detected in the cells. The latter observations led to the conclusion that prostacyclin was either synthesized in the cell and rapidly released, or it was being formed at the endothelial cell surface. The enzymatic nature of the process was verified by incubating PGH$_2$ in empty flasks. Under these conditions no PGI$_2$ was measurable, although PGF$_{2\alpha}$, PGE$_2$, PGD$_2$, and HHT were detected. Results of an experiment wherein radiolabeled PGH$_2$ was incubated with endothelial cell suspensions are shown in Figure 1–2.

Since the endothelial cell monolayers rapidly and efficiently converted exogenous PGH$_2$ to PGI$_2$, and since the PGI$_2$ as well as other products appeared in the supernatant, it was of interest to determine whether the endothelial cells could synthesize prostacyclin from endoperoxides provided by a natural source—the stimulated platelet.[20]

PGI₂ Production From Platelet-Derived Endoperoxides by Endothelial Cells

Since previous experiments suggested the possibility that endothelial cells produce PGI_2 at or near the cell surface, we reasoned that an experimental system which brought stimulated platelets into close proximity with endothelial cells might allow for utilization of platelet endoperoxides by the endothelial cells for PGI_2 synthesis.[20] Platelets were prelabeled with ^3H arachidonic acid and then reacted with ionophore A23187, thrombin, or collagen in the presence of aspirin-treated endothelial cells in aggregometer cuvettes. This technique permitted thin-layer radiochromatographic quantitation of radiolabeled PGI_2 as ^3H 6-keto-$PGF_{1\alpha}$, as well as of radiolabeled TXA_2 as ^3H TXB_2. Platelet aggregation responses could also be analyzed in the same sample.

In the presence of ASA-treated endothelial cells, platelet aggregation in response to ionophore or thrombin or collagen was inhibited. ^3H 6-keto-$PGF_{1\alpha}$ was recovered from the supernatants of combined cell suspensions after stimulation by all three stimuli. The quantitative order of PGI_2 synthesis initiated in these systems was ionophore > thrombin > collagen.

Synthesis of radiolabeled thromboxane by platelets was always reduced in the presence of aspirin-treated endothelial cells. It is possible that the PGI_2 formed by the endothelial cells rapidly led to inhibition of further platelet aggregation, and thus to a decrease in thromboxane production. It is also plausible that platelet endoperoxides available at the surface were diverted to PGI_2 production by the aspirin-treated endothelial cells.

Radioimmunoassay for 6-keto-$PGF_{1\alpha}$ and TXB_2 was carried out in separate experiments. The results paralleled those obtained by thin-layer radiochromatography. Quantities of 6-keto-$PGF_{1\alpha}$ measured in the radioimmunoassay procedure represented amounts of PGI_2 sufficient to inhibit platelet aggregation.

Not only was the proximity of platelets to endothelial cells an important factor, but the ratio of platelets to endothelial cells was critical. When 200,000 platelets/μl were combined with 3,000 to 6,000 ASA-treated endothelial cells/μl, PGI_2 was detectable in the system. At higher platelet concentrations the proportion of measurable 6-keto-$PGF_{1\alpha}$ to TXB_2 decreased. This was accompanied by a normal platelet aggregation response rather than by the inhibition observed at platelet levels of 200,000/μl. It can be speculated that at high platelet concentrations the endoperoxides formed at the surface were utilized by other platelets in close proximity, so that larger quantities of thromboxane were generated.

The effectiveness of aspirin treatment was monitored at the beginning and end of each experiment. Thus, the endothelial cells were stimulated with thrombin first in the absence (Fig 1–3), then in the presence, of ASA. Measurements were then made for 6-keto-$PGF_{1\alpha}$ by radiolabeling and by radioimmunoassay. In no case did the ASA-treated cells synthesize measurable PGI_2. Therefore the results indicated that the endothelial cell suspensions could only have utilized endoperoxides from stimulated platelets for PGI_2 production. In radioimmunoassay experiments utilizing an aspirin-free system, it could also be shown that approximately half of the total 6-keto-$PGF_{1\alpha}$ produced in endothelial cell-platelet suspensions was actually derived from platelet endoperoxides.

As already mentioned, we believe that one of the major factors in demonstrating platelet endoperoxide transfer to endothelial cells was proximity. Thus, when radiolabeled platelets were added to ASA-treated endothelial cell monolayers, there was less PGI_2 production than that observed when platelets and ASA-treated endothelial cell suspensions were used. PGI_2 production from platelets could be in-

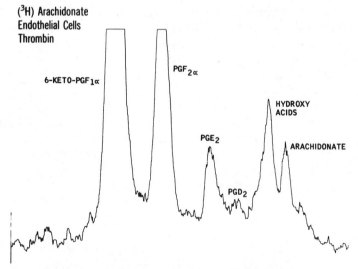

Fig 1–3.—Endothelial cell suspensions were incubated with ³H arachidonate and thrombin (5 U/ml) in the presence of 3 mM Ca^{++} for 5 minutes. Percent distribution of the metabolites depicted was: 6-keto-$PGF_{1\alpha}$ (PGI_2), 66%; $PGF_{2\alpha}$, 17%; PGE_2, 3%; PGD_2, 1%; hydroxy acids, 4%; arachidonic acid, 2%.[20]

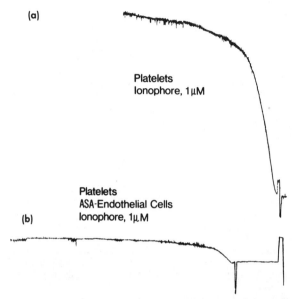

(a)

Platelets
Ionophore, 1 μM

Platelets
ASA-Endothelial Cells
(b)   Ionophore, 1μM

Fig 1–4.—a, aggregation response of washed platelets following stimulation with ionophore A23187 over a five-minute period. b, response of platelets to ionophore when aspirin-treated endothelial cells were included in the aggregometer cuvette. Platelets did not aggregate when stimulated in the presence of ASA-treated endothelial cells. PGI₂ synthesis was demonstrable in the supernatant fluid derived from these combined suspensions. (Courtesy of Marcus A.J., et al.: *J. Clin. Invest.* 66:979–986, 1980.)

creased in monolayers if thromboxane synthetase inhibitors, such as imidazole or U54701, were employed. The fact that PGI₂ was indeed synthesized when endoperoxides "piled up" in the presence of the TXA₂ synthetase inhibitors indicated to us that the transfer phenomenon could indeed occur under appropriate experimental conditions. When we used endothelial cell suspensions in preference to monolayers, platelet-endothelial cell proximity was enhanced, and the components of the system could be concentrated in a small volume.[20] This permitted efficient mixing of the combined suspensions as well. In order to study platelets in the range of 200,000/μl, it was necessary to utilize radiolabeled arachidonate of high specific activity. Thus, ³H arachidonate was used in preference to ¹⁴C 20:4. If labeling was carried out with ¹⁴C, it was necessary to increase platelet concentrations to a point where aggregation occurred and large quantities of thromboxane were produced relative to the synthesis of prostacyclin.[20] Results of experiments in which ionophore was used as stimulus are shown in Figures 1–4 and 1–5.

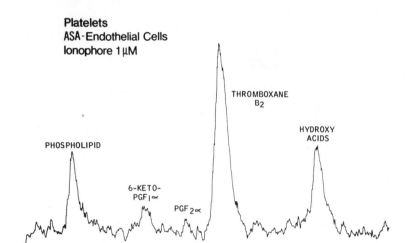

Platelets
ASA-Endothelial Cells
Ionophore 1 μM

Fig 1-5.—Scan of thin-layer radiochromatogram of lipids in supernatant fluid from incubation mixture depicted in Figure 1-4. Percent distribution of radioactivity was as follows: 6-keto-PGF$_{1\alpha}$ (prostacyclin), 5%; PGF$_{2\alpha}$, 4%; thromboxane B$_2$, 56%; PGE$_2$, 4%; PGD$_2$, 2%; hydroxy acids, 18%; arachidonic acid, 0.6%. It is of interest that no aggregation occurred in these combined suspensions despite formation of large quantities of thromboxane. The 6-keto-PGF$_{1\alpha}$ measurable in this system could only have originated from platelet endoperoxides, since the endothelial cells were not labeled and were unable to synthesize PGI$_2$ from endogenous sources. (Courtesy of Marcus A.J., et al.: *J. Clin. Invest.* 66:979–986, 1980.)

Summary

New insight into functions of essential fatty acids was provided by the demonstration that EFA were precursors for physiologically active metabolic products—the hydroxy acids, prostaglandins, thromboxane, and prostacyclin. It was already known that EFA were metabolized differently from the nonessential polyunsaturated fatty acids. The nonessential fatty acids are metabolized rapidly, and mammalian cells always attempt to conserve the stores of essential fatty acids. Whether the main purpose of this conservation mechanism is to maintain the arachidonic acid pathway intact is not clear. Apparently diminished prostanoid production per se is not accompanied by symptoms of EFA deficiency, since chronic aspirin ingestion is not associated with these symptoms. The effects of diminished hydroxy acid production in humans are not known because no therapeutic agent currently in use specifically inhibits their synthesis on a chronic basis. Therefore it can be speculated that other important functions of essential fatty acids have yet to be elucidated.

Prostaglandins, thromboxane A$_2$, and prostacyclin may be defined as autacoids derived from arachidonic acid, which appear to be important for the regulation of vascular tone, cell secretion, and contractile processes.[21] The hydroxy acid derivatives appear to function as chemotactic agents and also give rise to slow-reacting substances. Additional functions are not known, although this is an important area for research, since hydroxy acids are formed in relatively large amounts in patients who ingest aspirin and other nonsteroidal antiinflammatory agents. The endoperoxides PGG_2 and PGH_2 are the common intermediates for all prostanoid end products of arachidonic acid. Whenever a specific tissue is under study, the profile of endoperoxide transformation products should be established. This will help us to understand how the tissue will respond to stimuli that induce arachidonic acid release and transformation. Platelets and blood vessels are prime examples of this mechanism. In the platelet, endoperoxides are transformed mainly to TXA_2, which is a potent vasoconstrictor and inducer of platelet aggregation. In contrast, endothelial cells convert endoperoxides to PGI_2, which is a vasodilator and an inhibitor of platelet aggregation. In addition, under appropriate experimental conditions and possibly in vivo, endothelial cells can utilize endoperoxides from stimulated platelets to form prostacyclin. The finding that platelets and endothelial cells can share common precursors for the production of important autacoids may indicate that this interchange can occur with combinations of other cell types such as leukocytes and platelets, or leukocytes and endothelial cells.

ACKNOWLEDGMENTS

This work was supported by grants from the Veterans Administration, the National Institutes of Health (HL 18828 06 SCOR), the New York Heart Association, and the A.R. Krakower Foundation.

REFERENCES

1. Gurr M.I., James A.T.: *Lipid Biochemistry. An Introduction,* ed. 2. New York, John Wiley & Sons, Inc., 1975.
2. Broekman M.J., Ward J.W., Marcus A.J.: Phospholipid metabolism in stimulated human platelets. Changes in phosphatidylinositol, phosphatidic acid, and lysophospholipids. *J. Clin. Invest.* 66:275–283, 1980.
3. Marcus A.J., Ullman H.L., Safier L.B.: Lipid composition of subcellular particles of human blood platelets. *J. Lipid Res.* 10:108–114, 1969.
4. Marcus A.J., Ullman H.L., Safier L.B.: Studies on human platelet gangliosides. *J. Clin. Invest.* 51:2602–2612, 1972.
5. Alfin-Slater R.B., Aftergood L.: Essential fatty acids reinvestigated. *Physiol. Rev.* 48:758–784, 1968.

6. Hamberg M., Samuelsson B.: Detection and isolation of an endoperoxide intermediate in prostaglandin biosynthesis. *Proc. Natl. Acad. Sci. USA* 70:899–903, 1973.
7. Fukami M.H., Holmsen H., Bauer J.: Thrombin-induced oxygen consumption, malonyldialdehyde formation and serotonin secretion in human platelets. *Biochim. Biophys. Acta* 428:253–256, 1976.
8. Muenzer J., Weinbach E.C., Wolfe S.M.: Oxygen consumption of human blood platelets. I. Effect of thrombin. *Biochim. Biophys. Acta* 376:237–242, 1975.
9. Muenzer J., Weinbach E.C., Wolfe S.M.: Oxygen consumption of human blood platelets. II. Effect of inhibitors on thrombin-induced oxygen burst. *Biochim. Biophys. Acta* 376:243–248, 1975.
10. Mürer E.H.: Release reaction and energy metabolism in blood platelets with special reference to the burst in oxygen uptake. *Biochim. Biophys. Acta* 162:320–326, 1968.
11. Pickett W.C., Cohen P.: Mechanism of the thrombin mediated burst in oxygen consumption by human platelets. *J. Biol. Chem.* 251:2536–2538, 1976.
12. Marcus A.J.: The role of lipids in platelet function: with particular reference to the arachidonic acid pathway. *J. Lipid Res.* 19:793–826, 1978.
13. Bressler N.M., Broekman M.J., Marcus A.J.: Concurrent studies of oxygen consumption and aggregation in stimulated human platelets. *Blood* 53:167–178, 1979.
14. Bressler N.M., Broekman M.J., Marcus A.J.: In preparation.
15. Feinstein M.B., Becker E.L., Fraser C.: Thrombin, collagen and A23187 stimulated endogenous platelet arachidonate metabolism: Differential inhibition by PGE_1, local anesthetics and a serine-protease inhibitor. *Prostaglandins* 14:1075–1093, 1977.
16. Marcus A.J.: Pathways of oxygen utilization by stimulated platelets and leukocytes. *Semin. Hematol.* 16:188–195, 1979.
17. Marcus A.J., Silk S.T., Safier L.B., Ullman H.L.: Superoxide production and reducing activity in human platelets. *J. Clin. Invest.* 59:149–158, 1977.
18. Weksler B.B., Marcus A.J., Jaffe E.A.: Synthesis of prostaglandin I_2 (prostacyclin) by cultured human and bovine endothelial cells. *Proc. Natl. Acad. Sci. USA* 74:3922–3926, 1977.
19. Marcus A.J., Weksler B.B., Jaffe E.A.: Enzymatic conversion of prostaglandin endoperoxide H_2 and arachidonic acid to prostacyclin by cultured human endothelial cells. *J. Biol. Chem.* 253:7138–7141, 1978.
20. Marcus A.J., Weksler B.B., Jaffe E.A., Broekman M.J.: Synthesis of prostacyclin from platelet-derived endoperoxides by cultured human endothelial cells. *J. Clin. Invest.* 66:979–986, 1980.
21. Marcus A.J.: The role of prostaglandins in platelet function. *Progr. Hematol.* 11:147–171, 1979.

Blood Vessels, Platelets, and Prostaglandins: New Strategies for the Modification of Thrombotic Disorders

PHILIP NEEDLEMAN

Department of Pharmacology
Washington University Medical School
St. Louis, Missouri

Perusal of most current biomedical journals will quickly indicate the tremendous outpouring of papers that deal with prostaglandins (PG). Prostaglandins are synthesized by nearly every tissue in the body. The precursor for their production is the essential (essential since it or a related fatty acid must be ingested in the diet) 20-carbon fatty acid known as arachidonic acid. The rapid expansion of information has largely been based on the discovery of the synthesis, chemistry, and biologic properties of a number of new metabolites of arachidonic acid which are produced in the body. Since there are no preformed stores of the various PG in the body, the release of PG into the circulation reflects an immediate local production of this substance. The release of PG from tissues throughout the body (such as heart, blood vessels, kidney, platelets, etc.) can be stimulated by various means, such as hormones, nerve stimulation, decreased oxygen tension in the blood, or injury. The PG produced are released from the tissue involved and appear in the venous drainage of that tissue. Most prostaglandins are either destroyed in the lung or are labile and rapidly degraded; few, if any, are detected in arterial blood. Thus, PG could be considered largely as local hormones that are synthesized at or near their site of action.

As previously indicated, nearly all tissues in the body are capable of producing PG. The initial conversion of arachidonic acid is carried

15

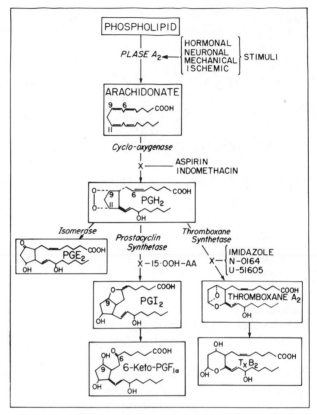

Fig 2–1.—Sequence of enzymatic steps (in italics) in the biosynthesis of the primary prostaglandins and related products (in boxes) as well as some of the known enzymatic inhibitors (site of action denoted with an X).

out by an enzyme called cyclo-oxygenase via the metabolic pathway shown in Figure 2–1. This enzyme converts the fatty acid into labile intermediates known as PG-endoperoxides (PGG_2 and PGH_2). Aspirin and numerous nonsteroid anti-inflammatory drugs (these drugs are often called PG-synthesis inhibitors or cyclo-oxygenase inhibitors) owe their effectiveness to their ability to block the enzyme cyclo-oxygenase. The labile endoperoxide is, in turn, enzymatically converted into any one of a variety of products. Different tissues use different enzyme(s) for this conversion. Therefore, in blood vessels the endoperoxide is converted primarily into prostacyclin (PGI_2); in the kidney it is normally converted to PGE_2 and, in platelets, to the very labile substance called thromboxane A_2. Whereas the three aforementioned tissues (blood vessels, kidney, platelets) have only one primary cyclo-oxygenase product (via the endoperoxide intermediate), some tissues, such as lung and spleen, possess several enzymes that use endoperoxide as a substrate. For example, the lung has been demonstrated to simultaneously produce PGE_2, prostacyclin, and thromboxane. Since the various PGs have different biologic actions, the ultimate response of an organ to activation of prostaglandin biosynthesis will be determined by which product or product(s) are produced.

The primary arachidonate metabolite produced both in isolated perfused hearts and in isolated coronary arteries (including those of human beings) is prostacyclin (PGI_2). In addition, the major site of cardiac prostacyclin synthesis appears to be in the coronary vasculature itself. The reaction sequence is arachidonic acid → PG endoperoxide → prostacyclin (Fig 2-1). The enzymatic synthesis of prostacyclin from the endoperoxides can be blocked in vitro by hydroperoxy fatty acids. All blood vessels readily synthesize prostacyclin from intrinsic arachidonate. Prostacyclin both relaxes blood vessels and is a potent inhibitor of platelet aggregation. The therapeutic potential of this recently discovered pathway is being rapidly evaluated. Exogenously administered prostacyclin is currently being tried in the treatment of patients with peripheral vascular disease and in those undergoing cardiac bypass surgery or hemodialysis. The evaluation of these trials will be detailed throughout this text.

Platelets also contain arachidonic acid-metabolizing enzymes, but the major arachidonic acid-endoperoxide product is thromboxane A_2. This labile compound (its half-life is 30 seconds in aqueous solution) is a potent vasoconstrictor that also causes platelet aggregation. Blood vessels lack the PG-endoperoxide-dependent enzyme to produce thromboxane, and platelets lack the enzyme that converts the precursor PG endoperoxide into prostacyclin. These two endoperoxide metabolites are obviously antagonists on both blood vessels and platelets, and they may interact when platelets adhere to damaged vessels. This interaction is illustrated in Figure 2-2. The prostacyclin produced by the blood vessels may normally protect intact blood vessels and help avoid platelet adherence. Damage of the vessel may reduce the vascular prostacyclin production and facilitate the adherence of the platelet to the damaged area. The attachment of platelets to the damaged vessels leads to the production of thromboxane by the platelets, which in turn would facilitate the local vascular constriction around the thrombus, and the released thromboxane would also aggregate surrounding platelets. This kind of thrombotic event would be of importance in such clinical situations as coronary thrombosis

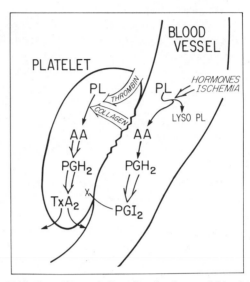

Fig 2-2.—Arachidonic acid metabolism by platelets and blood vessels. **PL,** phospholipid; **AA,** arachidonic acid; **PG,** prostaglandin; **TxA$_2$,** thromboxane A$_2$; and **PGI$_2$,** prostacyclin.

(e.g., myocardial infarction), ischemia (e.g., angina pectoris), and possibly coronary vasospasms, as well as in cerebral thrombosis (e.g., stroke or transient ischemic attacks). Indeed, a prevailing hypothesis suggests that the initial event in atherosclerosis involves platelets. Platelets stick to damaged blood vessels and elaborate a mitogen that causes an intimal hyperplasia. In some cases this hyperplasia does not regress, foam cells accumulate, and an atherosclerotic lesion is initiated. Thus, an ability to manipulate platelet aggregation and adhesion may ultimately be pertinent to the treatment of atherosclerosis.

An obvious extension of this research is the quest for therapeutic agents or strategies that would interfere with platelet thromboxane production and the resultant thrombosis. Numerous clinical trials are under way to evaluate the effect of aspirin on the thrombotic disorders. Aspirin blocks the initial enzyme (cyclo-oxygenase) that begins the process of converting arachidonic acid into thromboxane. Unfortunately, as already indicated, the cyclo-oxygenase enzyme is common to all tissues, and aspirin, if given in high enough doses, would abolish the production of all PGs including prostacyclin, which is a natural endogenous antithrombotic agent. A new strategy, which has greater potential for specificity, is the development of drugs that only block the conversion of the endoperoxide into thromboxane (e.g., imidazole in Fig 2–1) and no other endoperoxide-dependent enzymes. Indeed, we initially discovered agents that blocked the isolated enzyme and now have succeeded in proving that a newer agent (OKY-1581) is capable of blocking thromboxane production in intact tissues. Platelets, when activated by thrombin or collagen, initiate arachidonic acid metabolism, which culminates primarily in the synthesis and release of thromboxane A_2. It should be remembered that thromboxane production only occurs during aggregation and especially during adhesion to an injured blood vessel. During thrombosis there is a tight contact between the platelet and the blood vessel. In this situation we have shown that a thromboxane synthetase inhibitor will not only abolish the synthesis of the vasoconstrictor-aggregator thromboxane A_2, but such an inhibitor will now cause the accumulation and release of the PG-endoperoxides. Since the platelet is adherent to the blood vessel at the injury site, the released PG-endoperoxide is then readily converted by the vascular smooth muscle cells into prostacyclin. The thromboxane synthetase inhibitor thus abolishes the aggregator-constrictor and enhances the antithrombotic dilator (prostacyclin) right at the critical site of injury. These findings suggest a promising new approach to the treatment of thrombosis.

An alternative approach for the treatment of chronic thrombotic disorders could rely on a dietary strategy that alters the availability of precursor arachidonic acid for thromboxane production. We discovered that a novel fatty acid eicosapentaenoic acid (EPA), which is present in large quantities in cold water fish, is readily incorporated in platelet lipid membranes in place of arachidonic acid. When the platelets are stimulated, this novel fatty acid proves to be an effective competitive antagonist in platelets and prevents the conversion of any remaining arachidonic acid into thromboxane A_2. People who either naturally (e.g., Greenland Eskimos or Japanese fishermen) or experimentally ingest a diet that substitutes EPA for arachidonic acid have been found by numerous investigators to have suppressed thromboxane A_2 production and a suppressed ability to aggregate their platelets. This approach, perhaps in combination (Fig 2–3) with a thromboxane synthetase inhibitor (thereby allowing a more modest dietary EPA supplement), might be usefully employed in transient ischemic attacks or coronary patients.

In summary, as an outgrowth of some critical fundamental investigations, several strategies for the therapeutic manipulation of thrombotic and vasospastic disorders have emerged. These include:

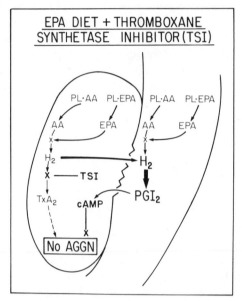

EPA DIET + THROMBOXANE SYNTHETASE INHIBITOR (TSI)

Fig 2–3.—Schematic diagram of the potential antithrombotic effectiveness of the combination of dietary supplementation with 5,8,11,14,17-eicosapentaenoic acid (EPA) and a thromboxane synthetase inhibitor (TSI). The following additional abbreviations were employed: **PL·AA**, arachidonate-containing phospholipids; **PL·EPA**, eicosapentaenoate-containing phospholipids; **AGGN**, aggregation; **cAMP**, 3'5'-cyclic adenosine monophosphate (which inhibits platelet aggregation).

(1) prostacyclin and related analogues; (2) thromboxane synthetase inhibitors; and (3) dietary manipulation with novel fatty acids that reduce intrinsic thromboxane synthesis. To this list could be added the emerging possibility of specific receptor blocking agents, or agents that may enhance the action or delay the destruction of beneficial arachidonate metabolites. These discoveries are the stimulus for active drug development and testing. Indeed, we are in the midst of studies to establish dosage forms, treatment strategies, and therapeutic potential of prostacyclin. The near future should see the development and testing of other agents of the nature described. I view with anticipation and some excitement their development as therapeutic agents.

Mechanism of Action of Prostacyclin and Thromboxane A_2

ROBERT R. GORMAN

Department of Experimental Biology
Upjohn Company, Kalamazoo, Michigan

Introduction

In the early 1930s it was known that some substance in seminal fluid could contract or relax human uterine tissue, depending on the gestational state of the uterus.[1-3] Later this substance was identified as an acidic lipid by Von Euler and named prostaglandin.[4] Thirty years later the actual crystalline compounds were isolated by Bergstrom and Sjovall,[5] and the structural determinations made by Bergstrom et al.[6] and Samuelsson.[7] Since these early basic studies, literally thousands of papers dealing with prostaglandins and/or thromboxanes have been published, but a single concise mechanism of action for all prostaglandins and thromboxanes has not been elucidated. Most, if not all, of the biology of prostaglandins and thromboxanes appears to be associated with changes in calcium metabolism and adenosine $3',5'$-cyclic monophosphate levels. Since this symposium is concerned with cardiovascular disease, we will principally use the human platelet as a model for the mechanism of action of TXA_2 and PGI_2. The physiology and biochemistry of the platelet has been rigorously studied with respect to prostaglandins and thromboxanes, and the regulation of platelet adenylate cyclase by these agents is well delineated.

Materials and Methods

Prostaglandins E_1, 6-keto-E_1, D_2, I_2, 9,11-azoprosta-5,13 dienoate (azo analogue I), and (E)-2-methyl-3-[4-(3-pyridinylmethyl)phenyl]-2-propenoic acid (MPPA) were all obtained from Experimental Chem-

istry, The Upjohn Company, Kalamazoo, MI. The complete radioimmunoassay kit for cyclic AMP was purchased from Collaborative Research, Waltham, MA. 1-Methyl-3-isobutylmethylxanthine (MIX)
was purchased from Aldrich Chemical Company, Milwaukee, WI.

Human platelet-rich plasma (PRP) was prepared by withdrawing
blood directly into 3.8% (v/v) trisodium citrate, followed by centrifugation at 200 × g for 10 minutes at room temperature. Platelet cyclic
AMP was measured by radioimmunoassay,[8] with the incorporation of
the acetylation modification.[9] The superfusion technique of Vane was
used to assay the vasodilatory potencies of prostaglandins.[10]

Results and Discussion

Human platelet homeostasis is controlled by the "reciprocal regulation" of cyclic AMP levels by PGI_2 and TXA_2.[11] Agents that elevate
cyclic AMP, such as PGE_1 or PGI_2, block both primary (noncyclo-ox-

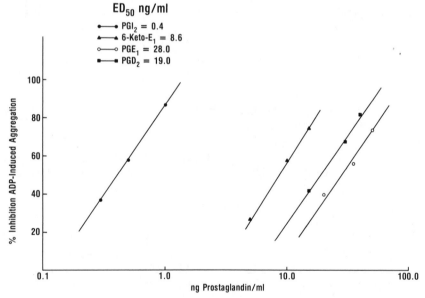

Fig 3–1.—Inhibition of ADP-induced human platelet aggregation by prostaglandins that stimulate adenylate cyclase. Human platelet-rich plasma (PRP) was incubated for 1 minute at 37°C with the appropriate concentration of prostaglandin and
was then challenged with 8 μM ADP. The resulting aggregation was then compared
to the control ADP aggregation response. Data are plotted as percent inhibition vs log
dose prostaglandin. The inhibitory potency of prostaglandins is directly related to the
ability of these compounds to stimulate platelet adenylate cyclase.[12] (Courtesy of
Miller O.V., Aiken J.W., Shebuski R.J., Gorman R.R.: *Prostaglandins* 20:391–400,
1980.)

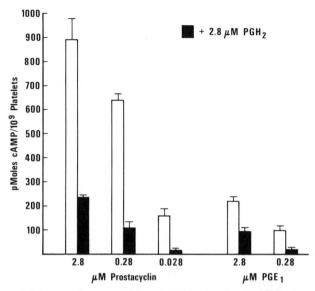

Fig 3–2.—Inhibition of prostacyclin and PGE_1-stimulated cAMP accumulation by PGH_2. One milliliter of PRP was incubated for 1 min at 37°C with either prostacyclin or PGE_1 at the indicated concentrations. Half the tubes contained 2.8 μM PGH_2. Incubations were terminated with 0.8 ml of 5% TCA and rapid freezing in liquid nitrogen. Data are presented as mean ± S.E.M. of triplicate samples. The basal level of cAMP (31 pmoles/10^9 platelets) has been subtracted from all values.

ygenase-dependent) and secondary (cyclo-oxygenase-dependent) aggregation. In fact, PGI_2 inhibits platelet aggregation regardless of the proaggregatory stimulus. The platelet inhibitory potency of prostaglandins can be directly correlated with their ability to stimulate platelet cyclic AMP levels. The data in Figure 3–1 show that when PGI_2, 6-keto-E_1, PGD_2 and PGE_1 are tested for their ability to block ADP-induced aggregation, PGI_2 is the most potent inhibitor with 6-keto-E_1>PGD_2>PGE_1. This rank order of potency is directly related to their ability to stimulate platelet adenylate cyclase.[12]

TXA_2 is a strong inducer of human platelet aggregation. Like PGI_2, TXA_2 is formed from the endoperoxides PGG_2 or PGH_2. In contrast to PGI_2, TXA_2 inhibits platelet adenylate cyclase.[13] The data in Figure 3–2 show that either PGE_1 or PGI_2 gives dose-dependent stimulations of human platelet cyclic AMP levels. However, if PGH_2 is added simultaneously with either PGE_1 or PGI_2, there is a marked inhibition of cyclic AMP accumulation. The actual inhibition of PGI_2-stimulated cyclic AMP levels by PGH_2 has been shown to be dependent upon TXA_2 synthesis, because TXA_2 synthetase inhibitors block the

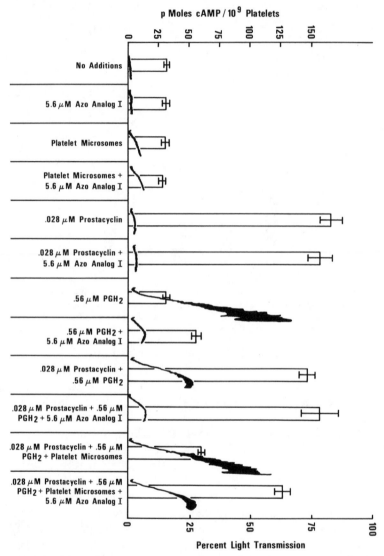

Fig 3–3.—Effect of azo analogue I on the cAMP-lowering activity of PGH₂. Aliquots (1 ml) of PRP (0.68 × 10⁹ platelets/ml) were preincubated for 2 minutes at 37°C, and then the appropriate compounds were added and platelet aggregation monitored for 1 minute. For the samples that contained azo analogue I, both the platelets and the microsomes were preincubated for 2 minutes with the inhibitor. At the end of 1 minute, the aggregations were stopped by the addition of 0.7 ml 10% TCA and freezing in liquid nitrogen. The samples were subsequently extracted with ether and the cAMP contents measured as described in the text. The platelet microsomal preparation (20 μl) used to generate TXA₂ contained 80 μg protein. Data are presented as mean ± S.E.M. of triplicate samples.

cyclic AMP-lowering activity of endoperoxides.[14] Not only do thromboxane synthetase inhibitors block the cyclic AMP-lowering activity of PGH_2, but they also inhibit PGH_2 or arachidonic acid-induced aggregation, indicating that the synthesis of TXA_2 is required for cyclooxygenase-dependent aggregation. The complete biologic and biochemical effects of a thromboxane synthetase inhibitor (9,11-azo-prosta-5,13 dienoic acid or azo analogue I), PGH_2, and PGI_2 are summarized in Figure 3–3.

Reading top to bottom (Fig 3–3), the basal level of cAMP (no additions) is not changed by 5.6 μM azo analogue I. The addition of platelet microsomes does not change the cAMP level, but induces a small aggregatory response. Azo analogue I does not alter the small aggregation caused by microsomes or change the basal cAMP levels. Prostacyclin (0.028 μM) induces a dramatic rise in cAMP, which is not antagonized by 5.6 μM azo analogue I. In this experiment, 0.56 μM PGH_2 induces a violent platelet aggregation without altering the basal level of cAMP, but 5.6 μM azo analogue I completely blocks the PGH_2-induced aggregation with only a small increase in cAMP levels, which is probably due to PGE_2 and PGD_2 formation from the endoperoxide. Coincubation of prostacyclin and 0.56 μM PGH_2 results in a partial inhibition of PGH_2-induced aggregation with a modest decrease in the prostacyclin-induced cAMP accumulation. Azo analogue I suppresses the PGH_2-induced aggregation further without a significant change in cAMP levels. However, if the same concentration of PGH_2 is incubated with 20 μl platelet microsomes (and TXA_2 formed), there is a potent aggregation, even in the presence of 0.028 μM prostacyclin. The generation of TXA_2 results in an essentially complete inhibition of the prostacyclin stimulation of cAMP levels. The addition of 5.6 μM azo analogue I, which blocks TXA_2 synthesis, inhibits both the aggregation and the cAMP-lowering activity caused by TXA_2 generation.

TXA_2 does not inhibit basal cyclic AMP levels in platelets. Such levels must be initially increased by PGE_1 or PGI_2 before the lowering effect of TXA_2 can be observed.[13] This suggests that TXA_2 might block cyclic AMP indirectly. Ca^{2+} is an integral part of the mechanism responsible for human platelet aggregation, and it has even been suggested that prostaglandins and/or TXA_2 may act as calcium ionophores.[15] If TXA_2 can induce translocation of Ca^{2+} from the bound to the free state and can inhibit adenylate cyclase, then inhibition of adenylate cyclase by TXA_2 should be antagonized by agents that inhibit Ca^{2+} mobilization. An agent known as TMB-8 is a Ca^{2+} antagonist that is thought to block Ca^{2+} release from membranes. When TMB-8 was tested in the presence of PGI_2 and PGH_2 (TXA_2), the cyclic AMP-lowering effect of TXA$_2$ was blocked, but the stimulatory activity of PGI$_2$ was not inhibited (Table 3–1). In fact, in some instances the stimulation of cyclic AMP accumulation was enhanced by TMB-8.[16] Recently Hathaway and Adelstein have shown that the phosphorylation of platelet myosin kinase by a cyclic AMP-dependent protein kinase decreases myosin kinase activity.[17] Phosphorylation decreases the ability of myosin kinase to bind calmodulin, and calmodulin, of course, regulates the expression of Ca^{2+} effects. Through such a series of events, an agent such as TXA$_2$, which would stimulate Ca^{2+} mobilization (and inhibit adenylate cyclase), should enhance the contraction of platelet actomyosin and induce platelet aggregation. An agent like PGI$_2$, which stimulates cyclic AMP levels, would enhance the phosphorylation of myosin kinase, which favors the unphosphorylated form of myosin, and platelet aggregation would be inhibited. Regardless of the exact mechanism(s) responsible for the inhibition of human platelet aggregation by PGI$_2$ or the stimulation of aggregation by TXA$_2$, it does appear that these two molecules oppose each other through the regulation of adenylate cyclase.[18] It should be noted that the vasodilatation induced by PGE$_1$ or PGI$_2$ has been shown to be associated with an elevation in cyclic AMP as

TABLE 3–1.—TMB AND PLATELET CYCLIC AMP LEVELS

TMB CONCENTRATION (μM)	ADDITIONS	CYCLIC AMP (pmol/10^9 platelets per 30s)	INHIBITION OF PGI$_2$ STIMULATION (%)
0	PGI$_2$	731.36 ± 109.70	
	PGI$_2$ + PGH$_2$	430.44 ± 30.90	41
	PGI$_2$ + ADP	397.39 ± 12.77	46
	PGI$_2$ + PGH$_2$ + ADP	119.23 ± 12.88	84
375	PGI$_2$	803.60 ± 120.72	
	PGI$_2$ + PGH$_2$	552.34 ± 80.63	31
	PGI$_2$ + ADP	535.66 ± 20.66	33
	PGI$_2$ + PGH$_2$ + ADP	181.77 ± 17.66	77
750	PGI$_2$	713.88 ± 32.89	
	PGI$_2$ + PGH$_2$	733.00 ± 58.51	0
	PGI$_2$ + ADP	725.62 ± 18.88	0
	PGI$_2$ + PGH$_2$ + ADP	297.14 ± 38.71	58
1250	PGI$_2$	497.63 ± 28.26	
	PGI$_2$ + PGH$_2$	541.39 ± 74.48	0
	PGI$_2$ + ADP	539.42 ± 13.01	0
	PGI$_2$ + PGH$_2$ + ADP	352.00 ± 17.21	29

Prostaglandin I$_2$ was tested at 0.14 μM, prostaglandin H$_2$ at 2.8 μM, and ADP at a concentration of 2.0 μM in all experiments. TMB was preincubated with the platelet-rich plasma for 2 minutes prior to the addition of prostaglandin I$_2$, prostaglandin H$_2$, or ADP. The basal level of cyclic AMP was 71.04 ± 3.20 pmol/10^9 platelets. All platelets were pretreated with 80 μM flurbiprofen, a potent cyclo-oxygenase inhibitor before being used.

TABLE 3-2.—DOSE RESPONSE OF PGI_2 STIMULATED CYCLIC NUCLEOTIDE ACCUMULATION IN DOG FEMORAL ARTERIES

	CONTROL	pMOLES CYCLIC NUCLEOTIDE/MG WET WT.				
		μM PGE_1			μM PGE_2	μM PGI_2
		0.84	2.8	8.4	2.8	0.84
cAMP	0.70 ± 0.06	0.99 ± 0.22	1.43 ± 0.23	2.36 ± 0.23	0.60 ± 0.09	2.29 ± 0.08
cGMP	0.025 ± 0.008	—	0.040 ± 0.07	—	—	0.031 ± 0.008

Dog femoral arterial rings were incubated for five minutes with 0.84, 2.8, or 8.4 μM PGE_1, 2.8 μM PGE_2, or 0.84 μM PGI_2 in the presence of the phosphodiesterase inhibitors. Data presented as mean ± S.E.M. of triplicate samples, and are representative of three confirmatory experiments.

well,[19] but no evidence of a TXA$_2$ inhibition of blood vessel adenylate cyclase has been obtained.

Interestingly, PGE$_2$ does not elevate cyclic AMP in dog femoral rings, whereas PGE$_1$ and PGI$_2$ give dose-dependent increases in cyclic AMP (Table 3–2). If the cyclic AMP data are correlated with the vasodilatory properties of PGE$_1$, PGE$_2$, and PGI$_2$ on bovine coronary arteries, the same relationships are observed. PGE$_1$ and PGI$_2$ relax arteries (elevate cyclic AMP), but PGE$_2$ actually gives mild contractions of the artery, and no increase in cyclic AMP (Fig 3–4).

The in vitro effects of PGE$_1$, PGI$_2$, and thromboxane synthetase inhibitors can also be readily demonstrated in vivo. In healthy human volunteers, intravenous infusions of PGI$_2$ produced dose-dependent inhibition of ADP-induced aggregation that were sustained until the infusions were terminated.[20] Some representative data are shown in

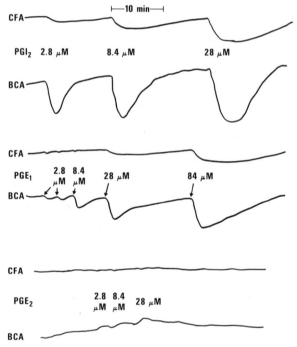

Fig 3–4.—Prostaglandin-mediated relaxation of canine femoral and bovine coronary arteries. Spirally cut strips of canine femoral *(CFA)* and bovine coronary artery *(BCA)* strips were superfused in cascade with Kreb's solution containing a mixture of antagonists and 2.8 μM indomethacin. Vascular tone was maintained by a constant infusion of 2.8 μM PGF$_{2\alpha}$. The prostaglandins tested were added as a single bolus dose in 0.1 ml of buffer at the indicated concentrations. Data are representative of 6 confirmatory experiments.

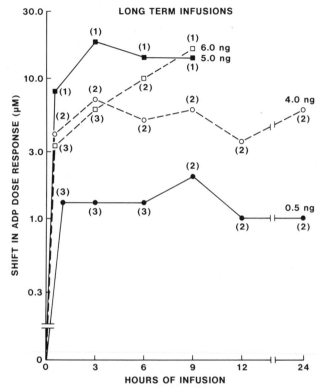

Fig 3-5.—Log shift in ADP dose-response curve during longer (up to 24 hours) infusions of prostacyclin sodium. Prostacyclin sodium was infused for 6 to 24 hours at rates of 0.5 to 6.0 ng/kg/min at the indicated times, the log shift in the ADP dose-response was determined and plotted against the time of infusion. Numerals in parentheses represent the number of subjects at each time point.

Figure 3-5. At an infusion rate of 0.5 ng/kg/min the ADP dose-response curve was shifted 1.0 μM to the right, 4.0 ng/kg gave a 4 to 7 μM shift, and finally 5.0 or 6.0 ng/kg/min produced greater than 10 μM shifts to the right in the ADP dose response curve (Fig 3-5). The inhibition of ADP-induced aggregation by PGI_2 shown in Figure 3-5 could be correlated with an increase in platelet cyclic AMP levels. A particularly good example is shown in Figure 3-6. When 10 ng/kg/min PGI_2 was infused into the human volunteer, there was an immediate rise in both total and intracellular platelet cyclic AMP levels (Fig 3-6). The peak cyclic AMP increase was obtained after 40 minutes of infusion, and was maintained until the infusion was terminated at the 60-minute point. After termination, there was an im-

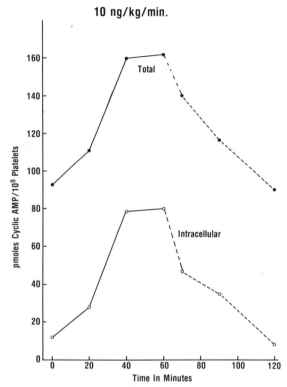

Fig 3-6.—Influence of 10 ng/kg/min infusion of prostacyclin sodium on human platelet cyclic AMP levels. At time zero and at 20, 40, and 60 minutes during the infusion of prostacyclin, cyclic AMP levels were determined in platelet-rich plasma as described in the Methods. Both the total (platelets and plasma) and intracellular (platelets) levels of cyclic AMP are plotted against time. Dotted lines show levels of cyclic AMP after infusion. Data are reported as pmoles cyclic AMP/10^9 platelets (average of two determinations).

mediate fall in cyclic AMP, and 60 minutes later control levels were re-established (Fig 3-6).

Finally, the antiaggregatory activity of a thromboxane synthetase inhibitor can also be demonstrated in vivo in the dog. Using the standardized model of partial obstruction of the circumflex coronary artery,[21, 22] one observes a series of cyclical coronary flow reductions on the polygraph recording (Fig 3-7). These decreases in flow are due to the formation of a platelet plug at the point of obstruction, and have been previously shown to be dependent on platelet cyclo-oxygenase activity (TXA$_2$ formation).[23] We have found that a single 1 mg/kg intravenous bolus injection of the thromboxane synthetase inhibitor

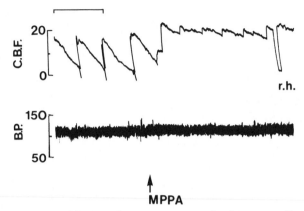

Fig 3–7.—In vivo inhibition of coronary artery platelet aggregation by MPPA. Polygraph recording shows circumflex blood flow (CBF) in ml/min, and arterial blood pressure (BP) in mm Hg. The cyclical declines in CBF represent the appearance of platelet thrombi in the coronary artery, and subsequent diminution of flow. Thrombi were mechanically shaken loose with forceps. After the intravenous administration of MPPA (1 mg/kg) the aggregation gradually disappeared, indicating that thromboxane synthetase inhibitors can block platelet aggregation in vivo. The letters rh represent the point at which reactive hyperemia was checked.

(E)-2-methyl-3-[4-(3-pyridinylmethyl)phenyl]-2-propenoic acid (MPPA) completely blocks any further cyclical flow reductions (Fig 3–7).[24] This inhibition of in vivo platelet aggregation in the coronary artery is directly related to the inhibition of the platelet thromboxane synthetase.[25]

A somewhat oversimplified working model of platelet homeostasis is depicted in Figure 3–8. The blood vessel wall contains the enzyme prostacyclin synthetase, but not thromboxane synthetase. The platelet contains a thromboxane synthetase, but not the prostacyclin synthetase. When platelets are stimulated they produce TXA_2, which causes aggregation of other platelets and induces vasoconstriction. When vascular endothelium is stimulated (e.g., by thrombin), PGI_2 is produced, which elevates cyclic AMP, inhibits platelet aggregation, and induces vasodilatation. In the presence of a thromboxane synthetase inhibitor, platelet endoperoxide (PGH_2) is diverted away from the thromboxane synthetase toward the blood vessel prostacyclin synthetase. This so-called "steal" of platelet endoperoxide by the blood vessel is one of the principal advantages of a thromboxane synthetase inhibitor over a cyclo-oxygenase inhibitor.[25] This balance between the proaggregatory activity of TXA_2 and the antiaggregatory activity of PGI_2 appears to control human platelet aggregation.

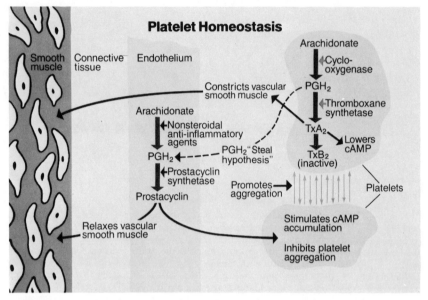

Fig 3–8.—Model of platelet and vascular homeostasis. Platelet aggregation and vascular tone are regulated by a balance between the proaggregatory and vasoconstricting actions of TXA_2 and the vasodilating and antiaggregatory actions of PGI_2. The mechanism responsible for these activities is probably the reciprocal regulation of cAMP levels. TXA_2 lowers and PGI_2 stimulates cAMP levels.

In summary, the reciprocal regulation of cyclic AMP levels by PGI_2 and TXA_2 may not explain all of the actions of prostaglandins and thromboxanes, but when considering cardiovascular actions of these agents, cyclic AMP-regulated systems are clearly dominant.

REFERENCES

1. Kurzrok R., Lieb C.C.: Biochemical studies of human semen. II. The action of semen on the human uterus. *Proc. Soc. Exp. Biol. Med.* 28:268–273, 1930.
2 Goldblatt M.W.: Properties of human seminal fluid. *J. Physiol.* (London) 84:208–216, 1935.
3. von Euler U.S.: Zur kenntnis der pharmakologischen accesorischen geschlechtsdrunsen. *Arch. Exp. Pathol. u Pharmakol.* 175:78–89, 1934.
4. von Euler U.S.: On the specific vasodilating and plain muscle stimulating substance from accessory genital glands in man and certain animals (prostaglandin and vesiglandin). *J. Physiol.* (London) 88:213–221, 1937.
5. Bergstrom S., Sjovall J.: The isolation of prostaglandin E from sheep prostate glands. *Acta Chem. Scand.* 14:1701–1705, 1960.
6. Bergstrom S., Ryhage R., Samuelsson B., Sjovall J.: Prostaglandins and

related factors. 15. The structures of prostaglandin E_1, $F_{1\alpha}$ and $F_{1\beta}$. *J. Biol. Chem.* 23:3555–3564, 1963.

7. Samuelsson B.: Prostaglandins and related factors. 17. The structure of prostaglandin E_3. *J. Am. Chem. Soc.* 85:1878–1879, 1963.

8. Steiner A.L., Parker C.W., Kipnis D.M.: Radioimmunoassay for cyclic nucleotides. I. Preparation of antibodies and iodinated cyclic nucleotides. *J. Biol. Chem.* 247:1106–1113, 1972.

9. Harper J.F., Brooker G.: Femtomole sensitive radioimmunoassay for cyclic AMP and cyclic GMP after 2'0 acetylation by acetic anhydride in aqueous solution. *J. Cyclic Nucl. Res.* 1:207–218, 1975.

10. Vane J.R.: Use of isolated organs for detecting active substances in the circulating blood. *Br. J. Pharmacol.* 23:360–368, 1964.

11. Gorman R.R., Fitzpatrick F.A., Miller O.V.: Reciprocal regulation of human platelet cAMP levels by thromboxane A_2 and prostacyclin, in George W.J., Ignarro L.J. (eds.): *Advances in Cyclic Nucleotide Research,* vol. 9. New York, Raven Press, 1978, pp. 597–609.

12. Miller O.V., Aiken J.W., Shebuski R.J., Gorman R.R.: 6-Keto-Prostaglandin E_1 is not equipotent to prostacyclin (PGI_2) as an antiaggregatory agent. *Prostaglandins* 20:391–400, 1980.

13. Miller O.V., Gorman R.R.: Modulation of platelet cyclic nucleotide content by PGE_1 and the prostaglandin endoperoxide PGG_2. *J. Cyclic Nucl. Res.* 2:79–87, 1976.

14. Gorman R.R., Fitzpatrick F.A., Miller O.V.: A selective thromboxane synthetase inhibitor blocks the cAMP lowering activity of PGH_2. *Biochem. Biophys. Res. Commun.* 79:305–313, 1977.

15. Gerrard J.M., Butler A.M., White J.G.: Calcium release from a platelet calcium-sequestering membrane fraction by arachidonic acid and its prevention by aspirin. *Prostaglandins* 15:703, 1977. (Abstract)

16. Gorman R.R., Wierenga W., Miller O.V.: Independence of the cyclic AMP lowering activity of thromboxane A_2 from the platelet release reaction. *Biochim. Biophys. Acta* 572:95–104, 1979.

17. Hathaway D.R., Adelstein R.S.: Human platelet myosin light chain kinase requires the calcium binding protein calmodulin for activity. *Proc. Nat. Acad. Sci. USA* 76:1653–1657, 1979.

18. Gorman R.R., Bunting S., Miller O.V.: Modulation of human platelet adenylate cyclase by prostacyclin (PGX). *Prostaglandins* 13:377–388, 1977.

19. Miller O.V., Aiken J.W., Hemker D.P., Shebuski R.J., Gorman R.R.: Prostacyclin stimulation of dog arterial cyclic AMP levels. *Prostaglandins* 18:915–925, 1979.

20. Data J.L., Molony B.A., Meinzinger M.M., Gorman R.R.: Intravenous infusion of prostacyclin sodium in man. Clinical effects and influence on platelet adenosine diphosphate sensitivity and adenosine 3':5'-cyclic monophosphate levels. *Circulation* 64:4–12, 1981.

21. Folts J.D., Crowell E.D., Rowe G.G.: Platelet aggregation in partially obstructed vessels and its elimination by aspirin. *Circulation* 54:365–370, 1976.

22. Aiken J.W., Gorman R.R., Shebuski R.J.: Prevention of blockage of partially obstructed coronary arteries with prostacyclin correlates with inhibition of platelet aggregation. *Prostaglandins* 17:483–494, 1979.

23. Aiken J.W., Shebuski R.J., Gorman R.R.: Blockage of partially obstructed coronary arteries with platelet thrombi: comparison between its prevention with cyclo-oxygenase inhibitors *versus* prostacyclin, in *Advances in Prostaglandin Thromboxane Research*, vol. 7. Samuelsson B., Paoletti R. (eds.): New York, Raven Press, 1980, pp. 635–639.
24. Miyamoto T., Tanaguchi K., Tanouchi T., Itirata F.: Selective inhibitor of thromboxane synthetase: pyridine and its derivatives, in Samuelsson B., Paoletti R. (eds.): *Advances in Prostaglandin Thromboxane Research,* vol. 6. New York, Raven Press, 1980, pp. 443–445.
25. Aiken J.W., Shebuski R.J., Miller O.V., Gorman R.R.: Endogenous prostacyclin contributes to the efficacy of a thromboxane synthetase inhibitor for preventing coronary artery thrombosis. *J. Pharmacol. Exp. Ther.* 219:299–308, 1981.

The Analytical Process for Eicosanoid Determinations

F. A. FITZPATRICK AND M. A. WYNALDA

Drug Metabolism Research
Upjohn Company, Kalamazoo, Michigan

Introduction

Discussions on analytic methods for prostaglandins, thromboxanes, and other eicosanoid metabolites usually focus on the abstract merits of different techniques. Depending on a blend of subjective factors such as bias, enthusiasm, novelty, accessibility, convenience and whimsy; and objective factors such as sensitivity, selectivity, reproducibility, accuracy, reliability, applicability, and cost, different techniques are ranked according to their alleged value. For example, it remains fashionable to discredit radioimmunoassay and bioassay, and to dignify gas chromatography/mass spectroscopy as a "better" technique. These distinctions are seldom accurate or helpful because they fail to address the question: Better for what?

A more progressive approach to the selection of analytic methods for eicosanoid determinations could focus on the analytic process itself.[1] This process can be conveniently divided into six stages: (1) define the problem, (2) sample, (3) eliminate interferences, (4) measure, (5) process the data, and (6) solve or redefine the problem. The first stage, defining the problem, offers little opportunity to judge the superiority or inferiority of any technique without some concrete link to the problem itself and the subsequent stages of the process. If one defines the problem as the measurement of certain biologic activities, then bioassay may be appropriate; if one defines the problem as a search for the structure of an unidentified, biologically active factor, then GC/MS may be appropriate; if one defines the problem as a search for a few selective enzyme inhibitors from a field of thousands of candidates, then RIA may be appropriate. The value of a technique exists, principally, in the context of its intended applications. Until the application is clearly defined, discussions about methods are pointless. It is self-evident that inaccuracy or imprecision at the problem definition stage (1) can multiply during the four subsequent operational stages: (2) sampling, (3) eliminating interferences, (4) measuring, and (5) processing the data. These stages are noted in a temporal sequence, but the boundaries between them are vague. During stage 2, sampling, it is vital to know: What can the sample be? How large can it be? How heterogeneous/homogeneous can it be? How many samples must be analyzed? How will the analysis of certain samples help to solve the problem? For example, if the problem is to monitor the rate of in vivo biosynthesis and disposition of a prostaglandin, determination of peripheral plasma levels may seem appropriate. However, if the samples come from small experimental animals or infants, the determination of urinary prostaglandins may be more appropriate.[2] Stage 3, eliminating interferences, may restrict the sampling options, or vice versa. Certainly one can eliminate urinary interferences by using another type of sample.

Typically, however, one considers the ancillary techniques, such as extraction and chromatography, that can be implemented in this stage; or the alternative compounds that can be measured with fewer interferences and yet still solve the problem. Simple chemical treatments are often overlooked, but they provide a powerful weapon to eliminate interferences. For example, cross reaction of PGE_1 or PGE_2 with 6-keto-$PGF_{1\alpha}$ is minimized by treating samples with 1/10 volume of 10% w/v sodium carbonate for 24 hours at 37°C. This converts PGE_2 into PGB_2, which interferes much less in subsequent radioimmunoassays. In this case, chemical treatment alters interferences without altering the compound being analyzed. It may be advantageous to alter the compound being analyzed, deliberately, as a way of eliminating interferences. Assays for TXA_2, 6-keto-$PGF_{1\alpha}$ and PGE_2 have been based on this concept.[3-5]

Note that we have proceeded halfway through the analytic process without selecting any particular analytic method. The goal to this point has been the accumulation of several strategic options dependent solely on the problem. The list of options includes the possible compounds, the possible samples, and the possible manipulations that are compatible with stage 4, measurement, and the ultimate solution of the problem. Above all, the problem governs the process. Eventually, in stage 4 we consider the specific merits of different techniques, but we consider them in relation to the concrete options provided by stages 1, 2, and 3. Comprehensive reviews of the different techniques such as radioimmunoassay,[6, 7] gas chromatography/mass spectroscopy,[8] and others[9] have already been published. Since one of our aims is to stress the critical importance of selecting methods to fit well-defined problems we refer the reader to the reviews to learn how problems fit well-defined methods. Although one repeatedly hears that ". . . prostaglandin measurements are difficult," in the restricted sense intrinsic to the analytic process, the actual measurement is usually the simplest step.

Data processing, for the analytic chemist, is both a mathematical operation and a judgment on his skill in using the analytic process, which gives him five uniquely different ways to fail or succeed.

Radioimmunoassay for Thromboxane B₂

Some examples illustrate the consequences of emphasizing the problems rather than the processes. Radioimmunoassay has been

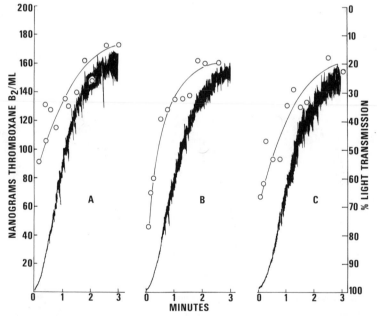

Fig 4–1.—Typical results from the aggregation of washed human platelets (10^9 platelets/ml) induced by PGH_2 (1 μg/ml). Platelet suspension (2.0 ml, 37°C) was transferred to a cuvette containing PGH_2 (2 μg). Aggregation was followed by monitoring the decrease in light transmission through the cuvette. Samples (20 μl) were withdrawn at the times indicated by circles; transferred to a test tube containing 2 M citric acid (10 μl); and frozen immediately. The TXB_2 content of the sample was measured by radioimmunoassay.[11, 18] A, B, C represent three different experiments. Note that TXB_2 formation parallels the aggregation response and accumulates during the experiment.

used extensively to quantitate thromboxane B_2.[10-14] Its sensitivity, selectivity, reliability, reproducibility, and convenience are compatible with the problem of determining TXB_2 levels during in vitro platelet experiments. Available information about the enzymatic and chemical processes suggested that such an approach was reasonable.[10, 15-17] As expected, in most experiments, thromboxane B_2 accumulated as aggregation proceeded (Fig 4-1) regardless of the aggregatory stimulus (arachidonic acid, collagen, thrombin) or the type of platelet preparation (platelet-rich plasma, washed and resuspended platelets). However, for one unique case the results were unexpected. When human platelet-rich plasma was aggregated by the direct addition of PGH_2, exogenously, the TXB_2 levels were maximal the instant after the addition of PGH_2, and they declined as the aggregation proceeded (Fig 4-2). If one emphasizes the procedure rather than the problem, such results would be attributed to an assay artifact. By emphasizing the problem, rather than the procedure, alternative explanations

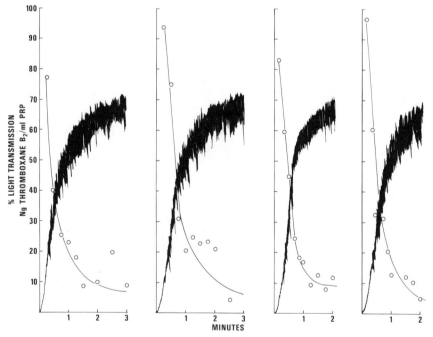

Fig 4-2. —Typical results from the aggregation of human platelet-rich plasma with PGH_2 (1 μg/ml). Procedure and assay are identical to those in Figure 4-1. Four panels indicate typical results from 4 distinct volunteers. Note the inverse relationship between measurable TXB_2 and the aggregation response, and note that, apparently, TXB_2 disappears during the experiment, in contrast to Figure 4-1.

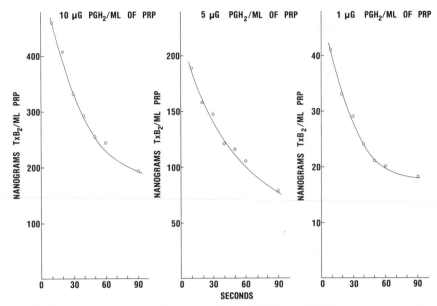

Fig 4–3.—Dose-dependent transformation of PGH₂ into TXB₂ by human platelet-rich plasma. Conditions as in Figure 4–2. Increased addition of PGH₂ to human platelet-rich plasma results in increased formation of measurable TXB₂.

must be considered. Are the results truly artifactual? If they are artifactual, how valid are the so-called acceptable data of other experiments?

In the context of the analytic process new experiments are required to redefine the problem. Are we studying TXB₂ formation? Evidently yes, because the TXB₂ produced was related to the concentration of PGH₂ used for aggregation (Fig 4–3); different selective thromboxane synthetase inhibitors effectively suppressed its formation (Fig 4–4); and agents that elevated intracellular cyclic 3′:5′ adenosine monophosphate did not suppress its formation.[18] What is unique to the sample? First, the stimulus is unique. Aggregations with PGH₂, added exogenously, bypass the phospholipase enzyme and the cyclooxygenase enzyme that are involved with other aggregatory stimuli. Experiments to test the possibility that PGH₂ or its decomposition products caused the problems were negative. For example, when PGH₂ was added to platelet-depleted plasma there was no measurable "TXB₂" derived from unexpected chemical or enzymatic transformations. Addition of platelets showed that they were the source of the enzyme and PGH₂ was the source of the TXB₂. Thus, the concentra-

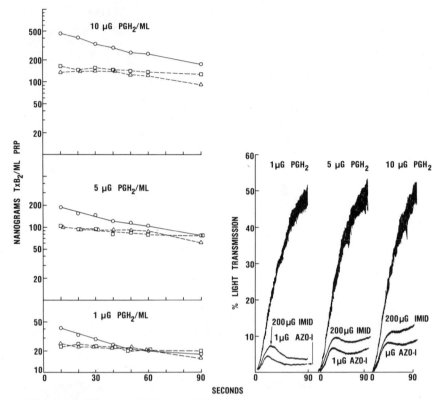

Fig 4–4.—Selective inhibition of TXB$_2$ formation during the incubation of PGH$_2$ with human platelet-rich plasma.

tion-time relationship of TXB$_2$ formation had to be unique to another element of the sample. Since aggregations of washed platelets with PGH$_2$ gave a conventional pattern of accumulation of TXB$_2$, it appeared that plasma was responsible for the unconventional results. We traced our procedure to isolate places where plasma could affect the results.

During the radioimmunoassay for TXB$_2$, samples (50 to 100 μl) were removed from the aggregometer and transferred immediately to another tube that contained acid (10 μl of 2 *M* citric acid). The instantaneous acid "quench" aimed to prevent any further enzymatic transformations of residual PGH$_2$ into TXA$_2$ once the sample was withdrawn from the aggregometer, and to hydrolyze all TXA$_2$ into TXB$_2$. The last point led to an understanding of the problem. TXB$_2$ measurements have always been based on the assumption that all

WHAT IS THE FATE OF THROMBOXANE A$_2$ IN PLATELET RICH PLASMA?

CASE I: THROMBOXANE A$_2$ "DISAPPEARS" BY HYDROLYSIS ONLY

TIME	AMOUNT OF TxA$_2$ IN PRP	AMOUNT OF TxA$_2$ CONVERTED TO TxB$_2$ BY HYDROLYSIS WITHIN THE PRP DURING AGGREGATION	AMOUNT OF TxB$_2$ IN PRP AFTER ACID QUENCHING: MEASURABLE TxB2 FORMED BY FORCED HYDROLYSIS
0	0	0	0
1	20	0	20
2	100	0	100
3	80	20	100
4	60	40	100
5	40	60	100
6	20	80	100
7	0	100	100
8	0	100	100

WHAT IS THE FATE OF THROMBOXANE A$_2$ IN PLATELET RICH PLASMA?

CASE II: THROMBOXANE A$_2$ "DISAPPEARS" BY HYDROLYSIS AND COVALENT BINDING TO PROTEINS

TIME	AMOUNT OF TxA$_2$ IN PRP	AMOUNT OF TxA$_2$ CONVERTED TO TxB$_2$ BY HYDROLYSIS WITHIN PRP DURING AGGREGATION	AMOUNT OF TxA$_2$ "MASKED" OR "REMOVED" BY COVALENT BINDING TO PROTEINS WITHIN THE PRP DURING AGGREGATION	AMOUNT OF MEASURABLE TxB$_2$: COMPOSITION OF PRP AFTER ACID QUENCH	
0	0	0	0	0	
1	20	0	0	20	
2	100	0	0	100	
3	80	10	10	90	10
4	60	20	20	80	20
5	40	30	30	70	30
6	20	40	40	60	40
7	0	50	50	50	50
8	0	50	50	50	50
9	0	50	50	50	50

Fig 4–5.—Proposed reconciliation of the different results of Figure 4–1 and Figure 4–2.

TXA$_2$ must eventually transform into TXB$_2$. Control experiments with quenching agents (acetone) that precipitated the plasma proteins showed that this assumption was faulty. They led to the proposal that during aggregations induced in platelet-rich plasma by PGH$_2$, unusually high levels of TXA$_2$ appear nearly instantaneously and TXA$_2$ binds covalently to proteins at a rate equalling or exceeding its hydrolysis rate under this particular set of experimental conditions. Figure 4–5 shows a tabular explanation of two possible results in terms of the conventional wisdom that TXA$_2$ disappeared by hydrolysis alone, and our proposal that TXA$_2$ disappeared by covalent protein binding and hydrolysis.[19] Subsequently, Maclouf et al. identified albumin as the protein involved,[20] and Eling has found that PGH_2 and TXA_2 can also bind covalently to platelet membranes.[21]

High-Performance Liquid Chromatography of PGI_2

Analyses that are developed according to the multistage analytic process can be used with confidence. Confidence in these analyses prevents the automatic rejection of unusual results. Acceptance of the results can then contribute to the solution of other problems. The uncertain role of albumin in prostaglandin analysis and biochemistry may be such a problem, especially with unstable compounds like PGI_2 and TXA_2.

Pederson has suggested that blood protects PGI_2 from degradation in vitro.[22] Jorgensen has suggested that plasma inhibits phosphodiesterase enzymes. This maintains the elevation of intracellular cAMP by PGI_2 and, consequently, prolongs the antiaggregatory effect.[23] Gimeno et al. claimed that plasma converts PGI_2 into a new, stable antiaggregatory factor.[24] All three groups agree that plasma prolongs the biologic activity of PGI_2, but their selection of analytic methods is inappropriately matched to solve the problem: How does plasma prolong the biologic activity of PGI_2? Bioassays measure biologic activity exclusively; therefore, they cannot validate any of the proposed mech-

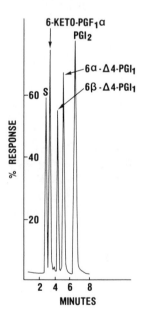

Fig 4–6.—High performance liquid chromatographic separation of PGI_2 from related compounds.

anisms for the prolonged activity of PGI$_2$ in plasma. Other methods are required.

Despite its instability under usual conditions, PGI$_2$ is sufficiently stable at high pH ($\geq$ 9) that it can be chromatographed and separated from its hydrolysis product, 6-keto-PGF$_{1\alpha}$, and quantitated.[25] Figure 4–6 shows the chromatographic resolution of PGI$_2$·Na from 6-keto-PGF$_{1\alpha}$ on a μBondapak C18 column (300 × 4 mm) with the mobile phase acetonitrile: water, 200:800 v/v containing 1.2 gm of sodium borate and 0.75 gm of boric acid. Compounds were detected by monitoring the ultraviolet absorbance (λ = 214 nanometers) of the column effluent. This chromatographic method provides a chemical analysis for PGI$_2$ in its biologically active form. The method is compatible with the problem of defining the mechanism of the prolonged PGI$_2$ activity.

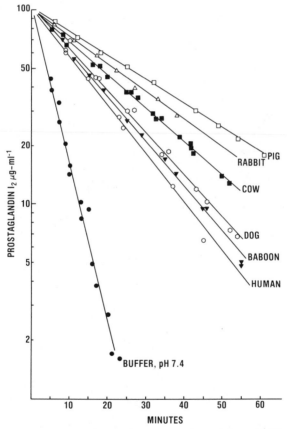

Fig 4–7.—Influence of vertebrate albumins on the stability of PGI$_2$ at pH 7.4.

We monitored the effect of albumin on the stability of PGI_2 under conditions resembling those reported by Pederson,[22] Jorgenson,[23] and Gimeno.[24] Crystalline albumin was dissolved in 0.1 M pH 7.4 phosphate buffer containing 0.9% w/v NaCl. After incubation to fix the temperature at 4°, 25°, or 37°C, the buffer alone or buffered albumin solutions were added to volumetric flasks (10.0 ml) containing crystalline PGI_2·Na (1.0 mg). An initial sample (20 μl) was injected directly onto the chromatographic column within 5 seconds after mixing the buffer with the PGI_2·Na. Chromatography was carried out under the conditions seen in Figure 4–6.

Results show that albumin prolonged the half-life of PGI_2 compared to its half-life in otherwise equivalent albumin-free buffers. The stabilization by albumin was evident at 25°C ($t^{1/2}$ = 12.2 ± 0.3 minutes in pH 7.4 buffer with 50 mg/ml human albumin versus $t^{1/2}$ = 3.8 ± 0.2 minutes in pH 7.4 buffer alone); at 37° ($t^{1/2}$ = 5.6 ± 0.4 minutes in pH 7.4 buffer with 50 mg/ml human albumin versus 2.1 ± 0.2 minutes in pH 7.4 buffer alone); and at 4°C ($t^{1/2}$ = 57.6 minutes in pH 7.4 buffer containing 50 mg/ml human albumin versus 20.9 minutes in pH 7.4 buffer alone).

Vertebrate albumins differed quantitatively in their ability to sta-

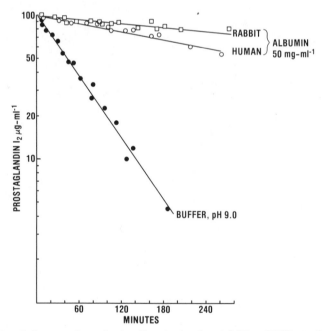

Fig 4–8.—Influence of vertebrate albumins on the stability of PGI_2 at pH 9.0.

bilize PGI_2 (Fig 4–7). At 24 ± 2°C, pH 7.4, the half-lives (minutes) of PGI_2 in the presence of vertebrate albumins were: pig, 25.2 ± 0.3 > rabbit, 20.1 ± 0.9 > cow, 17.7 ± 0.5 > dog, 15.0 ± 0.7 > baboon, 13.7 ± 0.1 > human, 12.2 ± 0.3 >> albumin free buffer, 3.8 ± 0.2 minutes. PGI_2 hydrolysis followed first-order kinetics for all vertebrate albumins.

Above pH 7.0 albumin undergoes a change in conformation designated the N → B transition. This pH-induced conformation change may augment the effect of albumin. For instance, at pH 7.4, 25°C, human albumin (50 mg/ml) increased the half-life of PGI_2 three-fold compared to its half-life in buffer. At pH 9.0, 25°C, human albumin (50 mg/ml) increased the half-life of PGI_2 by nine-fold compared to its half-life in pH 9.0 buffer alone (Fig 4–8).

Conclusions

Current problems in eicosanoid research usually require an eclectic approach for their solution. We rely on six points that stress the paramount importance of the problem instead of the method. We acknowledge that there are limitations to this approach. The examples cited in this text support two conclusions relevant to the so-called analytic process:

1. Unusual results are not necessarily due to deficient analyses. For example, TXB_2 radioimmunoassays can reflect the actual status of TXA_2 under unusual conditions.

2. Assays that are useful for one purpose are not necessarily useful for another purpose. Bioassays for PGI_2 indicate its biologic activity. High performance liquid chromatographic assays for PGI_2 indicate its stability.

In summary, the only generalization that seems appropriate to the status of analytic methods for eicosanoid analysis is: much has been done, much remains to be done.

REFERENCES

1. Lucchesi C.A.: The analytical chemist as problem solver. *Am. Lab.* 113–119, 1980.
2. Seyberth H.W., Mueller H., Erlenmaier T., Mrongovius R.: Mass spectrometric determination of urinary prostaglandins in preterm infants. *Eur. J. Clin. Pharmacol.* 18:89–93, 1980.
3. Oliw E.: A radioimmunoassay for 6-keto-prostaglandin $F_{1\alpha}$ utilizing an antiserum against 6-methoxime-prostaglandin $F_{1\alpha}$. *Prostaglandins* 19:271–284, 1980.
4. Granstrom E., Kindahl H., Samuelsson B.: A method for measuring the

unstable thromboxane A_2: radioimmunoassay of the derived mono-o-methyl thromboxane B_2. *Prostaglandins* 12:929–941, 1976.

5. Lindgren J.A., Kindahl H., Hammarström S.: Radioimmunoassay of prostaglandin E_2 and $F_{2\alpha}$ in cell culture media utilizing antisera against prostaglandins $F_{2\beta}$ and $F_{2\alpha}$. *FEBS Letters* 48:22–25, 1974.
6. Granstrom E., Kindahl H.: Radioimmunoassay of prostaglandins and thromboxanes, in Frölich J.C. (eds.): *Advances in Prostaglandin and Thromboxane Research*, vol. 5. New York, Raven Press, 1978, pp. 119–210.
7. Granstrom E.: Radioimmunoassay of prostaglandins. *Prostaglandins* 15:3–17, 1978.
8. Green K., Hambert M., Samuelsson B., Smigel M., Frölich J.C.: Measurement of prostaglandins, thromboxanes, prostacyclin and their metabolites by gas liquid chromatography-mass spectrometry, in Frölich J.C. (ed.): *Advances in Prostaglandin and Thromboxane Research*, vol. 5. New York, Raven Press, 1978, pp. 39–118.
9. Andersen N., Wilson C.H., De B., Tynan S., Watkins J., Callis J., Giannelli M., Harker L., Hanson S., Eggerman T.: Analytical methodology in the cardiovascular and platelet areas, in Hegyeli R.J. (ed.): *Atheroslcerosis Reviews*, vol. 8. New York, Raven Press, 1981, pp. 1–38.
10. Granstrom E., Kindahl H., Samuelsson B.: Radioimmunoassay for thromboxane B_2. *Anal. Lett.* 9:611–627, 1976.
11. Fitzpatrick F., Gorman R., McGuire J., Kelly R., Wynalda M., Sun F.: A radioimmunoassay for thromboxane B_2. *Anal. Biochem.* 82:1–7, 1977.
12. Anhut H., Bernauer W., Peskar B.A.: Radioimmunological determination of thromboxane release in cardiac anaphylaxis. *Eur. J. Pharmacol.* 44:85–88, 1977.
13. Sors H., Pradelles P., Dray F., Rigaud M., Maclouf J., and Bernard P.: Analytical methods for thromboxane B_2 measurement and validation of radioimmunoassay by gas liquid chromatography-mass spectrometry. *Prostaglandins* 16:217–227, 1978.
14. Lewy I., Smith J.B., Silver M.J., Saia J., Walinsky P., Wiener L.: Detection of thromboxane B_2 in peripheral blood of patients with Prinzmetal's angina. *Prostaglandins and Medicine* 2:243–248, 1979.
15. Smith J.B., Ingerman C., Kocsis J., Silver M.: Formation of prostaglandins during the aggregation of human blood platelets. *J. Clin. Invest.* 52:965–969, 1973.
16. Hamberg M., Svensson J., Samuelsson B.: Thromboxanes: A new group of biologically active compounds derived from prostaglandin endoperoxides. *Proc. Natl. Acad. Sci. USA* 72:2994–2998, 1975.
17. Diczfalusy U., Falardeau P., Hammarström S.: Conversion of prostaglandin endoperoxides to C17 hydroxy acids catalyzed by human platelet thromboxane synthetase. *FEBS Letters* 84:271–274, 1977.
18. Fitzpatrick F., Gorman R.: Regulatory role of cyclic adenosine $3':5'$ monophosphate on the platelet cyclooxygenase and platelet function. *Biochim. Biophys. Acta* 582:44–58, 1979.
19. Fitzpatrick F., Gorman R.: Platelet-rich plasma transforms exogenous prostaglandin endoperoxide H_2 into thromboxane A_2. *Prostaglandins* 14:881–889, 1977.
20. Maclouf J., Kindahl H., Granstrom E., Samuelsson B.: Interactions of

prostaglandin H_2 and thromboxane A_2 with human serum albumin. *Eur. J. Biochem.* 109:561–566, 1980.

21. Wilson A., Kung H., Anderson M., Eling T.: Covalent binding of intermediates formed during the metabolism of arachidonic acid by human platelet subcellular fractions. *Prostaglandins* 18:409–422, 1979.
22. Pederson A.: Untitled letter. *Lancet* ii:270, 1978.
23. Jorgenson K., Stoffersen E., Dyerberg, J.: Stability of prostacyclin in plasma. *Lancet* i:1352, 1979.
24. Gimeno M., Sterin-Borda L., Borda E., Lazzaii M., Gimeno A.: Human plasma transforms prostacyclin (PGI_2) into a platelet antiaggregatory substance which contracts isolated bovine coronary arteries. *Prostaglandins* 19:907–916, 1980.
25. Wynalda M., Fitzpatrick F.: High performance liquid chromatographic assay for prostacyclin. *J. Chromatogr.* 176:413–417, 1979.

Prostaglandin Effects on Platelets

GIOVANNI DE GAETANO, VITTORIO BERTELÉ,
CHIARA CERLETTI, GIOVANNI DI MINNO
Laboratory of Cardiovascular Clinical Pharmacology
Mario Negri Institute for Pharmacological Research
Milan, Italy

Introduction

Several investigators demonstrated that certain long chain saturated or unsaturated fatty acids induced aggregation of washed human platelets, but were poor aggregating agents in platelet-rich plasma (PRP).[1-4] In view of the fact that albumin at physiologic concentrations prevented aggregation of washed platelets by fatty acids,[2,4] the physiologic significance of this phenomenon was questioned.[2] However, Hoak et al. had shown that the marked elevation of plasma free fatty acids (FFA) in rabbits given ACTH was associated with thrombotic phenomena.[5] This suggested that under some conditions plasma FFA might not be fully or effectively bound by albumin and that the action of FFA on platelets could have pathologic significance.[2,5]

In 1972 it was reported that a commercial cephalin prepared as an ether extract of acetone-dried brain (Thrombofax-Ortho) induced rapid, irreversible aggregation in normal PRP, but not in the PRP obtained from individuals after the ingestion of aspirin or indomethacin.[6] Aggregation normally occurred after a latent period, but was immediate if Thrombofax was preincubated with PRP. In contrast, preincubation with albumin prevented the induction of aggregation by Thrombofax. If the supernatant of a Thrombofax-PRP mixture was added to another PRP sample, aggregation was immediate. On the basis of these and other data, it was suggested that FFA, which constituted about one third of the total lipid content of Thrombofax, were responsible for the aggregating activity of Thrombofax, which appeared to be mediated by a transferable substance generated or released during aggregation.[7] Evidence was obtained that this mediator

49

might be ADP extruded from the platelets during the release reaction.

Silver et al. unequivocally showed that arachidonic acid (AA) was the only known unsaturated fatty acid producing rapid, irreversible aggregation in human PRP.[8] They also suggested that intermediate metabolites formed after the addition of AA to PRP could be the actual mediators of AA-induced platelet aggregation and release.[8, 9] The discovery of the platelet-aggregating property of AA, also reported by Vargaftig and Zirinis,[10] extended the fundamental observation by Smith and Willis that washed human platelets treated with thrombin formed two stable prostaglandins (PG): PGE_2 and $PGF_{2\alpha}$.[11] Aspirin and indomethacin inhibited such platelet PG production both in vitro and in vivo. Since both drugs inhibited platelet aggregation and prolonged the bleeding time,[12-14] a relationship between these phenomena and platelet PG synthesis was suggested. However, neither PGE_2 nor $PGF_{2\alpha}$ directly affected platelet function.[15]

Exposure to aspirin or indomethacin prevented both platelet aggregation and PG synthesis initiated by AA.[8] This indicated that AA-induced aggregation and release had to involve an aspirin-sensitive intermediate step in platelet PG synthesis. Intermediate steps in PG synthesis had just been demonstrated in seminal vesicles,[16, 17] and the labile products formed were named PGG_2 and PGH_2 (PG cyclic endoperoxides). These products, derived from sheep vescicular glands[18] or formed during platelet aggregation,[9, 19, 20] were in fact shown to induce platelet aggregation.[21] Shortly thereafter Hamberg et al. presented evidence that the cyclic endoperoxides gave rise to another labile intermediate, named thromboxane A_2 (TXA_2), which was proposed as the actual inducer of platelet aggregation initiated by AA.[22] TXA_2, which is also a potent vasoconstrictor, very rapidly decomposes to TXB_2 which is stable and inactive. The existence of a feedback mechanism limiting the aggregating effect of AA was postulated by Smith et al.,[23] who showed that human platelets may also form PGD_2, a potent inhibitor of platelet aggregation, from added PGH_2.

Prostaglandin Endoperoxides, Thromboxane A₂, and Platelet Aggregation

The relative roles of PG endoperoxides and TXA_2 in platelet aggregation have not yet been clearly established. The involvement of endogenous PG endoperoxides in secondary platelet aggregation was suggested by the fact that aspirin and other nonsteroidal anti-inflammatory drugs inhibit both PG synthesis and the second phase of platelet aggregation. When added to PRP, exogenous PGG$_2$ almost instantaneously induces aggregation and release.[24] In addition, some synthetic analogues of PGH$_2$, such as U-46619 [(15S)-hydroxy-11-alpha, 9-alpha (epoxymethano)-prosta (5 Z, 13 E) dienoic acid], are potent inducers of platelet aggregation, which is neither preceded by a latent period nor accompanied by TXA$_2$ generation.[25] Thus, the assumption that PG endoperoxides have no proaggregatory activity in their own right may be incorrect. TXA$_2$ has neither been isolated nor shown to be the only aggregant present in TXA$_2$-generating systems. A possible resolution of the relative roles of PG endoperoxides and TXA$_2$ in platelet aggregation could be obtained by the use of TXA$_2$ sythetase inhibitors. However, the results so far obtained with these compounds have been inconsistent. Using as platelet stimulants endoperoxides derived from different precursors[26] or imidazole as a TXA$_2$ synthesis inhibitor,[27] Needleman et al. concluded that TXA$_2$ formation is not necessary for human platelet aggregation. In contrast, Gorman et al.,[28] using a synthetic prostaglandin analogue (9,11-azoprosta-5,13-dienoic acid, azo I analogue) as a TXA$_2$ synthesis inhibitor, concluded that PGH$_2$ must be converted to TXA$_2$ in order to induce platelet aggregation. However, imidazole can affect platelet

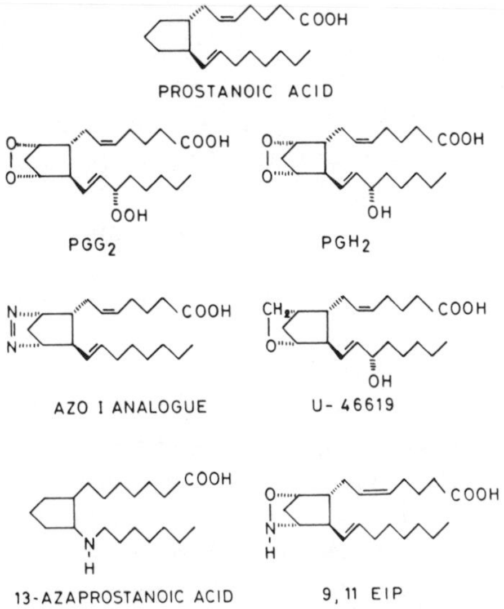

Fig 5–1.—Chemical structures of prostanoic acid, prostaglandin endoperoxides (PGG$_2$, PGH$_2$), and of other synthetic derivatives which interfere with platelet aggregation.

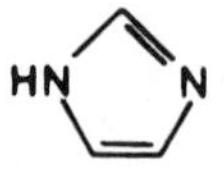

IMIDAZOLE

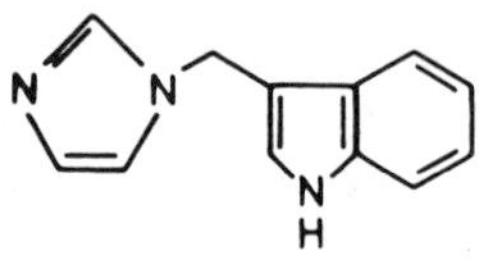

UK-34,787 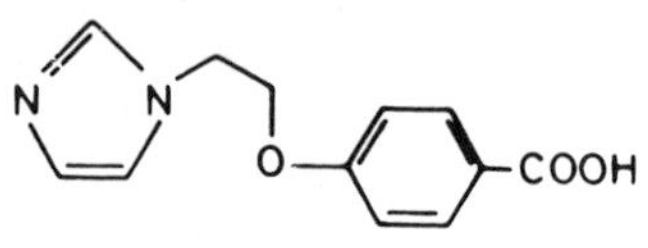   UK-37,248

Fig 5–2.—Chemical structures of imidazole and of two derivatives endowed with thromboxane A_2-synthetase inhibitory activity.

function by more than one mechanism,[29] while the azo I analogue is structurally very similar to endoperoxides (Fig 5–1) and may act as a receptor antagonist.[29, 30] Using imidazole derivatives, which were more potent and selective in their inhibition of TXA_2 synthesis (Fig 5–2), Heptinstall et al.[31] and Bertelé et al.[32] observed a clear dissociation between the inhibition of TXB_2 generation and the platelet aggregation induced by AA. Both UK-34387 (2-isopropyl-3(1-imidazolylmethyl)indole) and UK-37,248-01 (4-(2-[IH-imidazole-1-yl] ethoxy) benzoic acid) at micromolar concentrations effectively prevented TXB_2 generation in PRP from all individuals tested. However, platelet aggregation was inhibited only in some samples (responders) but not in others (nonresponders). As shown in Fig 5–3, UK-37,248-01 failed to prevent aggregation at the minimal concentration which totally inhibited TXB_2 generation and only slightly reduced the aggregating response at millimolar concentrations. Heptinstall et al. suggested that in the presence of UK-34787, platelets may generate significant quantities of PGD_2 in samples from responders, but not in those from nonresponders.[31] If true, then inhibition of TXA_2 synthesis would not be sufficient per se to block the aggregating response to AA and would require accompanying modifications of platelet biochemistry, such as an increase in PGD_2. However, the PGD_2 peaks following ^{14}C-AA tagging and incubation with UK 37,248-01 were similar in platelets obtained from a responder and a nonresponder (Fig 5–4 and 5–5). Moreover, platelets from responders and nonresponders were equally sensitive to the inhibitory activity of exogenous PGD_2.

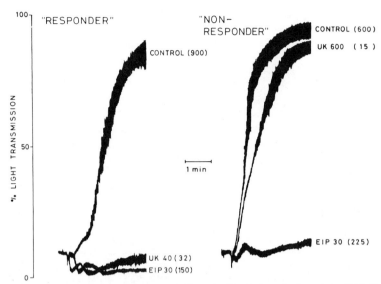

Fig 5–3.—Effect of UK 37,248-01 (UK) and of 9,11-epoxyiminoprosta-5,13-dienoic acid (EIP) on platelet aggregation and TXB₂ generation in response to threshold aggregating concentration of AA (0.4 mmoles/L) in PRP from a "responder" and a "nonresponder." The concentrations (μmoles/L) of both inhibitors are shown. Values of TXB₂ (nmoles/L) are indicated in brackets.

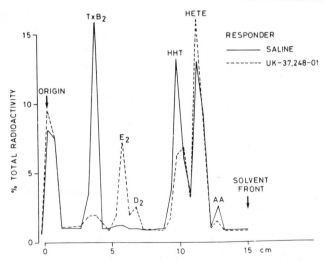

Fig 5–4.—¹⁴C-arachidonic acid metabolism in thrombin-stimulated washed platelets from a "responder" to UK-37248. The radioactive peaks in ethylacetate extracts of platelets were separated by thin-layer chromatography using the following solvent system: chloroform:methanol:acetic acid:water (90:8:1:0.8).

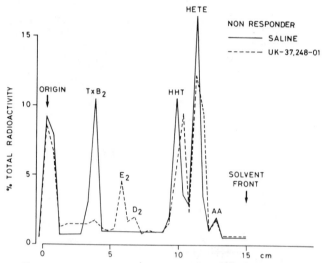

Fig 5-5.—[14]C-arachidonic acid metabolism in thrombin-stimulated washed platelets from a "nonresponder" to UK-37248. Methodologic details as in Figure 5-4.

PG endoperoxides, generated through the intact cyclo-oxygenase pathway, could replace TXA_2 as mediators of platelet aggregation. This could be accomplished by PGH_2 potentiated by a concomitant increase in production of PGE_2.[33] It has been suggested that PGH_2 and TXA_2 act at the same platelet level.[34, 35] The aggregating receptor site requires a molecule with an α-chain containing a double bond two carbons from the ring and an ω-chain without additional unsaturation (Fig 5-6). PGH_2 and TXA_2 both fulfill these requirements, whereas TXA_1 has no double bond on the α-chain and TXA_3 contains an additional double bond on the ω-chain at C_{17}. Other structural determinants, however, seem essential for induction of platelet aggregation since carbocyclic TXA_2, a stable analogue of TXA_2, does not induce platelet aggregation,[36] though both its side chains are identical to TXA_2. The carbon substitutions for the oxane ring oxygens in the currently proposed structure of TXA_2 might account for this difference (Fig 5-6).

The observation that carbocyclic TXA_2 antagonizes the aggregatory action of AA and endoperoxide analogues suggests that either the receptors for endogenous TXA_2 and endoperoxides are identical, or endoperoxide analogues mimic TXA_2. It is also worth noting that dissociation of the vasoconstrictor and platelet aggregatory activities of thromboxanes has been established.[26, 36] Several antagonists of the

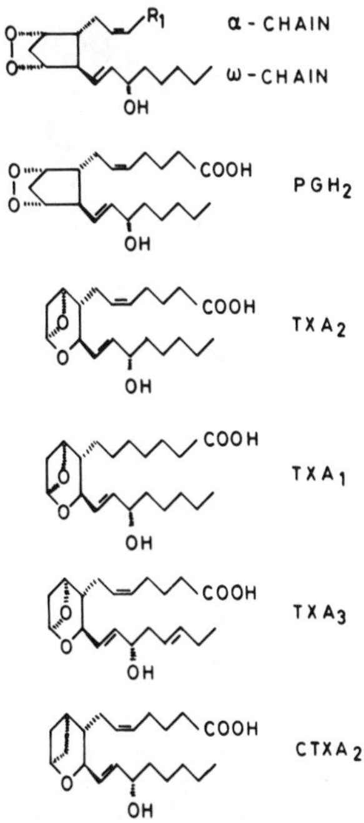

Fig 5–6.—Chemical structures of PGH₂ and some thromboxanes. The structural requirements for platelet aggregation are indicated in the general structure shown on top of the figure: an α-chain containing a double bond two carbons from the ring and an ω-chain with only one unsaturation.

PGH_2-TXA_2 platelet receptor have been described. Some of them (see Fig 5–1) such as the azo analogue I,[28] 9,11-azo-13-oxa-15-hydroxy-prostanoic acid,[35] and carbocyclic TXA_2,[36] are also inhibitors of TXA_2 synthetase. Others, such as 9,11-epoxyiminoprosta-5,13-dienoic acid (9,11 EIP), exhibit activities in systems other than platelets, such as inhibition of PGI_2 synthesis and stimulation of coronary smooth muscle, that are inconsistent with selective TXA_2 receptor antagonism.[37]

13-Azaprostanoic acid appears to be a specific receptor antagonist for platelets and also coronary muscle preparations.[34] It has recently been observed[32] that 9,11 EIP, a proposed platelet PGH_2-TXA_2 receptor antagonist, prevented AA-induced aggregation in PRP obtained from normal individuals who appeared to be nonresponders to UK 37,248-01, an inhibitor of TXA_2 synthesis (see Fig 5–3). Aggregation induced by U-46619, a stable analogue of PGH_2 and TXA_2 mimic, was prevented by 9,11 EIP, but was unaffected by UK37,248-01 (Fig 5–7). These studies suggest that inhibition of TXA_2 synthetase does not

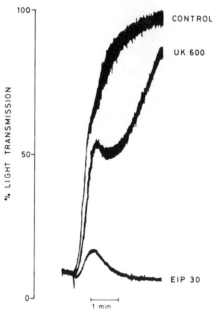

Fig 5–7.—Effect of UK 37,248-01 (UK) and 9,11-epoxyiminoprosta-5,13-dienoic acid (EIP) on platelet aggregation in response to threshold aggregating concentration of U-46619 (0.45 μmoles/L) in PRP from the "nonresponder" presented in Figure 5–5. The concentrations (μmoles/L) of both inhibitors are shown. No TXB_2 was detected during aggregation induced by U-46619.

necessarily result in the prevention of platelet aggregation and that receptor antagonists have a greater potential as antiaggregating compounds.

PGH_2-TXA_2 Induce Platelet Aggregation Without the Intervention of ADP

It is still uncertain whether PGH_2-TXA_2 stimulate platelet aggregation through the release of intraplatelet constituents, such as ADP. Evidence for and against this contention has recently been reviewed.[30, 33] It is likely that ADP (and possibly serotonin) released during AA-, PGH_2- or TXA_2-induced aggregation potentiates and amplifies the aggregating response. As for TXA_2 synthesis, however, ADP release appears to be *sufficient* but not *necessary* to trigger aggregation. As an example, U-46619 induced platelet aggregation at concentrations that were unaccompanied by serotonin release.[38] Moreover, U-46619-induced platelet aggregation and release were not prevented by aspirin. This suggests that U-46619 has mechanisms for aggregation and release unrelated to arachidonate metabolism. Fibrinogen is essential for ADP-induced platelet aggregation. This was also found to be true for U-46619 tested on washed platelets resuspended in a Ca^{++}-Mg^{++} rich milieu. However, when Mg^{++} was omitted from the suspending medium, platelet aggregation was induced by U-46619 even in the absence of fibrinogen. Thus the effect of this endoperoxide is not strictly dependent on fibrinogen and may be influenced by the ionic composition of the external milieu.

Role of Arachidonic Acid Pathway in Platelet Aggregation Induced by Physiologic Stimuli

It has long been known that physiologic stimuli such as thrombin, collagen, and epinephrine induce platelet aggregation which is propagated by the release from platelets of endogenous substances such as ADP. The reaction is prevented by aspirin and other inhibitors of cyclo-oxygenase.[12] More recently it has been found that TXA_2 synthetase inhibitors, as well as receptor antagonists, prevent secondary platelet aggregation by ADP or epinephrine.[34, 36, 37] It is therefore generally accepted that the release reaction is dependent upon endogenous AA metabolism. This is not inconsistent with the concept that PGH_2/TXA_2-induced aggregation can occur independent of ADP release. As shown in Figure 5–8, AA metabolites may be viewed as intracellular messengers amplifying the platelets' response to physiologic inducers such as thrombin and collagen. ADP would act as a second messenger, amplifying the effect of AA metabolites. Platelet-activating factor (PAF), or 1-lysophosphatidylcholine, which induces aggregation independent of both ADP and AA, has also been proposed as a messenger of platelet response.[39] Both thrombin and collagen stimulate PAF availability, whereas ADP and AA do not.[40] ADP, however, again appears to act as an amplifier of PAF activity. The existence of the PAF pathway had been foreshadowed by the fact that both ADP dephosphorylating enzymes and cyclo-oxygenase inhibitors failed to prevent platelet aggregation by thrombin or by high concentrations of collagen.[41] Possibly all three messengers ultimately act through calcium mobilization from intracellular stores, a phenomenon reportedly regulated by the levels of cyclic AMP.[42, 43]

The hypothetical scheme presented in Figure 5–8 shows some similarity to the "cascade" leading to fibrin formation. Indeed an "intrinsic" (thrombin) or an "extrinsic" (collagen) stimulus may initiate two biochemical pathways (PAF and AA), both leading to activation of a

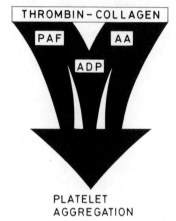

Fig 5–8.—Simplified scheme of the biochemical pathways of platelet aggregation stimulated by thrombin or collagen. PAF: platelet activating factor (L-lyso(2-acyl)-glycerophospholipid). AA: arachidonic acid. For detailed explanation, see the text.

"common" pathway (ADP) and eventually to platelet aggregation. Ca^{++} ions are essential for most of the reactions involved. Thrombin, which induces formation of platelet aggregates, may also trigger the generation of PGI_2. This could be considered analogous to the activation of protective fibrinolysis, which is triggered by fibrin formation.

Arachidonic Acid Metabolites and Platelet-Clot Retraction

Platelet aggregation is usually studied in an aggregometer requiring continuous stirring of the test sample.[44] This facilitates the platelet-platelet interactions which culminate in platelet aggregation in the presence of an appropriate stimulus. However, cell-cell contact itself favors platelet activation,[45] thus complicating the evaluation of the effects of different chemical stimuli. Experimental systems in which agonists and antagonists interact with platelets not stimulated by contact with other platelets would, therefore, be of interest. We have approached this problem by the use of the Reptilase Clot Retraction test.[46] Reptilase is the commercial name for the reagent containing *batroxobin,* a thrombin-like enzyme that clots fibrinogen without causing concomitant platelet activation. Because of this, reptilase clots, in contradistinction to thrombin clots, do not retract. Reptilase clots do retract, however, if a platelet stimulus is added to the

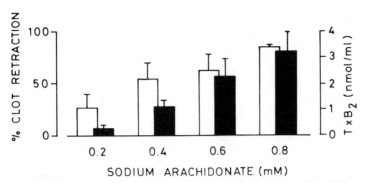

Fig 5-9.—Clot retraction and thromboxane B_2 production induced by different concentrations of arachidonic acid in human PRP clotted by reptilase. (Adapted from de Gaetano G. et al., in Forster W. (ed.): *Prostaglandins and Thromboxanes.* Proc. Third International Symposium on Prostaglandins and Thromboxanes in the Cardiovascular System. Halle/Saale, GDR, May 5–7, 1980. Jena, G. Fischer Verlag, 1981, pp. 173–176.)

system prior to clotting. ADP, epinephrine, and collagen have all been shown to stimulate reptilase clot retraction, an effect not prevented by aspirin or indomethacin.[46] More recently we have found that AA,[47] but not two closely related fatty acids (eicosatrienoic acids), also stimulates the retraction of reptilase induced clots. This phenomenon is accompanied by TXB_2 generation (Fig 5–9) and is completely blocked by aspirin (Fig 5–10), indicating that an intact cyclo-oxygenase pathway is essential for the effect of AA. None of the three stable PGs (PGE_2, $PGF_{2\alpha}$, and PGD_2) induced retraction, but all inhibited the AA-induced phenomenon. Two other naturally occurring PGs (PGE_1 and PGI_2), which are not synthesized by platelets but, like PGD_2, increase intracellular cyclic AMP levels, appeared to be potent inhibitors of AA-induced clot retraction. 4-Methyl-imidazole

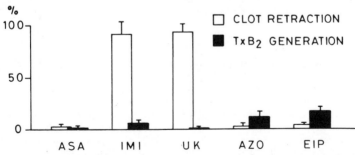

Fig 5-10.—Effect of different compounds on clot retraction and thromboxane B_2 generation induced by 0.6 mM arachidonic acid.

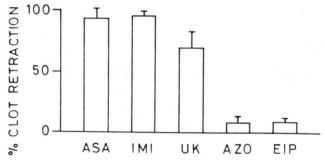

Fig 5–11.—Effect of different compounds on clot retraction induced by 0.6 μM U-46619.

and UK 37,248-01 prevented TXB_2 formation but not clot retraction, whereas the azo I analogue and 9,11 EIP suppressed both phenomena (Fig 5–10). These results could be interpreted as evidence that TXA_2 generation is not essential for clot retraction stimulated by AA. On the other hand, U-46619 stimulated clot retraction without detectable TXB_2 generation. Aspirin, 4-methyl-imidazole, and UK 37,248-01 did not affect U-46619-induced retraction, whereas both the azo I analogue and 9,11 EIP prevented it (Fig 5–11). These data support the suggestion that endoperoxides and TXA_2 may share a common platelet receptor and that U-46619 acts as a TXA_2 mimic (Fig 5–12).

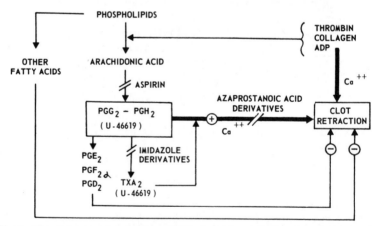

Fig 5–12.—Scheme of platelet arachidonic acid metabolism in relation to clot retraction. Parallel bars indicate the level at which different compounds may block formation and/or effects of arachidonic acid metabolites. The sign ⊕ indicates the final pathway through which arachidonic acid stimulates platelet aggregation. Thrombin, collagen, and ADP may act through activation of arachidonate metabolism, but this is not a necessary prerequisite for their effect. The sign ⊖ indicates an inhibitory effect not directly related to the enzymatic transformation of arachidonic acid.

The failure of apyrase, an ADP scavenger, to modify clot retraction stimulated by AA or U-46619 supports the concept that regulation of platelet function by AA metabolites is not necessarily through endogenous ADP release. Although functionally intact cyclo-oxygenase activity and PGH_2/TXA_2 receptors are essential for AA-induced clot retraction, neither TXA_2 synthetase activity nor nucleotide secretion are required. Clot retraction induced by stimuli other than AA is independent of AA metabolism, as shown by aspirin's failure to counteract the activity of ADP or thrombin.[46] The mechanisms involved in clot retraction induced by different stimuli are set out schematically in Figure 5–12.

Prostaglandins as Inhibitors of Platelet Aggregation and of Other Platelet Functions

Three naturally occurring PGs are potent inhibitors of platelet aggregation: PGE_1,[48] PGD_2,[23] and PGI_2.[49] While their precise mechanisms of action are unknown, all raise intracellular levels of cyclic AMP.[30]

PGD_2 is a potent inhibitor of the aggregation of human platelets but not of rat or rabbit platelets.[23] PGI_2, like PGE_1 inhibits aggregation of sheep, horse, human, rabbit, and rat platelets.[50] Variation in the effects of inhibitors on platelets from different species suggest that there may be corresponding variation in the platelet receptors from the various species. Similarities and differences between PGE_1, PGI_2, and PGD_2 have been reported concerning their antiaggregating profile, their interaction with platelet receptors that regulate adenylate cyclase activity, and their binding to platelet receptors. PGE_1 inhibited the formation of cAMP by human platelets in response to PGI_2 while PGD_2 did not.[51] Moreover, PGE_1 inhibited the binding of radioactive PGI_2 to its high affinity binding site, but PGD_2 was unable to do so, even at very high concentrations.[52] MacIntyre and Gordon showed that the compound N-0164 antagonized the inhibitory effect of PGD_2, but not that of PGE_1.[53] Di Minno et al. reported that epinephrine overcame the inhibitory activity of PGD_2, but not that of PGE_1 or PGI_2.[54] These findings suggest that receptors for PGD_2 are different from those for PGE_1 or PGI_2 (Fig 5–13).

Assessment of the relative potencies of these prostaglandins as inhibitors of aggregation must also take into account the particular aggregating agent used. For example, PGI_2 is six times more potent than PGD_2 in inhibiting aggregation induced by epinephrine, but only 1.3 times more potent than PGD_2 when tested against AA. The average inhibitory concentration for the three PGs in vitro varies

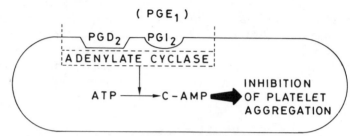

Fig 5–13.—Schematic representation of separate platelet receptors for PGD_2 on one hand and PGI_2 and PGE_1 on the other. All three prostaglandins stimulate adenylate-cyclases, thus increasing the intracellular level of cAMP.

between 4 and 160 nanomolar. However, inhibition may be overcome by relatively small increases in aggregating stimuli. In order to compare the antiaggregating potency of PGs, we first determined the "threshold aggregating concentration" (TAC), which is the minimum amount of aggregant required to produce more than 80% light transmittance (AA and collagen) or two waves of aggregation (ADP and epinephrine).[54] A "threshold inhibiting concentration" (TIC) can then be defined as the smallest amount of PG causing more than 90% inhibition of the aggregation induced by each aggregant at its TAC. TAC and TIC values obtained in a group of normal individuals are reported in Table 5–1 and Figure 5–14. All three PGs appeared to be particularly potent against AA-induced aggregation. To examine the effects of PGs on the first wave of aggregation alone, we suppressed the formation of the second wave by aspirin ingestion. This demonstrated that all three PGs at nanomolar concentrations were potent inhibitors of the first wave of aggregation induced by ADP, epinephrine, and collagen. However, while the TICs against the first wave of

TABLE 5–1.—THRESHOLD
AGGREGATING CONCENTRATIONS (TAC)
OF FOUR AGENTS*

AGGREGATING AGENT	TAC (RANGE)
ADP (μM)	0.25–4.0 (n = 16)
Epinephrine (μM)	2.5–20.0 (n = 25)
Collagen (μg/ml)	0.6–4.0 (n = 21)
Arachidonic acid (mM)	0.4–0.6 (n = 8)

*PRP from normal individuals who had not ingested aspirin was used.
Adapted from *Br. J. Haematol.* 43:637–647, 1979.

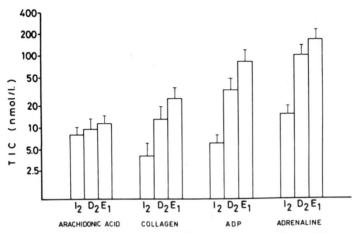

Fig 5–14.—Threshold inhibitory concentrations (TIC) of PGI_2, PGD_2, and PGE_1 against four aggregating agents at their TACs. PRP from 7 individuals who had not ingested aspirin was used. Means ± SEM are indicated. (Adapted from Di Minno G. et al.: *Br. J. Haematol.* 43:637–647, 1979.)

aggregation were never below 10 nM, 50% of the TICs against the second wave were less than 10 nM. Thus, the second wave of aggregation appears to be more easily inhibited by PGs than the first wave. The relative resistance of the first wave of aggregation in "aspirinated" PRP to inhibition by PG might be explained by the fact that cyclo-oxygenase inhibitors can also suppress the formation of endogenous PGD_2 by platelets.[55] Thus, without aspirin, endogenous PGD_2 formed during aggregation may contribute to inhibition so that less exogenous PG is required.

PGE_1, PGD_2, and PGI_2 may also influence other aspects of platelet function. All three PGs are potent inhibitors of reptilase clot retraction initiated by thrombin or by AA.[46, 47] In addition, they may prevent the associated development of "platelet factor 3" activity.[56] PGE_1 and PGI_2 have also been reported to inhibit platelet adhesion to subendothelial structures and to collagen-coated glass surfaces. However, much higher concentrations of PGs were required to inhibit adhesion and they did not prevent release of ^{14}C-serotonin from adhering platelets.[57–59] When infused into animals[60] or humans,[61] PGI_2 prolongs the bleeding time. This effect is unlikely to be secondary to hypotension since it outlasts the vascular effect.[60] In patients with uremia a positive association has been found between bleeding times and the amounts of PGI_2 released from specimens of forearm vein.[62] However, platelet function in uremia is altered in such a complex way that it would be an oversimplification to ascribe the prolongation of bleeding time in this condition solely to increased PGI_2.[63]

PGE_1, PGD_2, and PGI_2 all stimulate platelet adenylate cyclase, and their inhibitory effect on platelet aggregation is markedly potentiated by inhibitors of phosphodiesterases such as methylxanthines and dipyridamole.[64-66] A potentiation between PGI_2 and phosphodiesterase inhibitors has also been observed on the bleeding time in rats.[60] These results indicate that PGs and phosphodiesterase inhibitors exert their effect upon platelet aggregation by a common mechanism involving intracellular cyclic AMP. However, Sinha and Colman demonstrated that PGE_1 induces either an alteration or formation of an inhibitory macromolecule in plasma which can regulate platelet function independently of platelet cyclic-AMP.[67]

Drugs That Modify Prostaglandin Effects on Platelets

A number of chemicals may interfere with prostaglandin effects on platelets. They can be classified as follows: (1) inhibitors of arachidonic acid metabolism; (2) receptor antagonists; (3) compounds potentiating the biologic effects and/or the availability of PGs; and (4) compounds modulating the activity of lipoxygenase.

Inhibitors of Arachidonic Acid Metabolism

Several compounds have been described which may inhibit AA metabolism at one or more enzymatic steps (phospholipases, cyclooxygenase, TXA_2 synthetase, PGI_2 synthetase). Since these compounds have been recently reviewed,[30, 33, 68] we shall only summarize some controversial aspects related to their potential use as antithrombotic drugs.

Aspirin and Inhibitors of Cyclo-oxygenase

Aspirin prevents platelet aggregation, release,[12] and PG synthesis.[11] Majerus' group demonstrated that aspirin irreversibly acetylates platelet cyclo-oxygenase[69] and prevents the formation of cyclic endoperoxides and TXA_2 from AA. Aspirin appeared, therefore, to be a promising antithrombotic agent and several large clinical trials were initiated in order to establish a new indication for this old drug. The discovery of PGI_2[30, 49] and the inhibition of its synthesis by aspirin[66] posed a "dilemma" that has not yet been resolved. Could the dual effect of aspirin—inhibited synthesis of the aggregants PGH_2

and TXA_2 on the one hand and of the aggregation inhibitor PGI_2 on the other—explain the rather modest beneficial effect of aspirin in the prevention of clinical thromboembolic disorders? This important question is still unanswered. The significance of the TXA_2-PGI_2 balance in hemostasis and thrombosis is still awaiting clarification, and the interpretation of its pathophysiologic relevance appears to be quite complex. Accordingly, its pharmacologic modulation may not have simple consequences. The assumption that platelet cyclo-oxygenase is more susceptible to aspirin inhibition than the vascular enzyme has proved to be too simplistic. Observations on cultured cells,[70] laboratory animals,[71] and human volunteers[72-74] have failed to show a clear dissociation between the effects of aspirin on cyclo-oxygenase in different cells. However, aspirin's inhibitory effect lasts longer in platelets than in vascular cells.[70-76] This is consistent with the recent demonstration of an effect of aspirin upon megakaryocytes.[77]

Aspirin is rapidly hydrolyzed to salicylates in the gastrointestinal tract and recent experimental work[78-80] has shown that salicylate may prevent the inhibitory effect of aspirin on both platelet and vascular cyclo-oxygenase activity. It has been suggested[81, 82] that salicylate interacts with a supplementary binding site not directly involved with the enzyme's activity, whose occupancy is, however, essential for the inhibitory activity of aspirin. If the salicylate-aspirin interaction also occurs in vivo in humans, results obtained with high-dose aspirin or during long-term treatment should be reinterpreted.

Inhibitors of TXA_2 Synthetase

The difficulties encountered with aspirin use have prompted an intensive search for inhibitors of TXA_2 synthetase. The rationale for this kind of inhibitor is that it would prevent the formation of TXA_2 while leaving intact the PGI_2 pathway. However, as already mentioned, evidence is now accumulating that even complete inhibition of TXA_2 does not necessarily result in the prevention of platelet aggregation.

Figure 5-15 presents data supporting the suggestion that TXA_2 synthesis is accompanied by an increased conversion of PGH_2 to PGE_2. The combined effect of PGH_2 and PGE_2 apparently causes aggregation. Inhibition to TXA_2 synthetase could paradoxically render platelets more reactive to aggregating agents by increasing the synthesis of PGE_2, which is known to potentiate platelet aggregation induced by different stimuli.[30] On the other hand, platelets treated with a TXA_2 synthetase inhibitor may provide endoperoxides for PGI_2 syn-

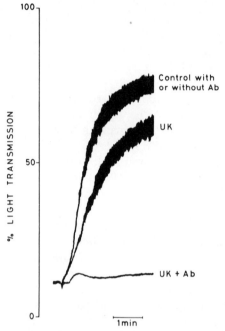

Fig 5–15.—Platelet aggregation induced by 0.6 mM arachidonic acid in a PRP sample "nonresponder" to UK-37,248-01(20 μM). Preincubation of PRP with 10 μl of an antiserum against PGE (Miles, Yeda Ltd., Israel) resulted in the prevention of platelet aggregation in the presence of UK-37,248-01. This implies a role for PGE_2 in platelet aggregation occurring when thromboxane A_2 synthetase is inhibited.

thesis by the vessel wall.[83] Clearly more work is needed to clarify the interactions of PGs and establish their relevance to in vivo situations. At this stage the use of selective TXA_2 synthetase inhibitors as potential antithrombotic drugs cannot be viewed as an obvious solution to the TXA_2-PGI_2 dilemma posed by aspirin-like compounds.

PGH_2-TXA_2 RECEPTOR ANTAGONISTS

This class of compounds appears to meet the major criteria for potential antithrombotic drugs. They appear to leave the metabolism of AA intact both in platelets and in vascular cells, and prevent only the aggregation induced by PGH_2 and TXA_2. However, such antagonists should be highly selective inhibitors of PGH_2-TXA_2 and not affect the action of other closely related compounds such as PGD_2 and PGI_2. Figure 5–16 offers experimental evidence that 9,11 EIP satisfies this requirement.

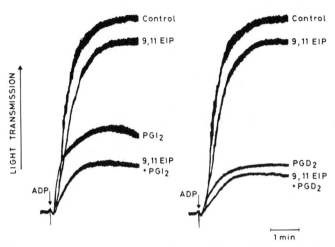

Fig 5–16.—Platelet aggregation induced in "aspirinated" PRP by 2 μM ADP. 9,11-Epoxyimino,prosta,5,13 dienoic acid (9,11 EIP) at 30 μM neither inhibited ADP-induced aggregation nor prevented the inhibitory effects of PGI_2 and PGD_2. This offers evidence that 9,11 EIP, a selective PGH_2/TXA_2 receptor antagonist, does not interact with platelet receptors for inhibitory prostaglandins.

The currently available receptor antagonists are azoprostanoic acid derivatives structurally related to PGH_2-TXA_2. As such they most likely act as *competitive* inhibitors. This implies that their concentration at the receptor level is critical and must be kept constant, a challenging task in clinical practice. TXA_2 is a potent vasoconstrictor, but very little is known[34] about similarities and differences between its vascular and platelet receptors. Consequently, the relative potency of TXA_2 antagonists as antiaggregating and vasoactive compounds remains to be established.

COMPOUNDS POTENTIATING THE BIOLOGIC EFFECTS AND/OR THE AVAILABILITY OF PLATELET INHIBITORY PROSTAGLANDINS

PGE_1, PGD_2, and PGI_2 may exert their inhibitory effect upon platelet aggregation through stimulation of adenylate cyclase and increase of cAMP levels. It is not surprising therefore that the antithrombotic activity of dipyridamole, an inhibitor of phosphodiesterase, has been linked to its ability to potentiate the PGI_2 system.[84] Though pharmacologically sound, this interpretation of the mechanism of action of dipyridamole has not received support from experimental models in vivo or from clinical experience.[60, 85] There are at least two possible explanations for the conflicting results reported by different investigators: first, dipyridamole exerts other pharmacologic actions, such as inhibition of adenosine uptake,[86] which might be relevant to its anti-platelet activity; second, the observation of an interaction between dipyridamole and *exogenously* administered PGI_2 does not necessarily mean that the same interaction occurs at the vascular level between dipyridamole and *endogenous* PGI_2.

Whether other drugs exert their antithrombotic effect by acting on the TXA_2-PGI_2 balance is not known. Studies with sulphinpyrazone in cultured endothelial cells[87] and in vivo in rats[88] suggest that this compound and its supposed metabolites have no effect on PGI_2 formation at doses inhibiting platelet function. The same is apparently true for ticlopidine[89] and for itanoxone[90] given orally to rats. A compound that might stimulate PGI_2 generation in humans after oral ingestion has also been reported.[91]

COMPOUNDS MODULATING THE ACTIVITY OF LIPOXYGENASE

Arachidonic acid released from platelet phospholipids is converted not only by cyclo-oxygenase, but also by lipoxygenase. The latter catalyzes the formation of a number of products, recently named "leukotrienes".[92] Very little is known about the effect of lipoxygenase products upon platelet function. However, modulation of the lipoxygenase pathway by pharmacologic or other means may result in alterations of the cyclo-oxygenase pathway. Whether such alterations would be due to altered substrate (AA) availability or to some direct interaction with lipoxygenase products is a question that will only be answered in the forthcoming years.

ACKNOWLEDGMENTS

This work was supported by the Italian National Research Council (CNR-80.01086.83 Progetto Finalizzato Medicina Preventiva-Aterosclerosi). The compounds U-46619, AZO I analogue and 9,11-epoxyimino-prosta-5,13-dienoic acid, PGE_1, PGD_2 and PGI_2 were provided by Upjohn Co., Kalamazoo, Michigan, USA. The compound UK-37,-248-01 was provided by Pfizer Ltd., Sandwich, Kent, U.K.

REFERENCES

1. Shore P.A., Alpers H.S.: Platelet damage induced in plasma by certain fatty acids. *Nature* 200:1331–1332, 1963.
2. Haslam R.J.: Role of adenosine diphosphate in the aggregation of human blood-platelets by thrombin and by fatty acids. *Nature* 202:765–768, 1964.

3. Kerr J.W., Pirrie P., MacAulay I., Bronte-Stewart B.: Platelet-aggregation by phospholipids and free fatty acids. *Lancet* I:1296, 1965.
4. Wagner E.D., Hoak J.C., Connor W.E.: The role of fatty acids in platelet aggregation and thrombosis. *Thromb. Diath. Haemorrh.* 26 (suppl.):249–259, 1967.
5. Hoak J.C., Poole J.C.F., Robinson D.S.: Thrombosis associated with mobilization of fatty acids. *Am. J. Pathol.* 43:987–998, 1963.
6. de Gaetano G., Vandenbussche A., Vermylen J.: Etude de l' agrégation plaquettaire par le Thrombofax. *Experientia* 28:1127–1128, 1972.
7. de Gaetano G., Vermylen J., Verstraete M.: Platelet aggregation by Thrombofax. Studies on the mechanism of action. *Experientia* 29:1136–1137, 1973.
8. Silver M.J., Smith J.B., Ingerman C., Kocsis J.J.: Arachidonic acid-induced human platelet aggregation and prostaglandin formation. *Prostaglandins* 4:863–875, 1973.
9. Smith J.B., Ingerman C., Kocsis J.J., Silver M.J.: Formation of an intermediate in prostaglandin biosynthesis and its association with the platelet release reaction. *J. Clin. Invest.* 53:1468–1472, 1974.
10. Vargaftig B.B., Zirinis P.: Platelet aggregation induced by arachidonic acid is accompanied by release of potential inflammatory mediators distinct from PGE_2 and $PGF_{2\alpha}$. *Nature N. Biol.* 244:114–116, 1973.
11. Smith J.B., Willis A.L.: Aspirin selectively inhibits prostaglandin production in human platelets. *Nature N. Biol.* 231:235–237, 1971.
12. O'Brien J.R.: Effects of salicylates on human platelets. *Lancet* I:779–783, 1968.
13. Mielke C.H. Jr., Kaneshiro M.M., Maher I.A., Weiner J.M., Rapaport S.I.: The standardized normal Ivy bleeding time and its prolongation by aspirin. *Blood* 34:204–215, 1969.
14. de Gaetano G., Donati M.B., Vermylen J.: Some effects of indomethacin on platelet function, blood coagulation and fibrinolysis. *Int. Z. Klin. Pharmakol. Ther. Toxikol.* 5:196–199, 1971.
15. Kloeze J.: Relationship between chemical structure and platelet-aggregation activity of prostaglandins. *Biochim. Biophys. Acta* 187:285–292, 1969.
16. Nugteren D.H., Hazelhof E.: Isolation and properties of intermediates in prostaglandin biosynthesis. *Biochim. Biophys. Acta* 326:448–461, 1973.
17. Hamberg M., Samuelsson B.: Detection and isolation of an endoperoxide intermediate in prostaglandin biosynthesis. *Proc. Natl. Acad. Sci. USA* 70:899–903, 1973.
18. Willis A.L., Kuhn D.C.: A new potential mediator of arterial thrombosis whose biosynthesis is inhibited by aspirin. *Prostaglandins* 4:127–130, 1973.
19. Hamberg M., Samuelsson B.: Prostaglandin endoperoxides. Novel transformations of arachidonic acid in human platelets. *Proc. Natl. Acad. Sci. USA* 71:3400–3404, 1974.
20. Willis A.L., Vane F.M., Kuhn D.C., Scott O.G., Petrin M.: An endoperoxide aggregator (LASS), formed in platelets in response to thrombotic stimuli: purification, identification and unique biological significance. *Prostaglandins* 8:453–507, 1974.
21. Hamberg M., Svensson J., Wakabayashi T., Samuelsson B.: Isolation and

structure of two prostaglandin endoperoxides that cause platelet aggregation. *Proc. Natl. Acad. Sci. USA* 71:345–349, 1974.

22. Hamberg M., Svensson J., Samuelsson B.: Thromboxanes: A new group of biologically active compounds derived from prostaglandin endoperoxides. *Proc. Natl. Acad. Sci. USA* 72:2994–2998, 1975.

23. Smith J.B., Ingerman C.M., Silver M.J.: Formation of prostaglandin D_2 during endoperoxide-induced platelet aggregation. *Thromb. Res.* 9:413–418, 1976.

24. Claesson H.E., Malmsten C.: On the interrelationship of prostaglandin endoperoxide G_2 and cyclic nucleotides in platelet function. *Eur. J. Biochem.* 76:277–284, 1977.

25. Di Minno G., Bertelé V., Bianchi L., Barbieri B., Cerletti C., Dejana E., de Gaetano G., Silver M.J.: Effect of an epoxymethano stable analogue of prostaglandin endoperoxides (U-46619) on human platelets. *Thromb. Haemost.* 45:103–106, 1981.

26. Raz A., Minkes M.S., Needleman P.: Endoperoxides and thromboxanes. Structural determinants for platelet aggregation and vasoconstriction. *Biochim. Biophys. Acta* 488:305–311, 1977.

27. Needleman P., Raz A., Ferrendelli J.A., Minkes M.: Applications of imidazole as a selective inhibitor of thromboxane synthetase in human platelets. *Proc. Natl. Acad. Sci. USA* 74:1716–1720, 1977.

28. Gorman R.R., Bundy G.L., Peterson D.C., Sun F.F., Miller O.V., Fitzpatrick F.A.: Inhibition of human platelet thromboxane synthetase by 9,11-azoprosta-5,13-dienoic acid. *Proc. Natl. Acad. Sci. USA* 74:4007–4011, 1977.

29. Fitzpatrick F.A., Gorman R.R.: A comparison of imidazole and 9,11-azoprosta-5,13-dienoic acid. Two selective thromboxane synthetase inhibitors. *Biochim. Biophys. Acta* 539:162–172, 1978.

30. Moncada S., Vane J.R.: Pharmacology and endogenous roles of prostaglandin endoperoxides, thromboxane A_2, and prostacyclin. *Pharmacol. Rev.* 30:293–331, 1979.

31. Heptinstall S., Bevan J., Cockbill S.R., Hanley S.P., Parry M.J.: Effects of a selective inhibitor of thromboxane synthetase on human blood platelet behaviour. *Thromb. Res.* 20:219–230, 1980.

32. Bertelé V., Cerletti C., Schieppati A., Di Minno G., de Gaetano G.: Inhibition of thromboxane synthetase does not necessarily prevent platelet aggregation. *Lancet* I:1057–1058, 1981.

33. Smith J.B., Araki H., Lefer A.M.: Thromboxane A_2, prostacyclin and aspirin: effects on vascular tone and platelet aggregation. *Circulation* 62(suppl V):19–25, 1980.

34. Le Breton G.C., Venton D.L., Enke S.E., Halushka P.V.: 13-Azaprostanoic acid: a specific antagonist of the human blood platelet thromboxane/endoperoxide receptor. *Proc. Natl. Acad. Sci. USA* 76:4097–4101, 1979.

35. Kam S.T., Portoghese P.S., Dunham E.W., Gerrard J.M.: 9,11-Azo-13-oxa-15-hydroxyprostanoic acid: a potent thromboxane synthetase inhibitor and a PGH_2/TXA_2 receptor antagonist. *Prostaglandins Med.* 3:279–290, 1979.

36. Lefer A.M., Smith E.F. III, Araki H., Smith J.B., Aharony D., Claremon D.A., Magolda R.L., Nicolaou K.C.: Dissociation of vasoconstrictor and

platelet aggregatory activities of thromboxane by carbocyclic thromboxane A_2, a stable analog of thromboxane A_2. *Proc. Natl. Acad. Sci. USA* 77:1706–1710, 1980.

37. Fitzpatrick F.A., Bundy G.L., Gorman R.R., Honohan T.: 9,11-Epoxyiminoprosta-5,13-dienoic acid is a thromboxane A_2 antagonist in human platelets. *Nature* 275:764–766, 1978.
38. O'Brien J.R., Finch W., Clark E.: A comparison of an effect of different anti-inflammatory drugs on human platelets. *J. Clin. Pathol.* 23:522–525, 1970.
39. Chignard M., Le Couedic J.P., Tence M., Vargaftig B.B., Benveniste J.: The role of platelet-activating factor in platelet aggregation. *Nature* 279:799–800, 1979.
40. Chignard M., Le Couedic J.P., Vargaftig B.B., Benveniste J.: Platelet-activating factor (PAF-Acether) secretion from platelets: Effect of aggregating agents. *Br. J. Haematol.* 46:455–464, 1980.
41. Kinlough-Rathbone R.L., Packham M.A., Reimers H-J., Cazenave J.P., Mustard J.F.: Mechanisms of platelet shape change, aggregation and release induced by collagen, thrombin, or A23,187. *J. Lab. Clin. Med.* 90:707–719, 1977.
42. Salzman E.W.: Platelets, prostaglandins, and cyclic nucleotides, in de Gaetano G., Garattini S. (eds.): *Platelets: A Multidisciplinary Approach.* New York, Raven Press, 1978, pp. 227–238.
43. White J.G., Gerrard J.M.: Platelet morphology and the ultrastructure of regulatory mechanism involved in platelet activation, in de Gaetano G., Garattini S. (eds.): *Platelets: A Multidisciplinary Approach.* New York, Raven Press, 1978, pp. 17–34.
44. Born G.V.R.: Aggregation of blood platelets by adenosine diphosphate and its reversal. *Nature* 194:927–929, 1962.
45. Massini P., Lüscher E.F.: On the mechanism by which cell contact induces the release reaction of blood platelets; the effect of cationic polymers. *Thromb. Diath. Haemorrh.* 27:121–133, 1972.
46. de Gaetano G., Bottecchia D., Vermylen J.: Retraction of reptilase-clots in the presence of agents inducing or inhibiting the platelet adhesion-aggregation reaction. *Thromb. Res.* 2:71–84, 1973.
47. de Gaetano G., Cerletti C., Bertelé V., Di Minno G.: Stimulation of human platelet fibrin clot retraction by arachidonic acid, in Forster W. (ed.): *Prostaglandins and Thromboxanes.* Proc. third International Symposium on Prostaglandins and Thromboxanes in the Cardiovascular System. Halle/Saale, GDR, May 5–7, 1980. Jena, G., Fischer Verlag, 1981, pp. 173–176.
48. Kloeze J.: Influence of prostaglandins on platelet adhesiveness and platelet aggregation, in Bergström S., Samuelsson B. (eds.): *Prostaglandins,* Proc. second Nobel Symposium. London, *Interscience,* 1967, pp. 241–252.
49. Moncada S., Gryglewski R., Bunting S., Vane J.R.: An enzyme isolated from arteries transforms prostaglandin endoperoxides to an instable substance that inhibits platelet aggregation. *Nature* 263:663–665, 1976.
50. Whittle B.J.R., Moncada S., Vane J.R.: Comparison of the effects of prostacyclin (PGI_2), prostaglandin E_1 and D_2 on platelet aggregation in different species. *Prostaglandins* 16:373–388, 1978.

51. Mills D.C.B., MacFarlane D.E., Nicolaou K.C.: Interaction of prostacyclin (PGI₂) with the prostaglandin receptors on human platelets that regulate adenylate cyclase activity. *Blood* 50(suppl 1):247, 1977.
52. Siegl A.M., Smith J.B., Silver M.J., Nicolaou K.C., Ahern D.: Selective binding site for (^{3}H) prostacyclin on platelets. *J. Clin. Invest.* 63:215–220, 1979.
53. MacIntyre D.E., Gordon J.L.: Discrimination between platelet prostaglandin receptors with a specific antagonist of bisenoic prostaglandins. *Thromb. Res.* 11:705–713, 1977.
54. Di Minno G., Silver M.J., de Gaetano G.: Prostaglandins as inhibitors of human platelet aggregation. *Br. J. Haematol.* 43:637–647, 1979.
55. Oelz O., Oelz R., Knapp H.R., Sweetman B.J., Oates J.A.: Biosynthesis of prostaglandin D₂-1. Formation of prostaglandin D₂ by human platelets. *Prostaglandins* 13:225–234, 1977.
56. Ehrman M., Jaffe E.A., Weksler B.B.: Prostacyclin (PGI₂) inhibits the development in platelets of ADP and arachidonate-mediated shape change and procoagulant activity. *Clin. Res.* 27:293A, 1979.
57. Higgs E.A., Moncada S., Vane J.R., Caen J.P., Michel H., Tobelem G.: Effect of prostacyclin (PGI₂) on platelet adhesion to rabbit arterial subendothelium. *Prostaglandins* 16:17–22, 1978.
58. Cazenave J.P., Dejana E., Kinlough-Rathbone R.L., Richardson M., Packham M.A., Mustard J.F.: Prostaglandins I₂ and E₁ reduce rabbit and human platelet adherence without inhibiting serotonin release from adherent platelets. *Thromb. Res.* 15:273–279, 1979.
59. Cazenave J.P., Dejana E., Kinlough-Rathbone R., Packham M.A., Mustard J.F.: Platelet interactions with the endothelium and the subendothelium: The role of thrombin and prostacyclin. *Haemostasis* 8:183–192, 1979.
60. Villa S., de Gaetano G.: Bleeding time in laboratory animals. IV. Effects of prostacyclin, pyrimido-pyrimidine compounds and aspirin in rats. *Thromb. Res.* 15:727–732, 1979.
61. Szczeklik A., Gryglewski R.J., Nizankowski R., Skawiński S., Gluszko P., Korbut R.: Prostacyclin therapy in peripheral arterial disease. *Thromb. Res.* 19:191–199, 1980.
62. Remuzzi G., Marchesi D., Livio M., Cavenaghi A.E., Mecca G., Donati M.B., de Gaetano G.: Altered platelet and vascular prostaglandin-generation in patients with renal failure and prolonged bleeding times. *Thromb. Res.* 13:1007–1015, 1978.
63. Remuzzi G., Benigni A., Dodesini P., Schieppati A., Gotti E., Livio M., Mecca G., Donati M.B., de Gaetano G.: Platelet function in patients on maintenance haemodialysis: depressed or enhanced? *Clin. Nephrol.* 17:60–63, 1982.
64. Mills D.C.B., Smith J.B.: The influence on platelet aggregation of drugs that affect the accumulation of adenosine 3',5'-cyclic monophosphate. *Biochem. J.* 121:185–196, 1971.
65. Mills D.C.B., MacFarlane D.E.: Stimulation of human platelet adenylate cyclase by prostaglandin D₂. *Thromb. Res.* 5:401–412, 1974.
66. Villa S., de Gaetano G.: Prostacyclin-like activity in rat vascular tissues. Fast, long-lasting inhibition by treatment with lysine acetylsalicylate. *Prostaglandins* 14:1117–1124, 1977.

67. Sinha A.K., Colman R.W.: Prostaglandin E₁ inhibits platelet aggregation by a pathway independent of adenosine 3',5'-monophosphate. *Science* 200:202–203, 1978.
68. Garattini S., Di Minno G., de Gaetano G.: Modulation of arachidonic acid metabolism: dietary and pharmacological perspectives, in Remuzzi G., Mecca G., de Gaetano G. (eds.): *Hemostasis, Prostaglandins and Renal Disease.* New York, Raven Press, 1980, pp. 217–233.
69. Roth G.J., Majerus P.W.: The mechanism of the effect of aspirin on human platelets. I. Acetylation of a particulate fraction protein. *J. Clin. Invest.* 56:624–632, 1975.
70. Jaffe E.A., Weksler B.B.: Recovery of endothelial cell prostacyclin production after inhibition by low doses of aspirin. *J. Clin. Invest.* 63:532–535, 1979.
71. Villa S., Livio M., de Gaetano G.: The inhibitory effect of aspirin on platelet and vascular prostaglandins in rats cannot be completely dissociated. *Br. J. Haematol.* 42:425–431, 1979.
72. Masotti G., Galanti G., Poggesi L., Abbate R., Neri Serneri G.G.: Differential inhibition of prostacyclin production and platelet aggregation by aspirin. *Lancet* II:1213–1216, 1979.
73. Pareti F.I., D'Angelo A., Mannucci P.M., Smith J.B.: Platelet and the vessel wall: how much aspirin? *Lancet* I:371–372, 1980.
74. Preston F.E., Whipps S., Jackson C.A., French A.J., Wyld P.J., Stoddard C.J.: Inhibition of prostacyclin and platelet thromboxane A₂ after low-dose of aspirin. *N. Engl. J. Med.* 304:76–79, 1981.
75. Burch J.W., Stanford N., Majerus P.W.: Inhibition of platelet prostaglandin synthetase by oral aspirin. *J. Clin. Invest.* 61:314–319, 1978.
76. Buchanan M.R., Dejana E., Cazenave J.P., Richardson M., Mustard J.F., Hirsch J.: Differences in inhibition of PGI₂ production by aspirin in rabbit artery and vein segments. *Thromb. Res.* 20:447–460, 1980.
77. Dejana E., Barbieri B., Cerletti C., Livio M., de Gaetano G.: Impaired thromboxane production by newly formed platelets after aspirin administration to thrombocytopenic rats. *Br. J. Haematol.* 46:465–469, 1980.
78. Vargaftig B.B.: The inhibition of cyclo-oxygenase of rabbit platelets by aspirin is prevented by salicylic acid and by phenanthrolines. *Eur. J. Pharmacol.* 50:231–241, 1978.
79. Merino J., Livio M., Rajtar G., de Gaetano G.: Salicylate reverses *in vitro* aspirin inhibition of rat platelet and vascular prostaglandin generation. *Biochem. Pharmacol.* 29:1093–1096, 1980.
80. de Castellarnau C., Cerletti C., Dejana E., Galletti F., Latini R., Livio M., de Gaetano G.: Salicylate-aspirin interaction and thrombosis prevention trials. *Thromb. Haemost.* 45:294, 1981.
81. Livio M., Rajtar G., Merino J., de Gaetano G.: Malondialdehyde formation in rat platelet-rich plasma. II. Modification of the reaction kinetics by aspirin and indomethacin. *Thromb. Haemost.* 44:52–55, 1980.
82. Humes J.L., Winter C.A., Sadowski S.J., Kuehl F.A. Jr.: Multiple sites on prostaglandin cyclo-oxygenase are determinants in the action of nonsteroidal antiinflammatory agents. *Proc. Natl. Acad. Sci. USA,* 78:2053–2056, 1981.
83. Needleman P., Wyche A., Raz A.: Platelet and blood vessel arachidonate metabolism and interactions. *J. Clin. Invest.* 63:345–349, 1979.

84. Moncada S., Korbut R.: Dipyridamole and other phosphodiesterase inhibitors act as antithrombotic agents by potentiating endogenous prostacyclin. *Lancet* I:1286–1289, 1978.
85. Di Minno G., Silver M.J., de Gaetano G.: Ingestion of dipyridamole reduces inhibitory effect of prostacyclin on human platelets. *Lancet* II:701–702, 1979.
86. Subbarao K., Rucinski B., Rausch M.A., Schmid K., Niewiarowski S.: Binding of dipyridamole to human platelets and to α_1 acid glyco-protein and its significance for the inhibition of adenosine uptake. *J. Clin. Invest.* 60:936–943, 1977.
87. Gordon J.L., Pearson J.D.: Effects of sulphinpyrazone and aspirin on prostaglandin I_2 (prostacyclin) synthesis by endothelial cells. *Br. J. Pharmacol.* 64:481–483, 1978.
88. Livio M., Villa S., de Gaetano G.: Long-lasting inhibition of platelet prostaglandin but normal vascular prostacyclin generation following sulphinpyrazone administration to rats. *J. Pharm. Pharmacol.* 32:718–719, 1980.
89. Ashida S.I., Abiko Y.: Effect of ticlopidine and acetylsalicylic acid on generation of prostaglandin I_2-like substance in rat arterial tissue. *Thromb. Res.* 13:901–908, 1978.
90. Livio M., Palmier C., Villa S., Maynadier B., Delhon A., Lauressergues H., de Gaetano G.: Differential effects of itanoxone—a new hypolipidemic and hypouricemic drug—on platelet and vascular prostaglandin generation in rats. *Atherosclerosis* 39:469–477, 1981.
91. Vermylen J., Chamone D.A.F., Verstraete M.: Stimulation of prostacyclin release from vessel wall by BAY g 6575, an antithrombotic compound. *Lancet* I:518–520, 1979.
92. Samuelsson B., Hammarström S.: Nomenclature for leukotrienes. *Prostaglandins* 19:645–648, 1980.

Nitroglycerin, Prostacyclin, and Platelet Function

ENNIO C. ROSSI, PETER R. LICHTENTHAL,
LAWRENCE L. MICHAELIS, HO-LEUNG FUNG

Departments of Medicine, Anesthesia, and Surgery,
Northwestern University School of Medicine, Chicago,
Illinois and Department of Pharmaceutics, School of
Pharmacy, SUNY, Buffalo, New York

In 1980, Schafer et al.[1] demonstrated that nitroglycerin (NTG) inhibited platelet aggregation in vitro. However, the concentration of NTG required to produce this effect was 800 μM, which exceeds by several orders of magnitude the concentration that can be achieved in vivo. More recently, Levin et al.[2] demonstrated that NTG also stimulates the synthesis of prostacyclin (PGI_2) by cultured human endothelial cells. This latter effect was observed with 0.1 to 10 ng/ml, which is well within the range that can be achieved in vivo. Since PGI_2 is a potent inhibitor of platelet aggregation, NTG in vivo could lead to impaired platelet function by stimulating the elaboration of PGI_2. In order to test this hypothesis, we measured changes in bleeding time and platelet aggregation in patients following intravenous infusion of NTG.

Methods

Nine patients scheduled to undergo cardiac surgery were the subjects of this study. Venous and arterial lines were put in place on arrival in the operating room. After this was completed, a bleeding time was performed and blood was drawn by venipuncture for platelet aggregation studies and determination of NTG plasma levels. An NTG infusion (30 mg in 250 cc 5% D/W; NTG obtained from American Critical Care, McGaw Park, IL.) was then initiated at 30 drops/minute and altered as needed to maintain systolic blood pressure at

120 mm Hg. Approximately five minutes after the start of the NTG infusion the bleeding time was repeated and a second venous sample was drawn for platelet aggregation studies and assay of NTG plasma level. Bleeding times were measured by Simplate II (General Diagnostics). The platelet aggregation response was quantitated by calculating the collagen concentration required to produce one-half maximum aggregation velocity.[3] NTG plasma concentrations were measured by the method of Yap et al.[4]

Results

The bleeding time and aggregation K_d for collagen observed prior to NTG infusion were 6.0 ± 1.9 minutes and 0.8 ± 0.5 µg/ml collagen, respectively. Following NTG infusion the bleeding time was prolonged to 8.0 ± 1.9 minutes and the platelet response to collagen was decreased as indicated by an increase in collagen K_d to 1.3 ± 0.8 µg/ml. When these data were analyzed as the differences between paired observations, statistical significance was demonstrated (bleeding time, "d" = 2.0 ± 0.4, p <0.001; collagen K_d, "d" = 0.50 ± 0.16 µg/ml, p <0.02) (Fig 6–1). However, there was no correlation between the differences in bleeding time and the differences in collagen K_d.

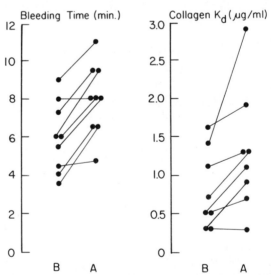

Fig 6–1.—Bleeding time and collagen K_d determinations before (B) and after (A) nitroglycerin infusion. One determination of collagen K_d could not be obtained for technical reasons.

The amount of NTG required to maintain systolic blood pressure at the desired level varied markedly between patients and resulted in NTG plasma levels which ranged between 0.2 and 54 ng/ml. The plasma NTG levels did not correlate with either the differences in bleeding time or the differences in collagen K_d. However, since the NTG infusion rate was subject to constant alteration, plasma levels reflected primarily the flow rate at the time of the second venipuncture and bore little relationship to the total NTG doses which ranged from 7 to 51 μg/kg. When the logs of the total NTG doses were plotted against the differences in bleeding time a statistically significant positive correlation was achieved ($r = 0.66$, $p < 0.05$, one tail). A similar plot of log total NTG dose against the differences in collagen K_d yielded a correlation coefficient of 0.15, which was not statistically significant.

Discussion

The administration of NTG intravenously led to a prolongation of bleeding time and a diminution of the platelet response to collagen. These changes were associated with NTG plasma levels which did not exceed 54 ng/ml (0.2 μM). Since the concentration of NTG required to produce a direct inhibitory effect upon platelet aggregation is 1000-fold greater,[1] it is not reasonable that the changes we observed are due to a direct effect of NTG. Moreover, the lack of correlation between these changes and NTG plasma levels would also rule against a direct effect. However, NTG could have produced these changes indirectly by stimulating the elaboration of PGI_2.

Levin et al.[2] demonstrated that endothelial cells incubated in the presence of 0.1 to 10 ng/ml NTG produced sufficient PGI_2 to inhibit collagen-induced platelet aggregation. Since plasma concentrations of NTG observed in this study were within this range, it seems likely that our patients received NTG in amounts sufficient to stimulate PGI_2 production. Unfortunately, efforts to obtain direct evidence for an increase in PGI_2 were unsuccessful. 6-Keto-$PGF_{1\alpha}$ could not be detected in the plasma of our patients before or after NTG infusion (assays performed by Dr. C. H. Ts'ao using radioimmunoassay, New England Nuclear Corp.). However, recently Patrono et al. presented evidence that suggests that the plasma level of 6-keto-$PGF_{1\alpha}$ may not be the most reliable index of PGI_2 production.[5]

Other investigators have also measured the effect of intravenous NTG on platelet function. Mehta and Mehta[6] were unable to detect any change in platelet aggregation in patients receiving 55 μg/min for 15 minutes. However, the total dose of NTG received by their patients (0.8 mg) was significantly less than the doses employed in this study (0.6 to 3.8 mg) and may explain the discrepancy in results. Moreover, if the effect of intravenous NTG is mediated by PGI_2, the bleeding time would be the more sensitive indicator of PGI_2 activity.

Ubatuba et al.[7] noted that perceptible prolongation of the bleeding time in rats was achieved with 10 ng PGI_2/kg/min, while the threshold intravenous dose for platelet aggregation inhibition was 200 ng/kg/min. They concluded that the relative insensitivity of platelet aggregation to intravenous PGI_2 was an artifact caused by the PGI_2 degradation, which occurred during the delay required to prepare platelet-rich plasma. Thus, the bleeding time performed during PGI_2 infusion might reflect the PGI_2 effect more accurately than aggregation studies conducted later at a time when the PGI_2 effect may have been dissipated. The statistically significant positive correlation we observed between NTG total dose and "d" in bleeding time (but not with "d" in collagen K_d) is concordant with the observation of Ubatuba et al. and strengthens the hypothesis that the effect of intravenous NTG upon the bleeding time and platelet aggregation may be mediated by PGI_2. However, this hypothesis will remain unproven until there is direct evidence linking NTG infusion with an increase in PGI_2 production.

ACKNOWLEDGMENTS

This study was supported by a grant from Blood Systems Inc. and NIH grant GM 20852.

REFERENCES

1. Schafer A.I., Alexander R.W., Handin R.I.: Inhibition of platelet function by organic nitrate vasodilators. Blood 55:649–654, 1980.
2. Levin R.I., Jaffe E.A., Weksler B.B., Tack-Goldman K.: Nitroglycerin stimulates synthesis of prostacyclin by cultured human endothelial cells. J. Clin. Invest. 67:762–769, 1981.
3. Rossi E.C., Louis G.: Kinetic parameters of platelet aggregation as an expression of platelet responsiveness. Thromb. Haemost. 37:283–290, 1977.
4. Yap P.S.K., McNiff E.F., Fung H.L.: Improved GLC determination of plasma nitroglycerin concentrations. J. Pharm. Sci. 67:582–584, 1978.
5. Patrono C., Ciabattoni G., Peskar B.M., Pugliese F., Peskar B.A.: Is plasma 6-keto-prostaglandin $F_{1\alpha}$ a reliable index of circulating prostacyclin? Clin. Res. 29:276A, 1981.

6. Mehta J., Mehta P.: Comparative effects of nitroprusside and nitroglycerin on platelet aggregation in patients with heart failure. *J. Cardiovas. Pharmacol.* 2:25–33, 1980.
7. Ubatuba F.B., Moncada S., Vane J.R.: The effect of prostacyclin (PGI_2) on platelet behavior, thrombus formation in vivo, and bleeding time. *Thromb. Haemost.* 41:425–435, 1979.

Bleeding Disorders Due to Abnormalities in Platelet Prostaglandins

KENNETH K. WU

Department of Medicine, Rush Medical College
Rush-Presbyterian-St. Luke's Medical Center
Chicago, Illinois

Introduction

The blood platelet plays a crucial role in hemostasis.[1] Platelets do not adhere to intact endothelium; but, when the blood vessel is injured they adhere to the subendothelium, where they undergo a series of cellular changes. First, platelets adhere to collagen and possibly other components in the subendothelium. This process requires the presence of plasma factor VIII—von Willebrand factor (VWF).[2] Second, platelets secrete (release) several types of granules, of which the dense granules appear to be of major importance. The released adenosine diphosphate (ADP) induces primary aggregation, which requires the presence of plasma fibrinogen.[3] Third, activated platelets provide the membrane surface needed for the blood coagulation cascade. Recently, it has been shown that the rate at which prothrombin is converted to thrombin is increased by a complex of factors Xa, Va, and calcium ion on this activated platelet surface.[4] Once thrombin is generated it enhances both the primary aggregation and the secretory function of platelets. Finally, the enzymes of the arachidonic acid metabolic pathway are activated and thus a number of biologically important metabolites are produced. Among these metabolites are the prostaglandin (PG) endoperoxides (PGG_2 and PGH_2), which are potent inducers of the platelet release reaction.[5,6] In fact, TXA_2 has been regarded as being the key mediator of platelet release reaction.[7] This entire series of cellular changes occurs rapidly and are interrelated.

TABLE 7–1.—CONGENITAL
PLATELET DYSFUNCTION

I. Defective platelet adhesion
    Bernard-Soulier syndrome
    von Willebrand's disease
II. Defective primary aggregation
    Glanzmann's thrombasthenia
    Congenital afibrinogenemia
III. Defective release reaction
    Primary release defect
    Storage pool deficiency
IV. Defective platelet procoagulant
    activity
    Isolated platelet factor III deficiency
    Congenital factor V deficiency

Defects in any of the processes result in defective platelet function and lead to significant bleeding problems in patients with functional disorders of platelets. Of relevance to this discussion is a group of congenital bleeding disorders with characteristic abnormalities in platelet function. They may be broken down into four sub-groups according to their primary defect (Table 7–1).[8] The disorders with a primary defect in platelet adhesion are due either to a lack of membrane receptors for VWF (Bernard-Soulier syndrome) or to a lack of VWF in plasma (von Willebrand's disease). Platelets from Bernard-Soulier syndrome have been shown to produce normal quantities of metabolites of arachidonate and respond normally to endoperoxides.[9] As anticipated, there are no prostaglandin abnormalities in these disorders. The disorders with characteristic abnormalities in the coagulant activity are due to either the inability of platelets to provide the necessary surface configuration or to factor V deficiency. These disorders are likely to have normal prostaglandin metabolism, although this has not been investigated. In contrast, primary release defects, storage pool deficiency and Glanzmann's thrombasthenia are all associated with major prostaglandin abnormalities.

Methodologic Considerations

Criteria for diagnosing the various congenital bleeding disorders have been well established and will not be described here. To investigate prostaglandin abnormalities in these disorders, assays of platelet prostaglandin metabolites may be performed by (1) radioimmunoassay, (2) radiochromatography, (3) biologic assay, and (4) gas chromatography and mass spectrometry. No matter which assay system is used, careful preparations of the samples are extremely important. The prostaglandin metabolites must be properly extracted from platelet preparations. As presented by Dr. Fitzpatrick in this symposium, the TXB_2 assay presents an additional problem in that the TXB_2 concentration measured will vary according to the time interval at which the samples are acidified and extracted for assay. In our experiments, platelet-rich plasma was obtained from patients or controls and incubated in an aggregometer cuvette while being stirred at 900 rpm at 37°C for 3 minutes. The reaction was then terminated by acidification, and the samples were extracted with ethyl acetate and chromatographed on silicic acid columns. The extracted TXB_2 has a recovery of approximately 80%. To study the response of platelets to various agonists, particularly arachidonic acid, endoperoxides, and endoperoxide analogue (i.e., U46619), platelet aggregation and release may be determined using a lumi-aggregometer. The release reaction can also be measured separately by the ^{14}C-serotonin release technique. In addition to these two commonly used parameters, platelet cyclic AMP levels in response to agonists may be useful. In this context, an adenylate cyclase stimulator (such as prostacyclin or PGE_1) and phosphodiesterase inhibitors (theophylline, for example) should be used.

Prostaglandin Abnormalities in Primary Release Defect

The platelet release disorder is a group of heterogeneous diseases characterized by a defect in the secretory function (Table 7–2). Through the work of Weiss, Holmsen, et al.,[10, 11] two distinct subgroups have been identified: (1) storage pool deficiency (SPD) and (2) primary release defect (PRD). The former is due to the lack of electron-dense granules, whereas the latter is related to an abnormal release mechanism per se, despite the presence of adequate dense granules. PRD is of particular interest here because it primarily reflects defects in platelet arachidonic acid metabolism (Fig 7–1). In the biosynthesis of TXA_2 in platelets, arachidonic acid is liberated from phospholipids by two alternate enzymic systems: (1) phospholipase A_2, and (2) phospholipase C and diglyceride lipase.[12, 13] Deficiency of either enzyme has not yet been identified and thus their role in causing bleeding remains unclear. By contrast, deficiency of cyclooxygenase, which converts arachidonic acid into PGG_2 and PGH_2, has been documented in several patients. Deficiency of thromboxane synthetase, which converts PGH_2 into TXA_2, has also been described. In

TABLE 7–2.—CLASSIFICATION OF PLATELET
RELEASE DISORDERS

I. Storage Pool Deficiency
   Congenital
      Hereditary storage pool disease
      Hermansky Pudlak syndrome
      Wiskott-Aldrich syndrome
      Thrombocytopenia with absence of radii (TAR)
   Acquired
      Acute leukemia
      Myeloproliferative disorders
      Cardiopulmonary bypass
      Immune complex disorders
      Drug-induced
II. Primary Release Defects
   Congenital
      Cyclo-oxygenase deficiency
      Thromboxane synthetase deficiency
      Abnormal response to thromboxane
   Acquired
      Drug-induced

---

addition, an abnormal response to TXA_2 has been described which represents another mechanism for primary release disorder.

Platelet Cyclo-oxygenase Deficiency

Cyclo-oxygenase is a rate-limiting enzyme in the arachidonic acid metabolism. It is present in many tissues, but has been purified primarily from seminal vesicles.[14, 15] Although it has not been purified from platelets, it is generally thought that the platelet cyclo-oxygenase is similar or identical in structure and function to the cyclo-oxygenase from seminal vesicles. It contains subunits of about 70,000 daltons. Its action requires oxygen and heme[16] and is enhanced by the availability of nonesterified substrate and hydroperoxide activator.[17] A deficiency of enzyme activity may, therefore, be due to a number of mechanisms. Malmsten et al. described the first patient with this enzyme deficiency.[18] The patient had a life-long mild bleeding tendency, a prolonged bleeding time, and an intrinsic defect in platelet release mechanism. Subsequently, three other patients have been reported.[19, 20] Their functional and clinical manifestations are similar (Table 7–3). They have a life-long history of mucocutaneous bleeding (easy bruising, epistaxis, and menorrhagia). Paradoxically, bleeding may not occur during major surgical procedures. The mode of inheritance has not been established. No morphologic abnormalities have

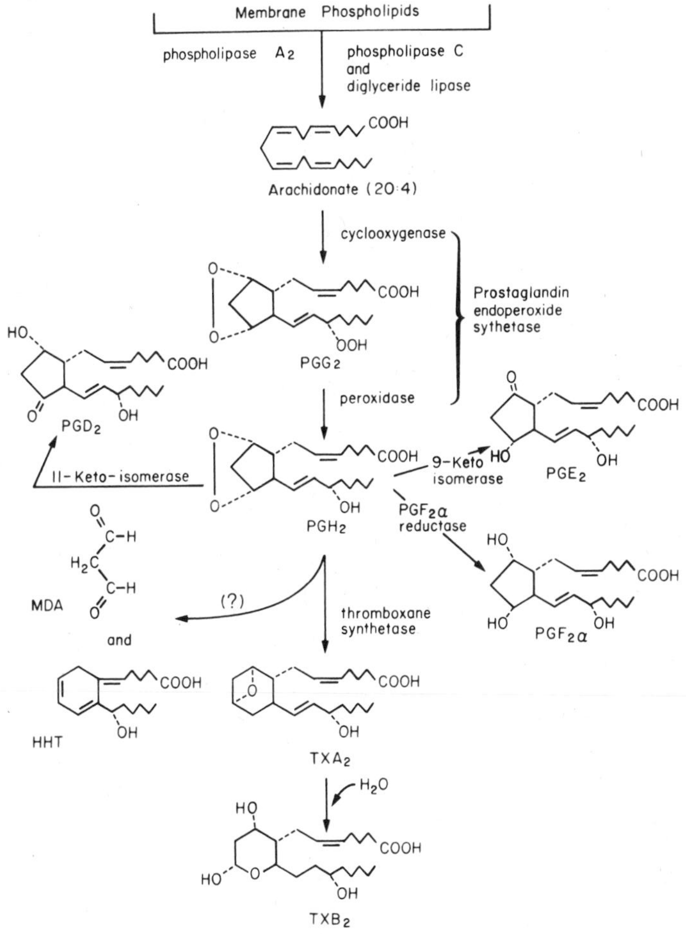

Fig 7-1.—Platelet arachidonic acid metabolism.

been reported in these cases; in fact, platelet diameter appeared normal in one study.[19] Besides the characteristic abnormalities in platelet release and aggregation in response to ADP, collagen, and epinephrine, platelets do not aggregate when arachidonic acid is added. Platelet release and aggregation are normal on the addition of prostaglandin endoperoxides (PGG_2). Platelet aggregation in response to thrombin and ristocetin is normal.[19] Biosynthesis of TXA_2 in patients' platelets, measured by bioassay,[19] thin-layer radiochromatography,[18] or radioimmunoassay,[20] is uniformly defective when arachidonic acid is added as a substrate. However, TXA_2 (or TXB_2) production is nor-

TABLE 7-3.—CYCLO-OXYGENASE DEFICIENCY:
CLINICAL DATA

PATIENT	AGE/SEX	MUCOSAL BLEEDING	SURGICAL BLEEDING	BLEEDING TIME (MIN)
1	30/F	+	−	9
2	33/F	+	−	
3	46/F	+	+	7
4	25/F	+	±	8

mal when PGG_2 is added. Thromboxane formation in response to platelet stimuli, such as ADP, collagen, epinephrine, and thrombin, is also reduced. Platelet $PGF_{2\alpha}$ evaluated in both patients reported by Lagarde et al. was significantly reduced.[19] Interestingly, prostacyclin formation in the venous ring of the patient reported by Pareti et al. was reduced.[20] It seems of little question that all four patients reported have a reduced cyclo-oxygenase activity, although further studies are needed to confirm this notion and to identify the mechanism(s) involved. These studies confirm that endoperoxides and TXA_2 are essential for normal hemostasis, and lack of normal production may lead to significant bleeding. The bleeding tends to involve small vessels in the skin and mucosa. The paradoxical absence of surgical bleeding in some of these patients may be explained by the formation of a significant amount of thrombin at the surgical sites, which can overcome the defect of TXA_2 and induce normal aggregation. This disease is similar to the acquired cyclo-oxygenase deficiency from aspirin ingestion,[21] and yet it is well recognized that aspirin ingestion seldom causes bleeding in normal individuals. The difference in the bleeding tendency between the inherent and drug-induced cyclo-oxygenase deficiency remains unclear. Prostacyclin synthesis by venous segments obtained from a patient with cyclo-oxygenase deficiency was found to be reduced, and yet the patient did not exhibit a thrombotic tendency. This puzzling phenomenon requires further investigation.

Thromboxane Synthetase Deficiency

This enzyme is present in the microsomal fraction of platelets.[22] It converts prostaglandin endoperoxides to thromboxane A_2. Deficiency of this enzyme may lead to the accumulation of endoperoxides and formation of increased quantities of classic prostaglandins, i.e., PGE_2, $PGF_{2\alpha}$, and PGD_2. PGD_2 is known to inhibit platelet aggregation,[23] while the effects of PGE_2 and $PGF_{2\alpha}$ on platelets remain uncertain.

Experimental studies have indicated that inhibition of this enzyme with selective inhibitors may provide endoperoxides for vascular prostacyclin synthetase to enhance the production of prostacyclin, the so-called "steal phenomenon."[24] Patients with this enzyme deficiency provide valuable clinical material for investigating these hypotheses. To date, only two brief reports have appeared in the literature.[25, 26] Of interest is the family reported by Machin et al.[25] Metabolic defects include reduced formation of TXB$_2$ and malondialdehyde in response to arachidonic acid challenge. On the other hand, PGE$_2$, PGF$_{2\alpha}$, PGD$_2$, and PGI$_2$ (measured as 6-keto-PGF$_{1\alpha}$) formation was increased. The affected family members have a moderate bleeding tendency and a prolonged bleeding time. However, it is uncertain whether this bleeding tendency is primarily due to reduced TXA$_2$ formation or increased PGI$_2$ production by the vessel wall.

Abnormal TXA$_2$ Response

A family with a mild bleeding disorder due to an abnormal response to TXA$_2$ has been studied in our laboratory.[27, 28] Several members of three generations have a life-long history of easy bruising and mucocutaneous bleeding. All of them were documented to have a primary defect in the release mechanism. Further investigation of the propositus' platelets revealed absent aggregation or release in response to arachidonic acid and U46619, a TXA$_2$ agonist. TXB$_2$ formation in response to arachidonate and other agonists was normal. Transfer of a fraction of the propositus' platelets treated with arachidonic acid induced normal PRP to aggregate, while transfer of normal PRP pretreated with arachidonate failed to aggregate the patient's platelets. To test the hypothesis that the abnormal response was due to abnormal membrane receptors for TXA$_2$/PGH$_2$, the suppression of platelet cyclic AMP (cAMP) by U46619 was investigated. Elevation of cAMP by prostacyclin was comparable between the propositus and normal controls.[28] However, this cAMP elevation in normal subjects was significantly reduced when platelets were pretreated with U46619, whereas in the propositus, U46619 had no effect on prostacyclin-induced cAMP elevation.[28] The lack of response to TXA$_2$ appeared specific rather than global, since platelets from the propositus respond normally to ristocetin, thrombin, and ionophore A23187. The propositus' platelets undergo normal shape change and primary aggregation when challenged by ADP or epinephrine. The defect is most likely due to a lack of TXA$_2$ receptors, which is being investigated. A patient reported by Lages and Weiss also appears to exhibit an abnormal TXA_2 response,[29] but the defect in that case appears to be related to defective intracellular calcium mobilization.

These studies support the concept that thromboxane A_2 plays an essential role in the platelet release reaction. Defects in thromboxane formation due to "enzymopathy" of the cyclo-oxygenase pathway or in platelet response to TXA_2 lead to an inherent defect in the release reaction and a significant though mild bleeding disorder. Thrombin, at sufficient concentrations, can cause these platelets to aggregate independently of TXA_2; therefore, patients may not bleed during major surgery because of significant thrombin formation at the damaged blood vessels. These patients are extremely valuable for increasing our understanding of the enzymes of the cyclo-oxygenase pathway and the membrane receptors for TXA_2/PGH_2.

Prostaglandin Abnormalities in Storage Pool Deficiency

The absence of electron-dense granules is the hallmark of storage pool deficiency (SPD). The SPD platelets take up exogenous ^{14}C-serotonin normally, but fail to release it.[30] The release of endogenous platelet factor 4 from alpha-granules[31] and acid hydrolases[32] from lysosomes is also defective. These studies suggest that SPD platelets have an intrinsic abnormality in the release mechanism as well. It remains uncertain whether the release defect is due to prostaglandin or other cellular abnormalities. Nevertheless, prostaglandin abnormalities have been reported in isolated SPD and in SPD associated with Hermansky-Pudlak syndrome. The abnormalities may be divided into two major categories: (1) impaired prostaglandin synthesis and (2) abnormal platelet response to arachidonate, endoperoxides, and other agonists. The data on prostaglandin synthesis in SPD are conflicting. Willis and Weiss demonstrated a reduced PGE_2 synthesis in response to connective tissue or thrombin stimulation in several members of a family with SPD.[33, 34] On the other hand, malondialdehyde formation by thrombin or sodium arachidonate was normal in another family with SPD.[35] Similarly, platelet TXB_2 synthesis induced by arachidonic acid and PGG_2 was normal in a patient with Hermansky-Pudlak syndrome.[9] Collagen-induced TXB_2 formation was slightly below one standard deviation of normal, but was within 2 standard deviations of the normal values. Differences in TXB_2 synthesis may reflect a heterogeneity in this disorder. However, it should be pointed out that these data are probably not directly comparable, since different methodologies were employed for determining the prostaglandin synthesis. Platelet aggregation in response to arachidonate and PGG_2 was normal, whereas arachidonate-induced ATP release was absent in the familial SPD of Ingerman et al.[32] By contrast, platelet aggregation in response to arachidonic acid and labile aggregation stimulating substance (LASS, consisting primarily of endoperoxides) was defective in the family described by Weiss et al.[36] The disparity of the results between these two families further suggests that SPD is a heterogeneous disorder. The prostaglandin abnormalities observed in these patients are different, yet each probably plays a role in the abnormal release reaction.

Prostaglandin Abnormalities in Glanzmann's Thrombasthenia

Thrombasthenic platelets fail to aggregate or undergo release reaction in response to stimulation by ADP.[37] This defect has been reported to be related to a lack of glycoprotein II_b-III_a.[38] Malmsten et al. showed that platelet aggregation in response to arachidonic acid and PGG_2 was subnormal, but not totally absent, in thrombasthenic platelets.[9] ADP-release by arachidonic acid and PGG_2 appeared normal, while ^{14}C-serotonin release was only slightly impaired. The synthesis of TXA_2 (measured as TXB_2), on the addition of arachidonic acid or PGG_2, was normal, but was reduced in response to ADP or collagen.[9] These findings suggest that membrane receptors for TXA_2 may be intact in these platelets and that the abnormal synthesis in response to ADP or collagen may be due to a defect in ADP's ability to make the fibrinogen receptor available.[39] This receptor interaction seems to be essential for the activation of the membrane phospholipase enzymes and therefore the cyclo-oxygenase pathway.

Conclusion

Bleeding disorders due to intrinsic platelet dysfunction represent unique experiments of nature which are extremely valuable for unraveling the mysteries surrounding platelet physiology and pathophysiology. They provide powerful tools for increasing our understanding of the role of prostaglandins in platelet function and disease. Prostaglandin abnormalities in congenital platelet dysfunction are summarized in Table 7–4. It is apparent that the primary release disorder is a heterogeneous group of diseases that may be due to a deficiency of platelet cyclo-oxygenase or thromboxane synthetase, a receptor abnormality to TXA_2, or an impaired calcium mobility. This group of diseases is of particular interest in the study of the arachidonate metabolic pathway and its regulation, and/or TXA_2 receptors.

TABLE 7–4.—Prostaglandin Abnormalities

| | PROSTAGLANDIN SYNTHESIS IN RESPONSE TO AA | | | | | | | PLATELET | | | |
	PGE_2	$PGF_{2\alpha}$	PGD_2	TXB_2	MDA	HHT	6-keto-$PGF_{1\alpha}$	AA	PGG_2/H_2	U46619	ADP
Cyclo-oxygenase deficiency	↓	↓		↓	↓	↓	↓	↓	↓	?	↓
Thromboxane synthetase deficiency	↑	↑	↑	↓	↓	↓	↑			?	
Abnormal TXA_2 response				N				↓		↓	↓
Storage pool disease				N				↓			
Glanzmann's thrombasthenia				N				N	N		↓
Bernard-Soulier syndrome				N				N	N		

The role of prostaglandin abnormalities in storage pool disease is less clear, but studies indicate that it too is a heterogeneous group of abnormalities, some accompanied by an intrinsic defect in the release mechanism and some not. Our understanding of the interrelationship of the release reaction and prostaglandin synthesis will be enhanced by further investigation of this group of disorders.

REFERENCES

1. Shattel S.J., Bennett J.S.: Platelets and their membranes in hemostasis—physiology and pathophysiology. *Ann. Intern. Med.* 94:108–118, 1980.
2. Tschopp T.B., Weiss H.J., Baumgartner H.R.: Decreased adhesion of platelets to subendothelium in von Willebrand's disease. *J. Lab. Clin. Med.* 83:296–300, 1974.
3. Bennett J.S., Vilaire G.: Exposure of platelet fibrinogen receptors by ADP and epinephrine. *J. Clin. Invest.* 64:1393–1401, 1979.
4. Kane W.H., Lindhout M.J., Jackson C.M., Majerus P.W.: Factor Va dependent binding of factor Xa to platelets. *J. Biol. Chem.* 255:1170–1174, 1980.
5. Hamberg M., Svensson J., Wakabayashi T., Samuelsson B.: Isolation and structure of two prostaglandin endoperoxides that cause platelet aggregation. *Proc. Natl. Acad. Sci. USA* 71:345–349, 1974.
6. Hamberg M., Svensson J., Samuelsson B.: Thromboxanes: A new group of biologically active compounds derived from prostaglandin endoperoxides. *Proc. Natl. Acad. Sci. USA* 72:2994–2998, 1975.
7. Marcus A.J.: The role of lipids in platelet function with particular reference to the arachidonic acid pathway. *J. Lipid Res.* 19:793–826, 1978.
8. Weiss H.J.: Platelet physiology and abnormalities of platelet function. *N. Engl. J. Med.* 293:531–541; 580–588, 1975.
9. Malmsten C., Kindahl H., Samuelsson B., Levy-Toledano S., Tobelem G., Caen J.P.: Thromboxane synthesis and platelet release reaction in Bernard-Soulier syndrome, thrombasthenia Glanzmann and Hermansky-Pudlak syndrome. *Br. J. Haematol.* 35:511–520, 1977.

IN CONGENITAL PLATELET DISORDERS

RELEASE		AGGREGATION			ADP					REFERENCE
Collagen	Thrombin	AA	PGG₂/H₂	U46619	1°	2°	Disag	Collagen	Thrombin	
↓	↓ , N	Abs	Abs		N	↓	+	↓	N	18, 19, 20
		Abs	↓		N	↓	+	↓		
↓	N	Abs		Abs	N	↓	+	↓	N	27, 28
		N to ↓	↓		N	↓	+	↓		33, 35, 36
		↓	↓							9, 36
		N	N		N	N	N	N	N	9

10. Weiss H.J., Rogers J.: Thrombocytopathia due to abnormalities in the platelet release reaction—Studies on six unrelated patients. *Blood* 39:187, 1972.
11. Holmsen H., Weiss H.J.: Further evidence for a deficient storage pool of adenine nucleotides in platelets from patients with thrombocytopathia—"storage pool disease." *Blood* 39:197–209, 1972.
12. Flower R.J., Blackwell G.J.: The importance of phospholipase A₂ in prostaglandin biosynthesis. *Biochem. Pharmacol.* 25:285, 1976.
13. Rittenhouse-Simmons S.: Indomethacin-induced accumulation of diglyceride in activated human platelets. *J. Biol. Chem.* 255:2259–2262, 1980.
14. Hemler M., Lands W.E.M.: Purification of the cyclo-oxygenase that forms prostaglandins. *J. Biol. Chem.* 251:5575–5579, 1976.
15. Roth G.J., Siok C.J., Ozols J.: Structural characteristics of prostaglandin synthetase from sheep vesicular gland. *J. Biol. Chem.* 255:1301–1304, 1980.
16. Yoshimoto A., Ito H., Tomita K.: Cofactor requirements of the enzyme synthesizing prostaglandin in bovine seminal vesicles. *J. Biochem.* 68:487–499, 1976.
17. Land W.E.M.: The biosynthesis and metabolism of prostaglandins. *Ann. Rev. Physiol.* 41:633–652, 1979.
18. Malmsten C., Hamberg M., Svensson J., Samuelsson B.: Physiologic role of an endoperoxide in human platelets: Hemostatic defect due to platelet cyclo-oxygenase deficiency. *Proc. Natl. Acad. Sci. USA* 72:1446–1450, 1975.
19. Lagarde M., Byron P.A., Vargaftig B.B., Dechavanne M.: Impairment of platelet TXA₂ generation and of the platelet release reaction in two patients with congenital deficiency of platelet cyclo-oxygenase. *Br. J. Haematol.* 38:251–266, 1978.
20. Pareti F.I., Mannucci P.M., D'Angelo A., Smith J.B., Santebin L., Galli G.: Congenital deficiency of thromboxane and prostacyclin. *Lancet* I:898–901, 1980.
21. Smith J.B., Willis A.L.: Aspirin selectively inhibits prostaglandin production in human platelets. *Nature New Biol.* 231:235–237, 1971.
22. Needleman P., Moncada S., Bunting S., Vane J.R., Hamberg M., Samuelsson B.: Identification of an enzyme in platelet microsomes which gen-

erates thromboxane A_2 from prostaglandin endoperoxides. *Nature* 261:558–560, 1976.

23. Cooper B., Ahern D.: Characterization of the platelet prostaglandin D_2 receptor: loss of PGD_2 receptors in platelets of patients with myeloproliferative disorders. *J. Clin. Invest.* 64:586–590, 1979.

24. Needleman P., Wych A., Raz A.: Platelet and blood vessel arachidonate metabolism and interactions. *J. Clin. Invest.* 63:345–349, 1979.

25. Machin S.J., Carreras L.O., Chamone D.A.F., Defreyn G., Danden M., Vermylen J.: Familial deficiency of thromboxane synthetase. *Br. J. Haematol.* 47:629, 1981.

26. Mester F., Oetliker O., Beck E., Felix R., Imbach P., Wagner H.P.: Severe bleeding associated with defective thromboxane synthetase. *Lancet* I:157, 1980.

27. Wu K.K., Minkoff I.M., Rossi E.C., Chen Y-C.: Hereditary bleeding disorder due to a primary defect in platelet release reaction. *Br. J. Haematol.* 47:241–249, 1981.

28. Wu K.K., LeBreton G.C., Tai H-H., Chen Y-C.: Abnormal platelet response to thromboxane A_2. *J. Clin. Invest.* 67:1801–1804, 1981.

29. Lages B., Malmsten C., Weiss H.J., Samuelsson B.: Impaired platelet response to thromboxane A_2 and defective calcium mobilization in a patient with a bleeding disorder. *Blood* 57:545–552, 1981.

30. Weiss H.J., Tschopp T.B., Rogers J., Brand H.: Studies of platelet 5-hydroxytryptamine (serotonin) in storage pool disease and albinism. *J. Clin. Invest.* 54:421, 1974.

31. Weiss H.J., Rogers J.: Platelet factor 4 in platelet disorders—storage location and the requirement of endogenous ADP for its release. *Proc. Soc. Exp. Biol. Med.* 142:30, 1973.

32. Holmsen H., Setkowsky C.A., Lages B., Day H.J., Weiss H.J., Scrutton M.C.: Content and thrombin-induced release of acid hydrolases in gel-filtered platelets from patients with storage pool disease. *Blood* 46:131–142, 1975.

33. Willis A.L., Weiss H.J.: A congenital defect in platelet prostaglandin production associated with impaired hemostasis in storage pool disease. *Prostaglandins* 4:783–794, 1973.

34. Weiss H.J., Chervenick P.A., Salusky R., Factor A.: A familial defect in platelet function associated with impaired release of adenosine diphosphate. *N. Engl. J. Med.* 281:1264–1270, 1969.

35. Ingerman C.M., Smith J.B., Shapiro S., Sedar A., Silver M.J.: Hereditary abnormality of platelet aggregation attributable to nucleotide storage pool deficiency. *Blood* 52:332–344, 1978.

36. Weiss H.J., Willis A.L., Kuhn D., Brand H.: Prostaglandin E_2 potentiation of platelet aggregation induced by LASS endoperoxide: absent in storage pool disease, normal after aspirin ingestion. *Br. J. Haematol.* 32:257–272, 1976.

37. Caen J.: Glanzmann's thrombasthenia. *Clin. Haematol.* 1:383–392, 1972.

38. Phillips D.R., Agin P.P.: Platelet membrane defects in Glanzmann's thrombasthenia. *J. Clin. Invest.* 60:535–545, 1977.

39. Hawiger J., Parkinson S., Timmons S.: Prostacyclin inhibits mobilization of fibrinogen binding sites on human ADP and thrombin treated platelets. *Nature* 283:195–197, 1980.

PART II

PHYSIOLOGIC EFFECTS OF PROSTAGLANDINS

The Toxicology of PGE_1 and PGI_2

JOHN E. LUND, W. P. BROWN, L. TREGERMAN

Pathology and Toxicology Research Unit
Upjohn Company, Kalamazoo, Michigan

Introduction

Prostaglandin E_1 (PGE_1) and prostaglandin I_2 (PGI_2) are being evaluated in clinical trials for potential use in the treatment of several cardiovascular disorders and to preserve platelet function in ex vivo manipulations. Toxicologic studies designed to evaluate potential toxicity of PGE_1 and PGI_2 include both the determination of the acute toxicologic potential and the effect of subacute exposure via the anticipated therapeutic route for human patients, continuous intravenous (IV) infusion. The purpose of this paper is to present the results of such studies performed to date.

Materials and Methods

LD_{50}

Stock solutions of PGE_1 and appropriate dilutions were prepared in absolute ethanol. Ten male and 10 female mice (Upj:TUC[CF₁]spf) and rats (Upj:TUC[SD]spf) were injected IV in the tail vein or subcutaneously (SC) with PGE_1. Mice were given 32, 50, 80, 125, and 200 mg/kg by both IV and SC routes; rats were given 12.5, 20, 32, 50, and 80 mg/kg by the IV route and 8, 12.5, 20, 32, and 50 mg/kg by the SC route.

The injection volume was 1 ml/kg for all animals except the mouse high-dose groups, which received 1.6 ml/kg. The time interval for IV injection was 40 to 60 seconds. Animals that died were examined for gross lesions. Surviving animals were killed and examined after 14 days' observation. The LD$_{50}$ values were estimated by the probit method of Finney.[1]

INTRAVENOUS INFUSIONS

Rats

The indwelling IV catheters and infusion apparatus, with slight modification, were described by Weeks.[2, 3] PGI$_2$, sodium salt, was diluted in glycine buffer (0.025M, pH 10.5). The continuous infusion apparatus utilized a displacement syringe, stored on crushed ice, to minimize PGI$_2$ degradation.[2] Stock solutions of PGE$_1$ in absolute ethanol were diluted in tris buffer (0.05M, pH 7.1) to contain 10% ethanol. The prepared dilutions were administered through the infusion apparatus directly from a plastic syringe mounted on a Razel pump. PGE$_1$ and PGI$_2$ dilutions were adjusted by group mean body weight (male and female separate) to deliver the desired amount. PGI$_2$ dilutions were prepared daily. PGE$_1$ dilutions were prepared every second day. The dose groups for the PGE$_1$ study were 0, 150, 475, and 1500 ng/kg/min continuously for 30 days. The dose groups for PGI$_2$ were 0, 56, 180, and 560 ng/kg/min continuously for 14 days. Each dose group consisted of 5 male and 5 female rats (Upj:TUC[SD]spf).

Dogs

Indwelling IV catheters, made of polyethylene tubing (PE 20) with a silastic terminal portion, were placed in the jugular vein with a dorsal exit just anterior to or between the scapulae. Mesh-top cages were fitted with a swivel holder, which allowed the infusion solutions to be transmitted from a pump through a waterproof cannula feed-through swivel to the dog. The dogs were fitted with a harness that was connected to the cannula feed-through swivel by a length of automobile choke cable, which protected the polyethylene tubing and transmitted rotary motion to the swivel. PGE$_1$ dilutions were prepared every 2 days, and the concentration was adjusted for the body weight of each dog to deliver the required amount of PGE$_1$. The dose groups were 0, 25, 80, and 250 ng/kg/min. Each dose group consisted of 2 male and 2 female dogs.

Results

LD_{50}

Following both IV and SC injection of PGE_1, rats and mice had rapid onset of diarrhea, reddening of the skin of the extremities, severe ocular tearing, difficult breathing, and inactivity. Most deaths occurred within the first 48 hours following injection. Lesions observed were pulmonary congestion and excess fluid and gas in the digestive tract.

Eleven of 19 male rats surviving 14 days following SC injection of PGE_1 had focal areas of ischemic testicular necrosis. Thirteen of 48 surviving mice following IV injection and 2 of 29 remaining alive after SC injection of PGE_1 had corneal opacities, which appeared to result from corneal edema and/or mineralization of Descemet's membrane. The mortality, estimated LD_{50} values, and 95% confidence limits are presented in Tables 8–1 and 8–2.

CONTINUOUS INTRAVENOUS INFUSION

Rats

Reddening of the non-fur-bearing epithelial surfaces of the paws and ears was observed on initiation of PGI_2 infusion in all rats in the high-dose group (560 ng/kg/min). This effect was persistent in the

TABLE 8–1.—MORTALITY, ESTIMATED LD_{50}, AND 95% CONFIDENCE INTERVAL FOR RATS INJECTED WITH PGE_1

Dose (IV) (mg/kg)	M	Sex F	Comb.	Dose (SC) (mg/kg)	M	Sex F	Comb.
			MORTALITY				
12.5	0/10	0/10	1/20	8	2/10	0/10	2/20
20	1/10	0/10	1/20	12.5	1/10	1/10	1/20
32	7/10	8/10	15/20	20	10/10	8/10	18/20
50	8/10	10/10	18/20	32	10/10	10/10	20/20
80	10/10	10/10	20/20	50	10/10	10/10	20/20
				LD_{50} (MG/KG)			
—	31.0	27.9	29.5	—	13.2	16.6	14.8
			CONFIDENCE INTERVAL (MG/KG)				
—	25.8	23.1	25.8	—	11.0	13.8	13.0
	to	to	to		to	to	to
	37.2	33.5	33.6		15.9	19.9	16.9

TABLE 8–2.—MORTALITY, ESTIMATED LD_{50}, AND 95% CONFIDENCE INTERVAL FOR MICE INJECTED WITH PGE_1

Dose (IV and SC) (mg/kg)	M	Sex F	Comb.	M	Sex F	Comb.
			MORTALITY			
32	0/10	0/10	0/20	1/10	1/10	2/20
50	1/10	3/10	4/20	6/10	5/10	11/20
80	7/10	3/10	10/20	9/10	9/10	18/20
125	9/10	9/10	18/20	10/10	10/10	20/20
200	10/10	10/10	20/20	10/10	10/10	20/20
			LD_{50} (MG/KG)			
—	73.1	78.4	75.8	48.1	50.1	49.1
			CONFIDENCE INTERVAL (MG/KG)			
—	59.4	63.7	65.5	38.0	39.9	42.4
	to	to	to	to	to	to
	89.9	96.3	87.7	58.4	61.9	56.4

male rats for the duration of the infusion, whereas it was less obvious in the female rats after day 6. However, the ears and extremities of all rats in the high- and mid-dose groups were consistently pink. The pink color was not out of range for that observed in the control group, but pale coloration as observed in the control group was never observed in these groups except when the infusion apparatus was being recharged. Swollen paws were also noted when the skin was reddened. Excessive tearing from both eyes was noted in 2 high-dose female rats during the first 24 to 48 hours. Lack of grooming, as evidenced by wet abdominal fur and/or soiled perianal area, was noted in 1 female and 1 male high-dose rat during the first 24 to 72 hours. Red crusty material, which was interpreted as dried porphyrin from excess tears, was noted on the external nares of 2 male rats on day 12. There were no deaths during the PGI_2 infusion. The mean food consumption value for the male high-dose group was significantly less than that of the control group (324 ± 31 vs. 414 ± 61 gm/rat/14 days).

Reddened ears and feet were observed in 3 of the 5 male rats in the 180 ng/kg/min group on days 6 to 13 after initiation of the infusion. Two male rats had wet abdominal fur during the first 24 hours of infusion. The low-dose groups (56 ng/kg/min) and control groups were similar in appearance. Ophthalmic examinations for rats in all groups were normal.

Six hours after initiation of PGI_2 infusion, there was a dose-related drop of the rectal temperature. The body temperatures returned to the control group level by 4 days post initiation for the male rats and 2 days for the female rats. Mean body temperatures were similar for all groups at the end of the study.

All treated male rats lost weight during the initial 48 hours of drug infusion. The 48-hour body weights for the low-, mid-, and high-dose groups were 97.9%, 94.5%, and 90.7% of the initial body weights, respectively. The weight loss in the low-dose group was transient. The mid- and high-dose groups equaled their starting weight by day 6 (mid-dose) and day 10 (high-dose). After 14 days of PGI_2 infusion, the mean weight of the high-dose group was less than that of the control group; however, the difference was not statistically significant.

The initial weight loss for the treated female rats was less severe and of shorter duration than that observed in the treated male rats. The final body weights for all groups were similar at the end of the study.

Hematologic results are presented in Table 8–3. There was a slight increase in circulating red blood cells (including Hgb and Hct) in the mid- and high-dose groups. The mean blood platelet level for the group receiving 560 ng/kg/min was approximately 50% of the control group value. The difference was statistically significant. The platelet count was also less then the control value for the low- and mid-dose groups for both sexes, indicating a probable dose response; however, these differences were not statistically significant.

The group mean clinical chemistry values are presented in Table 8–4. The creatine phosphokinase (CPK) level in the high-dose male rats was significantly less than that in the control group. Levels in the low- and mid-dose groups were also less than in the control group; however, these differences were not significant.

There were no gross or microscopic lesions that were attributable

TABLE 8–3.—HEMATOLOGY RESULTS, PGI_2 14-DAY
CONTINUOUS IV INFUSION IN SPRAGUE-DAWLEY RATS

| | | DOSE (NG/KG/MIN) | | |
	Control	56	180	560
RBC (/mm^3 × 10^6)	6.88	6.78	7.36*	7.04
Hemoglobin (gm/dl)	13.4	13.4	14.3*	14.2*
Hematocrit (%)	39.3	40.0	42.1*	42.4*
MCV (μ^3)	57.7	59.6	58.1	60.9
MCH (μμq)	19.3	19.7	19.5	20.1
MCHC (%)	33.8	33.5	33.9	33.5
WBC (/mm^3 × 10^3)	10.8	9.36	8.53	8.14
Neutrophil (/mm^3)	2672	2883	1987	2589
Lymphocyte (/mm^3)	7953	6346	6457	5389
Monocyte (/mm^3)	54	65	85	16
Eosinophil (/mm^3)	130	56	73	154
Platelets (/mm^3 × 10^3)	888	788	686	449*

*Significantly different from control group, $p < .05$.

TABLE 8–4.—CLINICAL CHEMISTRY RESULTS, PGI₂ 14-DAY
CONTINUOUS IV INFUSION IN SPRAGUE-DAWLEY RATS

	Control	DOSE (NG/KG/MIN) 56	180	560
Calcium (mg/dl)	9.7	9.6	10.0	9.7
Inorganic phosphorus (mg/dl)	6.9	6.5	7.0	6.6
Glucose (mg/dl)	183	175	183	164
Urea nitrogen (mg/dl)	21.1	18.8	18.9	19.9
Cholesterol (mg/dl)	39	41	42	47
Total protein (gm/dl)	5.8	5.8	6.0	6.0
Albumin (gm/dl)	3.8	3.8	4.2	4.2
Total bilirubin (mg/dl)	0.17	0.16	0.20	0.21
Alkaline phosphatase (mμ/ml)	164	171	175	187
AST‡ (mμ/ml)	163	153	147	138
ALT‡ (IU/ml)	16	18	16	15
CPK‡ (IU/ml)	222	120	119	100*
Na (mEq/L)	142	141	141	140
K (mEq/L)	4.47	4.22	4.35	4.03
Cl (mEq/L)	102	101	101	100

*Significantly different from control group, $p<.05$.
‡AST = aspartic transaminase; ALT = alanine transaminase;
CPK = creatine phosphokinase.

to PGI₂. Two lesions, however, were caused by an indwelling catheter that was too long and extended into the right heart in some of the rats. Mononuclear cell infiltrates were observed in the right AV valve, and endocardium and endocardial thrombosis was observed in 1/10, 1/10, 0/10, and 3/10 rats in control, low-, mid-, and high-dose groups, respectively. Organized thrombi were observed in the branches of the pulmonary artery in 4/10, 3/10, 4/10, and 4/10 rats in the groups just mentioned.

PGE₁ infusion in male and female rats at 1500 ng/kg/min resulted in flushing of the skin during the first day of treatment. Excessive ocular tearing and mucus were present by the second day of infusion. The eyelids appeared edematous by day 10. Distal limb edema was evident by day 6 and apparent limb pain on day 7. Twenty-four days following initiation of the infusion, one male rat had excessive fluid flowing from the ears, resulting in wet fur ventral to both ears. By the next day, excessive fluid production was evident in 4 of 5 male rats and 2 of 5 female rats in this dose group. The area ventral to the ears appeared slightly swollen. The rats receiving 475 ng/kg/min had excessive ocular tearing and mucus 48 hours after initiation of the infusion. Edema of the eyelids was evident by day 15. Three of 5 male rats had swollen ankles on day 10. This change was transient and was not evident after day 20.

The only clinical sign resulting from infusion at 150 ng/kg/min was the ocular response consisting of excessive tearing and mucus production.

Hematologic and clinical chemistry findings in the 30-day blood samples are presented in Tables 8–5 and 8–6. There were no statistically significant treatment-related changes.

Food and water consumption and weight gains were not affected by the PGE$_1$ infusion. Gross and microscopic changes were limited to the auditory sebaceous gland (Zymbal's gland) and the mammary gland.

TABLE 8–5.—HEMATOLOGY RESULTS, PGE$_1$ 30-DAY CONTINUOUS IV INFUSION IN SPRAGUE-DAWLEY RATS

| | | DOSE (NG/KG/MIN) | | |
	Control	150	475	1500
RBCs (/mm^3 × 10^6)	7.24	7.58	7.54	7.60
Hemoglobin (gm/dl)	14.0	14.6	14.3	15.0
Hematocrit (%)	37.8	38.8	38.5	40.4
MCV (μ^3)	52.4	51.5	52.3	53.5
MCH (pg)	19.3	19.2	19.3	19.8
MCHC (%)	37.0	37.5	37.2	37.2
WBCs (/mm^3 × 10^3)	10.6	8.9	9.7	8.4
Neutrophils (/mm^3)	3181	2315	2988	1964
Lymphocytes (/mm^3)	7075	6231	6227	6137
Monocytes (/mm^3)	297	321	262	219
Eosinophils (/mm)^3	74	63	116	101
Platelets (/mm^3 × 10^3)	934	922	864	847

TABLE 8–6.—CLINICAL CHEMISTRY RESULTS, PGE$_1$ 30-DAY CONTINUOUS IV INFUSION IN SPRAGUE-DAWLEY RATS

| | | DOSE (NG/KG/MIN) | | |
	Control	150	475	1500
Calcium (mg/dl)	9.8	9.7	9.8	9.6
Inorganic phosphorus (mg/dl)	7.1	7.1	7.1	7.3
Glucose (mg/dl)	139	154	154	144
Urea nitrogen (mg/dl)	19.6	18.6	18.5	18.2
Cholesterol (mg/dl)	53	49	58	52
Total protein (gm/dl)	6.3	6.1	6.0	6.1
Albumin (gm/dl)	4.4	4.2	4.2	4.4
Total bilirubin (mg/dl)	0.13	0.12	0.15	0.17
Alkaline phosphatase (mμ/ml)	200	219	228	216
AST† (mμ/ml)	194	184	192	163
ALT† (IU/L)	16	15	16	12
CPK† (IU/L)	253	197	221	198
Na (mEq/L)	142	142	141	141
K (mEq/L)	4.8	4.6	4.7	4.5
Cl (mEq/L)	102	102	101	101

†AST = aspartic transaminase; ALT = alanine transaminase; CPK = creatine phosphokinase.

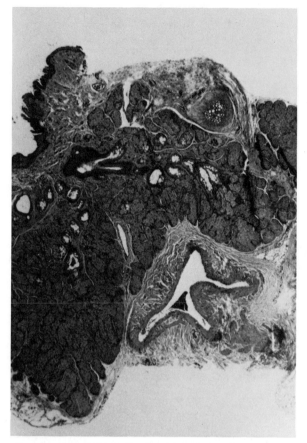

Fig 8–1.—Cross section of Zymbal's gland from a female rat in the control group. H&E; ×32.

There was a dose-response increase in the size and number of acinar cells in the Zymbal's gland (Figs 8–1 and 8–2). Two of 5 male rats receiving 1500 ng/kg/min, 2 of 5 receiving 475 ng/kg/min, and 1 of 5 receiving 150 ng/kg/min had moderate hypertrophy of the mammary gland acinar cells.

Dogs

Three of 4 dogs receiving 250 ng/kg/min PGE_1 developed moderate to severe scleral vascular congestion, tearing, excessive ocular mucus, ptosis of the inferior eyelid, swelling of the distal limbs, apparent

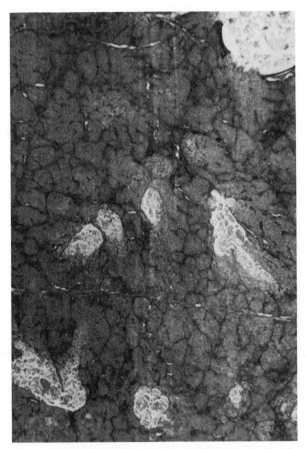

Fig 8–2.—Cross section of a portion of Zymbal's gland from a female rat receiving 1500 ng/kg/minute PGE₁. Note the large ducts filled with debris and enlarged glandular lobules. H&E; ×32.

muscular weakness and discomfort of the limbs, depressed level of activity, and anorexia. The clinical signs in the fourth dog, a female, were not as severe and were similar to those observed in the group receiving 80 ng/kg/min.

The dogs receiving 80 ng/kg/min had various degrees of scleral vascular congestion, tearing, excessive ocular mucus, ptosis of the inferior eyelid, and slight swelling of the distal limbs. The behavior and activity of the dogs was not affected. Clinical signs in the dogs receiving the low dose (25 ng/kg/min) were limited to intermittent tearing, slight scleral vascular congestion, and excessive ocular mucus.

The rectal body temperature and skin temperature on days 8 and 28 are presented in Table 8–7. Body temperature was only slightly elevated in the dogs in the high-dose group. Skin temperature was markedly elevated.

Food consumption during infusion was similar for control, low-dose, and mid-dose groups. The high-dose animals were anorexic, consistently refusing the dry dog chow. No differences were noted in mean water consumption values between the groups.

There was a dose-related loss in body weight in response to PGE_1 infusion. Low-, mid-, and high-dose group mean termination weights were 96.0%, 90.0%, and 85.8% of initial body weights.

The results of the hematologic examination are presented in Table 8–8. Treated dogs had decreased reticulocyte numbers and a normocytic, normochromic anemia that had a positive dose-response relationship. The dogs receiving 80 and 250 ng/kg/min had an increased sedimentation rate and high fibrinogen levels.

Significant changes in clinical chemistry values were: increased alkaline phosphatase and decreased calcium, glucose, BUN, total protein, albumin, AST, and ALT (Table 8–9). The serum CPK values were decreased in the treated groups; however, the differences were not statistically significant.

Gross changes observed in the skeletal system consisted of thickened, glistening, moist-appearing periosteum of the long bones of the limbs, with concomitant subperiosteal bone proliferation. In several areas, endosteal bone proliferation was also evident. Thickened, glistening periosteum was also observed over the nose of 1 high-dose (250 ng/kg/min) male dog. Microscopically, the subperiosteal osseous tissue was composed of poorly organized woven bone, more mature at the original periosteal surface with ample proliferative activity at the thickened periosteum (Fig 8–3). There were numerous resorption cavities in the remaining original cortical bone. Increased bone re-

TABLE 8–7.—Body Temperature and Skin Temperature* and Difference Between Core and Surface Temperature

		BODY TEMPERATURE	SKIN TEMPERATURE	Δ
Day 8	Control	101.6 ± 0.4	96.1 ± 3.0	5.6
	25 ng/kg/min	102.0 ± 0.8	97.0 ± 2.8	5.0
	80 ng/kg/min	101.7 ± 1.2	100.0 ± 0.6	1.6
	250 ng/kg/min	102.8 ± 1.3	101.6 ± 1.2	1.3
Day 28	Control	101.4 ± 0.4	93.7 ± 2.5	7.7
	25 ng/kg/min	101.8 ± 0.5	95.0 ± 2.5	6.8
	80 ng/kg/min	102.2 ± 0.6	96.6 ± 3.5	5.6
	250 ng/kg/min	102.4 ± 0.6	100.0 ± 3.8	2.4

*Measured between toe of forelimb.

TABLE 8–8.—HEMATOLOGY RESULTS, PGE$_1$ 30-DAY
CONTINUOUS IV INFUSION IN BEAGLE DOGS

		DOSE (NG/KG/MIN)		
	Control	25	80	250
RBCs (/mm^3 × 10^6)	7.33	7.26	6.41*	6.25*
Hemoglobin (gm/dl)	17.5	17.1	14.8*	14.3*
Hematocrit (%)	50.2	48.5	42.4*	40.8*
MCV (μ^3)	68.5	67.0	66.3	65.3
MCH (pg)	23.9	23.5	23.0	22.9
MCHC (%)	34.9	35.1	34.6	35.1
WBCs (/mm^3 × 10^3)	10.6	9.7	10.5	10.1
Neutrophils (/mm^3)	5138	5489	5605	5893
Lymphocytes (/mm^3)	3777	2703	3086	2517
Monocytes (/mm^3)	970	759	1440	1415
Eosinophils (/mm^3)	894	710	201	255
Platelets (/mm^3 × 10^3)	351	391	524	350
Prothrombin time (sec)	6.5	6.4	6.5	6.4
Fibrinogen (gm/dl)	0.24	0.22	0.51*	0.52*
Sedimentation rate (mm/hr)	0.25	0.25	9.75*	22.50*
Reticulocytes (/mm^3 × 10^3)	45.6	25.4	20.9*	7.7*

*Significantly different from control group, p<.05.

TABLE 8–9.—CLINICAL CHEMISTRY RESULTS, PGE$_1$ 30-DAY
CONTINUOUS IV INFUSION IN BEAGLE DOGS

		DOSE (NG/KG/MIN)		
	Control	25	80	250
Calcium (mg/dl)	10.7	10.5	9.9*	9.5*
Inorganic phosphorus (mg/dl)	4.4	4.4	4.7	5.3
Glucose (mg/dl)	115	108	104*	98*
Urea nitrogen (mg/dl)	15.3	12.5	10.8*	5.8*
Cholesterol (mg/dl)	117	112	137	111
Total protein (gm/dl)	5.6	5.7	5.9	5.2*
Albumin (gm/dl)	4.0	3.9	3.4	2.4*
Total bilirubin (mg/dl)	0.13	0.10	0.10	0.10
Alkaline phosphatase (mμ/ml)	53	66	135*	204*
AST† (mμ/ml)	37	36	25*	25*
ALT† (IU/ml)	22	21	14*	9*
CPK† (IU/ml)	99	51	36	74
Na (mEq/L)	148	148	146	147
K (mEq/L)	4.5	4.5	4.7	4.4
Cl (mEq/L)	111	113	109	113

*Significantly different from control group, p<.05.
†AST = aspartic transaminase; ALT = alanine transaminase; CPK
= creatine phosphokinase.

sorption was also evident in the ribs and vertebrae. Small areas of
subperiosteal bone proliferation were also present on the outer and
inner surface of the thoracic vertebrae. Subcutaneous edema and enlargement of the popliteal lymph nodes were also observed. The bone
and soft tissue changes had an obvious dose-response relationship,

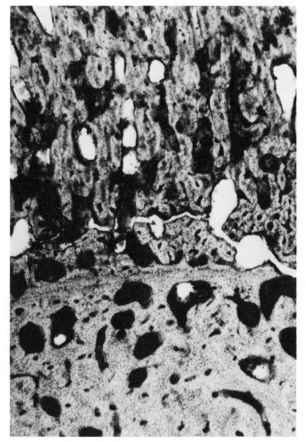

Fig 8–3.—Section of femur from a male dog receiving 250 ng/kg/minute. The original cortal bone is at the bottom of the picture. New bone is at the top. H&E; ×32.

with severe changes in the high-dose group and minimal microscopic changes in the low-dose group.

Other changes observed were: decreased muscle mass in dogs that were recumbent, thymic regression in the dogs receiving the high dose, and reduced spermatogenesis in the male dogs receiving the high dose.

Discussion

The acute LD_{50} for PGE_1 was less than that reported by Bergstrom et al.[4] but similar to those reported by Fujita et al.[5] The clinical signs following a single dose of PGE_1 were similar to those reported for

PGE_2 and $PGF_{2\alpha}$.[5, 6] The testicular necrosis observed in the rats surviving 14 days was presumed to have resulted from an acute vascular phenomenon because of the distribution and ischemic nature of the lesions. Degenerative lesions were not observed in the normal appearing testicular tissue adjacent to the necrotic areas. Degenerative testicular lesions have been observed in mature rats receiving 2.0 mg/kg body weight b.i.d. for 15 days.[7] The excessive ocular tearing in both rats and mice and corneal opacity in mice surviving 14 days may have been related to increased vascular permeability and increased intraocular pressure observed after local and intravenous administration of PGE_1.[8–12]

The slight sedative or tranquilizing effect of PGE_1 observed in the infusion studies as well as the clinical signs of ptosis, flushing of the extremities, and limb edema have been previously reported.[4, 13–15, 17]

The dogs receiving 250 ng/kg/min had responses resembling those observed in systemic disease, including elevated sedimentation rates with elevated fibrinogen and globulin levels, thymic regression, slight testicular degeneration, and slight nonregenerative anemia.[18–22] The foregoing responses may all be caused directly by PGE_1, indicating a potential role for PGE_1 as a mediator, or the responses may be part of a cascade of responses initiated but not directly mediated by PGE_1. One dog receiving 250 ng/kg/min, with the exception of bone changes, did not respond as did the others. This dog also consumed large quantities of water for several days following initiation of the infusion. The reason for the lack of response and increased water consumption is not known, but it may indicate a more efficient metabolism of PGE_1 in this one dog.

The subperiosteal bone formation observed in the dogs was similar in appearance to pulmonary and hepatic hypertrophic osteoarthropathy[23–25] and infantile cortical hyperostosis,[26] except for the presence of endosteal bone deposition. The observed increase in serum alkaline phosphatase and decreased serum calcium levels in the dogs receiving 80 and 250 ng/kg/min was attributed to the massive deposition of new bone.

The occurrence of hypertrophic osteoarthropathy has been attributed to increased blood flow to the affected limb(s).[25, 27] The latter was disputed by Riyami and Anderson[30] and Mukherjee.[31] Since PGE_1 stimulates release of growth hormone,[32, 33] and growth hormone administration to dogs results in a marked increase in new bone formation,[34] levels of growth hormone as well as parathyroid hormone were measured in serum taken from the dogs on the last day of infusion (day 30); neither hormone was elevated.

The dogs had apparent markedly increased blood flow to the limbs, evidenced by engorgement of the large veins with oxygenated blood and increased skin temperature as well as limb edema. Thus, the bone proliferation may simply have resulted from increased blood flow. However, prostaglandins of the E series as well as thromboxane A_2 have been reported to be involved in bone metabolism,[35-38] and therefore a direct effect of PGE_1 on bone formation cannot be eliminated. Similar bone changes have been observed in infants receiving long-term administration of PGE_1.[39, 40]

The effects of PGE_1 on the Zymbal's gland of male and female rats and mammary gland of male rats were similar in nature; however, the Zymbal's gland enlargement was much more pronounced. Similar cellular hypertrophy and hyperplasia of the Zymbal's gland in rats has been observed following administration of PGE_1 alcohol (D. Frank, G. Elliott, The Upjohn Co., unpublished observation). The mechanism of the stimulation is not known, but may be related to the effect on intracellular cyclic AMP. Prostaglandins play a role in cyclic mammary gland changes and have been reported to induce metaplastic changes in mammary tissue in vitro.[41, 42]

The acute IV toxicity of PGI_2 has been reported.[43] The LD_{50} was not determined, but was concluded to be above 10 mg/kg in mice.

The peripheral vascular dilatation and drop in body temperature, which were observed in our study in the rats receiving PGI_2 at 560 ng/kg/min, have been previously reported.[43] The possible effect of PGI_2 on behavior was difficult to assess, since all rats, including those receiving buffer, were inactive during the first several days following initiation of infusion due to the presence of the harness and connecting cable. Also, the initial weight loss during the first several days was attributed to decreased food consumption, both as a result of the reaction to the confinement associated with the infusion harness and the response to PGI_2.

There appeared to be a difference between the male and female rats in their clinical response to PGI_2. The drop in body temperature was less severe, and adaptation occurred earlier in the female rats. Flushing of the skin on the ears and feet was not as notable in the second week in the female rats as in the males, and the initial weight loss was less severe and recovery occurred sooner.

The pathogenesis of the decreased number of circulating platelets in the rats receiving 560 ng/kg/min is not known. Megakaryocyte abnormalities were not observed on bone marrow smears. An alternative to decreased platelet production would be increased peripheral utilization of platelets. Since PGI_2 has an apparent platelet-sparing effect, this mechanism would appear unlikely. However, the data available are not sufficient to support a definitive conclusion. The decreased serum CPK may indicate accelerated disappearance from the plasma, which has been reported to occur in hypermetabolic states.[44] However, since the platelet is one of the most probable sources of plasma CPK in the rat, the decreased level of CPK may simply result from the decreased platelet count.[45]

The endocardial lesions in the rats, consisting of valvular thickening, endocardial thrombosis, endocardial granulation tissue, and pulmonary artery thrombosis, were represented in all groups and were attributed to physical injury and hemodynamic abnormalities resulting from the presence of the catheter tip in the right heart. It was disappointing to find thrombosis occurring in the treated rats, because it would appear that the antiaggregatory[46, 47] and fibrinolytic[48] effects of PGI_2 did not protect against thrombus formation. However, many of the observed thrombi were well organized and may have formed during the recovery period following surgery, prior to initiation of PGI_2 infusion.

Further studies, including 30-day continuous IV infusion of PGI_2 in dogs, are in progress.

REFERENCES

1. Finney D.J.: *Statistical Methods in Biological Assay.* New York, Hafner Publishing Co., 1964.
2. Weeks J.R.: A method for administration of prolonged intravenous infusion of prostacyclin (PGI_2) to unanesthetized rats. *Prostaglandins* 17:495–499, 1979.
3. Weeks J.R.: Long-term intravenous infusion, in Meyers R.D. (ed.): *Methods in Psychobiology.* London, Academic Press, 1972, pp. 155–168.
4. Bergstrom S., Carlson L.A., Weeks J.R.: The prostaglandins: a family of biologically active lipids. *Pharmacol. Rev.* 20:1–48, 1968.
5. Fujita T., Suzuki Y., Yokohama H., Yonezawa H., Ozeki Y., Ichikawa Y., Yamamoto Y., Matsuoka Y.: Toxicity and teratogenicity of prostaglandin E_2. *Pharmacometrics* 8:787–796, 1973.
6. Matsuoka Y., Fujita T., Nozato T., Yokohama H., Onishi Y., Ohta K.: Toxicity and teratogenicity of prostaglandin $F_{2\alpha}$. *Iyakuhin Kenkyu* 2:403–413, 1971.
7. Ericsson R.J.: Prostaglandins (E_1 and E_2) and reproduction in the male rat. *Adv. Biosci.* 9:737–742, 1972.
8. Eakins K.E., Whitelocke R.A.R., Bennett A., Martenet A.C.: Prostaglandin-like activity in ocular inflammation. *Br. Med. J.* 3:452–453, 1972.
9. Pedersen O.O.: Electron microscopic studies on the blood-aqueous barrier of prostaglandin-treated rabbit eyes. 1. Iridial and ciliary processes. *Acta Ophthalmol. (Copenh.)* 58:685–698, 1975.
10. Waitzman M.B., King C.D.: Prostaglandin influences on intraocular pressure and pupil size. *Am. J. Physiol.* 212:329–334, 1967.
11. Chiang T.S.: Effects of epinephrine and progesterone on ocular hyperten-

sive response to intravenous infusion of prostaglandin A_2. *Prostaglandins* 4:415–419, 1973.

12. Beitch B.R., Eakins K.E.: The effects of prostaglandins on the intraocular pressure of the rabbit. *Br. J. Pharmacol.* 37:158–167, 1969.
13. Gilmore D.P., Shaikh A.A.: The effect of prostaglandin E_2 in inducing sedation in the rat. *Prostaglandins* 2:143–151, 1972.
14. Haubrich D.R., Perez-Cruet J., Reid W.D.: Prostaglandin E_1 causes sedation and increases 5-hydroxytryptamine turnover in rat brain. *Br. J. Pharmacol.* 48:80–87, 1973.
15. Potts W.J., Fast P.E., Mueller R.A.: Behavioral effects, in Ramwell P.W. (ed.): *The Prostaglandins.* New York, Plenum Press, 1974, pp. 157–172.
16. Rao K.S., Reno F.E.: Subacute toxicity studies with prostaglandin E_1 (PGE_1) in laboratory animal species. *J. Toxicol. Environ. Health* 1:495–504, 1976.
17. Smith E.R., Mason M.M.: Toxicology of the prostaglandins. *Prostaglandins* 7:247–268, 1974.
18. Henry J.B.: *Clinical Diagnosis and Management by Laboratory Methods.* Philadelphia, W.B. Saunders, 1979.
19. Chatten J.: The thymus in systemic disease. *Am. J. Med. Sci.* 248:715–727, 1964.
20. Finch C.A.: Anemia of chronic disease. *Postgrad. Med.* 64:107–113, 1978.
21. Barrett-Connor E.: Anemia and infection. *Am. J. Med.* 52:242–253, 1972.
22. Anderson W.A.D.: *Pathology.* St. Louis, C.V. Mosby Co., 1971, vol. 1.
23. Epstein O., Ajdukiewicz A.B., Dick R., Sherlock S.: Hypertrophic hepatic osteoarthropathy: clinical, roentgenologic, hormonal and cardiorespiratory studies, and review of the literature. *Am. J. Med.* 67:88–97, 1979.
24. Ginsburg J.: Observations on the peripheral circulation in hypertrophic pulmonary osteoarthropathy. *Q. J. Med.* 27:335–352, 1958.
25. Semple T., McCluskie R.A.: Generalized hypertrophic osteoarthropathy in association with bronchial carcinoma. A review based on 24 cases. *Br. Med. J.* 1:754–759, 1955.
26. Holman G.H.: Infantile cortical hyperostosis: a review. *Q. J. Pediatr.* 17:24–31, 1962.
27. Rosenthall L., Hawkins D., Chuang S.: Radionuclide demonstration of relative increased blood flow in uniappendicular secondary hypertrophic osteoarthropathy. *Clin. Nucl. Med.* 3:278–281, 1978.
28. Steiner H., Dahlbäck O., Waldenström J.: Ectopic growth-hormone production and osteoarthropathy in carcinoma of the bronchus. *Lancet* 1:783–785, 1968.
29. Greenberg P.B., Beck C., Martin T.J., Burger H.G.: Synthesis and release of human growth hormone from lung carcinoma in cell culture. *Lancet* 1:350–352, 1972.
30. Riyami A.M., Anderson E.G.: Hypertrophic pulmonary osteoarthropathy: a clinical and biochemical study. *Br. J. Dis. Chest* 68:193–196, 1974.
31. Mukherjee S.K.: Growth hormone secreting carcinoma of lung and hypertrophic osteoarthropathy. *Age Ageing* 4:95–98, 1975.
32. Hertelendy F., Todd H., Ehrhart K., Blute R.: Studies on growth hormone secretion: IV. In vivo effects of prostaglandin E_1. *Prostaglandins* 2:79–90, 1972.

33. Ito H., Momose G., Katayama T., Takagishi L.I., Nakajima H., Takei Y.: Effect of prostaglandin on the secretion of human growth hormone. *J. Clin. Endocrinol.* 32:857–859, 1971.
34. Harris W.H., Heaney R.P., Jowsey J., Cockin J., Akins C., Graham J., Weinberg E.H.: Growth hormone: the effect on skeletal renewal in the adult dog. I. Morphometric studies. *Calcif. Tissue Res.* 10:1–13, 1972.
35. Somjen D., Binderman I., Berger E., Harell A.: Bone remodelling induced by physical stress is prostaglandin E_2 mediated. *Biochim. Biophys. Acta* 627:91–100, 1980.
36. Heersche J.N.M., Vez D.H.: The effect of imidazole and imidazole analogues on bone resorption in vitro: A suggested role for thromboxane A_2. *Prostaglandins* 21:401–411, 1981.
37. Tashjian A.J. Jr., Voelkel E.F., Levine L., Goldhaber P.: Evidence that the bone resorption-stimulating factor produced by mouse fibrosarcoma cells is prostaglandin E_2. A new model for the hypercalcemia of cancer. *J. Exp. Med.* 136:1329–1343, 1972.
38. Sudmann E., Bang G.: Indomethacin-induced inhibition of haversian remodelling in rabbits. *Acta Orthop. Scand.* 50:621–627, 1979.
39. Ueda K., Saito A., Kakano H., Aushima M., Yukota M., Muraoka R., Iwaya T.: Cortical hyperostosis following long-term administration of prostaglandin E_1 in infants with cyanotic congenital heart disease. *J. Pediatr.* 97:834–836, 1980.
40. Sone K., Tashiro M., Fujinaga T., Tomomasa T., Tokuyama K., Kuroume T.: Long-term low-dose prostaglandin E_1 administration. *J. Pediatr.* 97:866–867, 1980.
41. Knazek R.A., Watson K.C., Lim M.F., Cannizzaro A.M., Christy R.J., Liu S.C.: Prostaglandin synthesis by murine mammary gland is modified by the state of the estrus cycle. *Prostaglandins* 19:891–897, 1980.
42. Schaefer F.V., Custer R.P., Sorof S.: Dibutyl cyclic AMP and prostaglandins induce epidermoid metaplasia in cultured mammary glands. *Fed. Proc.* 39:1748, 1980.
43. Creasy D.M., Follenfant M., James D.A., Dyan A.D.: Preliminary testing of prostacyclin, in Vane J.R., Bergstrom S. (eds.): *Prostacyclin*. New York, Raven Press, 1979, pp. 385–391.
44. Fleisher G.A., McConahey W.M., Pankow M.: Serum creatine kinase, lactic dehydrogenase and glutamic-oxalacetic transaminase in thyroid disease and pregnancy. *Mayo Clin. Proc.* 40:300–311, 1965.
45. Shibata S., Kobayashi B.: Blood platelets as a possible source of creatine kinase in rat plasma and serum. *Thromb. Haemost.* 39:701–706, 1978.
46. Armstrong J.M., Dusting G.J., Moncada S., Vane J.R.: Cardiovascular actions of prostacyclin (PGI_2), a metabolite of arachidonic acid which is synthesized by blood vessels. *Circ. Res.* 43 (suppl. 1):112–119, 1978.
47. Bayer B.L., Blass K.E., Förster W.: Anti-aggretory effect of prostacyclin (PGI_2) in vivo. *Br. J. Pharmacol.* 66:10–12, 1979.
48. Utsunomiya T., Krausz M.M., Valeri C.R., Shepro D., Hechtman H.B.: Treatment of pulmonary embolism with prostacyclin. *Surgery* 88:25–30, 1980.

Vascular Effects of Prostaglandins

DONALD W. DUCHARME, STEPHEN J. HUMPHREY,
GARRY L. DEGRAAF

Cardiovascular Diseases Research
Upjohn Company, Kalamazoo, Michigan

Introduction

Much attention has focused upon the local vascular effects of prostaglandins administered into isolated organ systems or directly into the arterial supply of specific vascular beds. When evaluated in this manner, prostaglandin E_1 (PGE_1) and prostacyclin (PGI_2) generally are potent vasodilators.[1, 2] These studies and others have stimulated great clinical interest in the use of PGE_1 and PGI_2, particularly to treat such clinical disorders as peripheral vascular disease, circulatory shock, stable and unstable angina, and acute myocardial infarction. A beneficial effect in these disorders is expected to result from an increased blood flow to the ischemic tissue. Because of technical and other complications, however, it is often not practical and frequently undesirable to administer the agent by intra-arterial infusions in patients. Consequently, most of the clinical evaluations employ intravenous infusions of the prostaglandins. When the entire cardiovascular system is exposed to a vasodilating agent, blood flow in a given regional vascular bed may or may not respond as in an isolated system. For these reasons, the present investigation was undertaken to determine the effects of systemically infused PGE_1 and PGI_2 on regional blood flows in the conscious dog.

Methods

The animals used for this study were beagle dogs of either sex which ranged from 7.8 to 11.6 kg in body weight. Cardiac output and

111

regional blood flows were determined by the radiolabeled tracer microsphere techniques. The technique used for these studies in general followed that described by Hoffbrand and Forsyth.[3] The radioactivity of the microsphere doses was determined from careful dilutions of the microsphere injectates to permit calculation of the cardiac output via the nonrecirculatable indicator-dilution principle as described by Archie et al.[4]

Dogs were anesthetized with sodium pentobarbital and indwelling arterial cannulae positioned. A PE-60 cannula was advanced from the femoral artery and positioned within the lower abdominal aorta at a point distal to bifurcation of the renal arteries. A double-lumen catheter was positioned within the left ventricle via the left common carotid artery. This cannula permitted simultaneous injection of the microspheres and infusion of the prostaglandin or vehicle. Both catheters were anchored to the muscle adjacent to the arterial entry point and led subcutaneously to a point between the shoulder blades where they exited through stab wounds. The animals were administered Penstrep intramuscularly to guard against infection during the recovery period.

The second day after cannulation, after an overnight fast with water ad lib, the dogs were brought into the laboratory and suspended in nylon body slings. Mean arterial blood pressure and heart rate were monitored from the aortic cannula with a Statham P23Db transducer coupled to a Grass 7D polygraph. One of the left ventricular catheters was connected to a Harvard model 940 syringe pump for drug or vehicle infusion. After a one-hour conditioning period, a 30-minute pretreatment control period began. Twenty minutes into the pretreatment period, the first blood flow determination was performed with ^{85}Sr, 15-μ diameter microspheres (3M Co.). Approximately 100,000 beads/kg were slowly and evenly injected (30 to 40 seconds) into the remaining left ventricular catheter and flushed with 2 ml of saline. Arterial sampling began prior to injection of the microspheres and continued for a total sampling time of 1.5 minutes. This dose of microspheres and the 4 ml/min sampling rate (Holter RL175 withdrawal pump) were selected to ensure approximately 2,000 beads within the reference arterial blood sample. The microspheres for this and all subsequent injections during the low, mid, and high drug infusion periods (^{51}Cr, ^{141}Ce, and ^{125}I, all 15 μ diameter) were prepared at a concentration of 1 million beads/ml in a 15% glucose, 1.5% NaCl vehicle, with a trace of zephiran chloride (0.005%) as a dispersant. The beads were kept in a sealed vial and mixed continuously for at least 30 minutes prior to injection. The injection syringe was weighed before and after injection to determine the net mg dose of the microsphere suspension. The reference arterial blood sample was pumped from the dog into a graduated 10 ml pipette at a constant rate. The volume of blood drawn during the reference sampling was replaced with isotonic saline.

All microsphere isotopes were calibrated prior to experimentation to provide a means to estimate cardiac output. A known weight of each microsphere suspension (0.5 to 1.0 gm) was diluted with 300 ml of 30% glucose and five 3- to 5-ml aliquots were carefully drawn during constant mixing. The count rate per milligram of the microsphere suspensions could thus be easily determined by counting these dilution standards. Multiplication of the count/milligram ratio by the weight of the microspheres injected yielded the total radioactivity administered to the dog. Simple division of this value by the specific activity of the reference arterial blood sample equaled cardiac output (dose counts ÷ counts/ml/min = cardiac output ml/min). Cardiac index was determined by dividing the cardiac output by body weight. Total peripheral resistance was calculated from the mean arterial blood pressure and cardiac index determined at the time of the microsphere injection. The reference arterial blood sample was also used to calculate regional blood flows.

After the initial 30-minute pretreatment interval, the low dose prostaglandin infusion began and continued for 30 minutes. The microsphere injection was performed at 20 minutes into the infusion exactly as during the pretreatment period. The identical procedure was again repeated with the mid- and high-dose prostaglandin infusions. The prostaglandin infusion rates were adjusted to achieve a minimal, moderate, and marked hemodynamic effect in each dog, and were administered in a stepwise, incremental manner.

After the last infusion interval the dogs were sacrificed with sodium pentobarbital and KCl, and the thorax was opened to ensure proper placement of the catheters. Samples were taken from all major tissues. Organ weights were recorded where possible. Skin, skeletal muscle, and fat were assumed to total 10%, 50%, and 5%, respectively, of total body weight. The dilutional standards, reference arterial samples, and various tissue samples were counted for 500 seconds on a Packard Auto-Gamma Scintillation Counter with the count data converted to paper tape for input into an IBM-370 computer for separation of the four microsphere isotopes, as detailed by Rudolph and Heymann.[5] Tissue sample and organ weights, the microsphere sequence and dose weights, and the mean arterial blood pressure and heart rate values were manually keypunched to permit computer calculation of whole body hemodynamics and tissue blood flow rates. Results were analyzed statistically by an unpaired t test. Differences were judged significant if $p \leq .05$.

Prostaglandin I_2 was dissolved in 50 mM *tris* buffer (pH = 8.0) at a concentration of 1 mg/ml and diluted in the same buffer to the appropriate concentration just prior to infusion. Prostaglandin E_1 was dissolved in 95% ethanol at a concentration of 10 mg/ml and diluted with physiologic saline to the appropriate concentration immediately prior to infusion. The mean dose levels and ranges in µg/kg/min for the low, mid and high infusion rates of PGE_1 were 0.0016 (0.001–0.004), 0.024 (0.02–0.04) and 0.14 (0.1–0.2), and of PGI_2 were 0.1 (0.1–0.1), 0.34 (0.3–0.5), and 1.2 (1.0–2.0).

Results

The changes in the hemodynamic parameters associated with the infusion of PGE_1 and PGI_2 are illustrated in Figure 9–1. Both PGE_1 and PGI_2 decreased mean arterial blood pressure in a dose-dependent manner. The cardiac index changed only slightly with the low and mid doses and decreased with the high dose of each compound. Cardiac rate was unchanged at the low dose of PGE_1, but increased at the mid dose and decreased at the high dose. A slowing of cardiac rate occurred with all three doses of PGI_2, with the greatest change associated with the highest level of infusion. Calculated total peripheral resistance (TPR) decreased with the low and mid doses of PGE_1, but increased markedly with the high dose. The TPR decreased during infusion of all three dose levels of PGI_2, but the greatest decrease occurred with the mid-dose level.

Changes in the regional blood flows associated with the infusion of PGE_1 and PGI_2 are illustrated by Figures 9–2 to 9–6. Figure 9–2 illustrates the blood flow changes determined for skin, skeletal muscle, bone, and spleen. Skin blood flow was essentially unchanged during the low- and mid-infusion levels of PGE_1, but decreased significantly during the high-dose infusion. Skin blood flow during infusion of PGI_2 was little changed with the low and mid doses and decreased significantly with the high dose. Skeletal muscle blood flow declined during infusion of both agents at all three dose levels; however, only the decreases associated with the mid and high doses of PGE_1 were statistically significant. Bone blood flow increased with the low- and mid-dose infusions of PGE_1, but decreased significantly with the high-dose infusion. Little change in bone blood flow occurred during the low- and mid-dose infusions of PGI_2, whereas a significant reduction

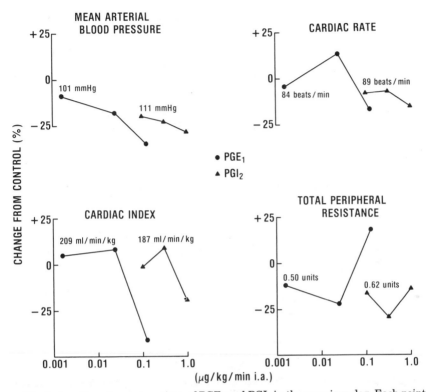

Fig 9–1.—Hemodynamic actions of PGE_1 and PGI_2 in the conscious dog. Each point represents the mean response of 6 dogs at each rate of infusion. The numbers associated with the first point of each dose-response curve are the pretreatment control values for each parameter illustrated.

in flow was associated with the high-dose infusion. Splenic blood flow decreased significantly with the high-dose infusion of both compounds.

The effect of PGE_1 and PGI_2 on the blood flow of selected regions of the gastrointestinal tract are illustrated by Figure 9–3. In the esophagus, stomach, small intestine, and large intestine the blood flows tended to increase at the low infusion rates of both agents and decrease at the highest infusion rate. Only the increase at the low dose of PGE_1 and the decrease at the high dose of PGE_1, however, reached statistical significance.

Figure 9–4 illustrates the changes in blood flow for the kidney, liver, lung, and pancreas. No significant change in renal blood flow occurred during infusion of PGE_1, but renal blood flow was signifi-

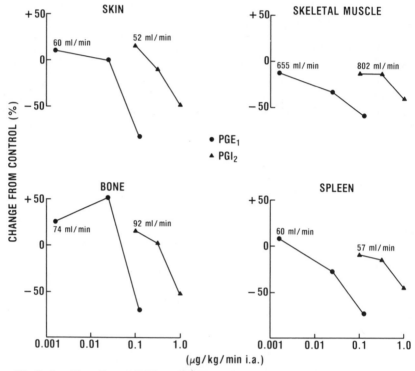

Fig 9-2.—The effect of PGE_1 and PGI_2 on skin, skeletal muscle, bone, and spleen blood flows. For additional details see Figure 9–1.

cantly increased during infusion of the mid and high doses of PGI_2. Liver blood flow tended to decrease with infusion of both agents, but the decrease was significant only during infusion of the high dose of PGI_2. Lung blood flow was not significantly altered by infusion of PGI_2, but increased significantly during infusion of PGE_1 at all dose levels. Blood flow to the pancreas decreased significantly at the high-dose infusion of both PGE_1 and PGI_2.

Changes in blood flow to the four major divisions of the heart during infusion of PGE_1 and PGI_2 are illustrated by Figure 9–5. Little change in coronary blood flow occurred with the low- and mid-infusion levels of PGE_1, and significant reductions were determined for the right atrium, left atrium, and right ventricle during infusion of the high dose. Blood flow to the right and left atria tended to increase during infusion of the lowest dose of PGI_2; however, only the decreased flow to the right and left ventricles during infusion of the highest dose reached statistical significance.

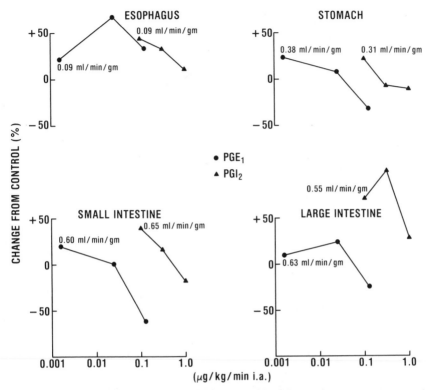

Fig 9-3.—The effect of PGE_1 and PGI_2 on the blood flows of various segments of the gastrointestinal tract. For additional details see Figure 9-1.

Blood flow changes determined for selected regions of the central nervous system are illustrated in Figure 9-6. No significant changes in blood flow to the cerebrum, midbrain, cerebellum or pons, and medulla were noted with infusion of PGI_2. A significant reduction in blood flow to the cerebrum and midbrain was associated with the high-dose infusion of PGE_1, and to the cerebellum with both the mid and high levels of infusion.

Discussion and Conclusions

The results of the present investigation point out many of the problems associated with the extrapolation of results obtained from isolated systems to the intact animal. It is widely recognized that both PGE_1 and PGI_2 are potent vasodilator agents, and many studies, both in vivo and in vitro, have demonstrated the ability of these agents to

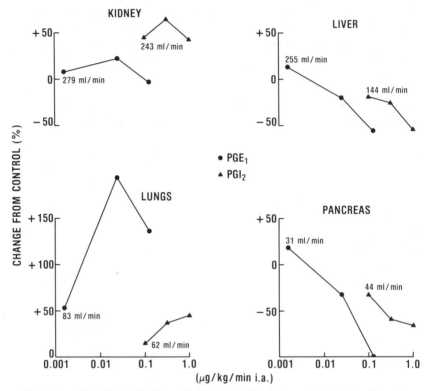

Fig 9–4.—The effect of PGE_1 and PGI_2 on the blood flows of the kidney, liver, lung, and pancreas. For additional details see Figure 9–1.

relax the smooth muscle of blood vessels in most vascular beds. The fact that both PGE_1 and PGI_2 are vasodilator agents, however, does not mean that blood flow will increase in all vascular beds when these agents are administered systemically. With systemic administration of a vasodilator agent, there are many factors that may alter the expected change in a specific regional blood flow. Among these factors are associated changes in cardiac output, neurogenic compensatory mechanisms, myogenic reactions of the blood vessels, metabolic demands of the perfused tissue, and simply the architecture of the vascular system. For these reasons, it was considered important for the future clinical development of PGE_1 and PGI_2 to determine the changes in regional blood flows associated with the systemic administration of these agents to the conscious dog. The compounds were infused continuously for 30 minutes at each dose level for a total of 90 minutes. This allowed sufficient time to reach a steady state at

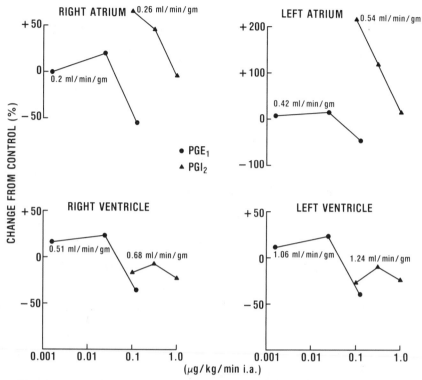

Fig 9–5.—The effect of PGE$_1$ and PGI$_2$ on the blood flows of the myocardium. For additional details see Figure 9–1.

each infusion level and sufficient time for the more rapid compensatory adjustments to occur. It obviously would be desirable in future studies to maintain the infusion for a much longer time at each dose level.

The present studies clearly demonstrate the relationship between regional blood flows and cardiac output. At the low and mid dose of PGE$_1$ and PGI$_2$ cardiac index was either maintained at the preinfusion level or slightly increased, and most regional blood flows followed. At the high-dose infusion level of both agents, cardiac output decreased as did most regional blood flows. A notable exception to the foregoing was the renal blood flow response. Renal blood flow during the high-dose infusions was maintained with PGE$_1$ and remained increased with PGI$_2$, in spite of the reductions in cardiac index. Thus, vascular resistance decreased disproportionately in the kidney relative to other vascular beds, so that the kidney received a greater per-

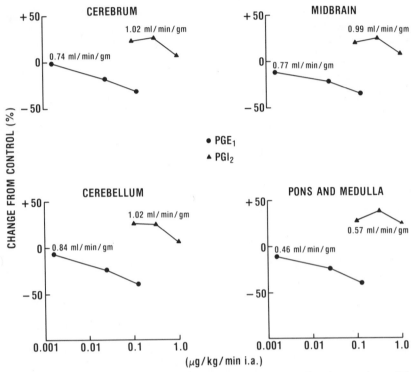

Fig 9–6.—The effect of PGE$_1$ and PGI$_2$ on the blood flows of various regions of the central nervous system. For additional details see Figure 9–1.

centage of the cardiac output during infusion of both PGE$_1$ and PGI$_2$. Pancreatic blood flow responded in the opposite manner, in that blood flow to the pancreas decreased to a greater extent than could be accounted for by the changes in cardiac index. The reason for the decrease in pancreatic blood flow is uncertain, but it may be related simply to the architecture of the vascular system. That is, the net vasodilatation associated with PGE$_1$ and PGI$_2$ may be less on the resistance vessels of the pancreas than on the resistance vessels of other parallel vascular beds, so that more blood is diverted to the beds with lower resistance at the expense of those with higher resistance.

Another factor that must be considered in relating experimental results from one preparation to another is the anesthetic employed. This appears to be particularly important with regard to some of the prostaglandins. As we reported previously,[6] a marked, dose-related increase in cardiac output was associated with the administration of PGI$_2$ in animals treated with morphine sulfate and anesthetized with a mixture of alpha-chloralose and urethane (MUC), whereas cardiac output increased minimally or declined in barbiturate or conscious dogs. Hintze et al.[7] have shown that PGI_2 stimulates a bradycardiac reflex. This reflex was not apparent in MUC-treated dogs, but may explain the decrease in cardiac output as well as cardiac rate associated with the high-dose infusions of PGI_2 in conscious dogs. Regardless, it is apparent that changes in regional blood flow associated with PGI_2 administration would be quite different in MUC-treated dogs as compared to conscious dogs.

It should also be kept in mind that the prostaglandins possess extremely diverse biologic actions, and frequently an unrelated biologic effect can significantly modify the blood flow response in a specific tissue. For example, PGE_1 stimulates gastrointestinal smooth muscle. Contraction of the gastrointestinal smooth muscle physically increases the resistance to blood flow and can counteract the vasodilator action of PGE_1 in this vascular bed. The prostaglandins also are known to stimulate many cellular metabolic pathways, and as metabolic requirements of a tissue increase, blood flow increases. Such an effect would be additive, of course, to a direct vasodilator action.

In view of the aforementioned, it was considered necessary to examine a portion of the dose-response curve for both PGE_1 and PGI_2. As shown by the results, the central hemodynamic and regional blood flow changes associated with PGE_1 and PGI_2 failed frequently to follow a linear dose relationship. This perhaps is not surprising when one considers that the result at any given level of infusion is the sum of the direct vascular action and all interacting pharmacologic effects of the prostaglandin plus the homeostatic compensatory adjustments.

In conclusion, the present study demonstrated that the systemic infusion of PGE_1 and PGI_2 resulted in a sustained, dose-related reduction in mean arterial blood pressure. Cardiac rate, cardiac index, and total peripheral resistance changes failed to follow a linear dose relationship. Cardiac rate and index were unchanged or slightly increased at low doses and decreased significantly at high doses. Total peripheral resistance declined at low doses and increased at the high doses, although with PGI_2 the resistance remained below the predrug level. Regional blood flows generally followed the changes in cardiac ouput, which suggests that both PGE_1 and PGI_2 relaxed the resistance vessels of most vascular beds uniformly. There were some notable exceptions, however. Renal blood flow was unchanged or increased even at the high doses of PGE_1 and PGI_2 in spite of the reduction in cardiac output; thus both PGE_1 and PGI_2 dilated the renal resistance vessels to a greater extent than the resistance vessels of other parallel vascular beds. Pancreatic blood flow decreased markedly during infusion of both PGE_1 and PGI_2. The decreased pancreatic blood flow was greater than could be accounted for by changes in cardiac output. Changes in regional blood flows associated with the infusion of prostaglandins reflect the sum of the direct vascular actions, the interacting pharmacologic actions, and the homeostatic compensatory adjustments.

REFERENCES

1. Nakano J.: Cardiovascular actions, in Ramwell P.W. (ed.): *The Prostaglandins*. New York, Plenum Press, 1973, pp. 238–316.
2. Moncada S., Vane J.R.: Prostacyclin, platelets and vascular disease, in *Prostaglandins in Cardiovascular and Renal Function*. Symposium, King of Prussia, Pennsylvania, May 8–9, 1978. New York, London, Spectrum Publications, 1980, vol. 6., pp. 241–263.
3. Hoffbrand B.I., Forsyth R.P.: Validity studies of the radioactive microsphere method for the study of the distribution of cardiac output, organ blood flow, and resistance in the conscious monkey. *Cardiovasc. Res.* 3:426–432, 1969.
4. Archie J.P. Jr., Fixler D.E., Ullgot D.J., Hoffman J.J.E., Uttey J.R., Carlson E.L.: Measurement of cardiac output with end organ trapping of radioactive microspheres. *J. Appl. Physiol.* 35:148–154, 1973.
5. Rudolph A.M., Heyman M.A.: Methods for studying distribution of blood flow, cardiac output, and organ blood flow. *Circ. Res.* 21:163–184, 1967.
6. DuCharme D.W., DeGraaf G.L., Humphrey S.J., Wendling M.G.: Hemodynamic activities of prostacyclin (PGI_2) as compared to other products of the arachidonic acid cascade, in *Prostaglandins in Cardiovascular and Renal Function*. Symposium, King of Prussia, Pennsylvania, May 8–9, 1978. New York, London, Spectrum Publications, 1980, vol. 6, pp. 265–277.
7. Hintze T.H., Martin E.G., Messina E.J., Kaley G.: Prostacyclin (PGI_2) elicits reflex bradycardia in dogs: Evidence for vagal mediation. *Proc. Soc. Exp. Biol. Med.* 162:96–100, 1979.

Hemodynamic Effects of PGE$_1$ and PGI$_2$ in Man

LENNART KAIJSER, BRITA EKLUND,
TORBJÖRN JORETEG

Department of Clinical Physiology
Karolinska Hospital, Stockholm, Sweden

Introduction

In the first reports on the pharmacologic effects of the newly discovered substance, prostaglandin, von Euler had already reported that it decreased the blood pressure, suggesting a vasodilatory effect.[1] After the clarification of the chemical structure and the identification of a whole family of prostaglandins, pharmacologic studies showed that among them were some of the most powerful vasodilators hitherto known. However, it was also shown that different prostaglandins had greatly different effects. Thus, while PGE$_1$ and PGE$_2$ were powerful vasodilators, PGF$_{2\alpha}$ was in most species found to be a vasoconstrictor. Furthermore, for some of the prostaglandins the effects differed between species, and for some of them effects differed between vascular beds even within the same species. Of the classic prostaglandins, those belonging to the E series seemed to be the most powerful vasodilators, with PGE$_1$ slightly more powerful than PGE$_2$. Infused intra-arterially, PGE$_1$, 10 ng/min, increased forearm blood flow in healthy volunteers tenfold.[2]

A few years ago a novel prostaglandin, prostacyclin or PGI$_2$, was identified.[3] In vitro experiments suggested that it relaxed coronary and mesentery arteries at least as potently as PGE$_1$, in addition to being a more powerful inhibitor of thrombocyte aggregation.[3-5] Vascular tissue of all species studied may generate PGI$_2$, and studies in our department, utilizing intra-arterial infusion of ^{14}C-labeled arachidonic acid, have shown that PGI$_2$ is the most common prostaglandin released into the vascular bed of heart and skeletal muscle in healthy men under resting conditions.[6, 7] We therefore considered it of interest to analyze the cardiovascular effects of PGI₂ in healthy men and, in doing so, to find out whether differences are at hand between effects in different vascular beds. Furthermore we wanted to compare the effects of PGI₂ with those of PGE₁.

Subjects and Methods

The effect of IV infusion of PGI₂ was measured in 25 subjects who took part in the different series of studies as follows:

Cardiac output, and pressures in the brachial artery, the pulmonary artery, and the right atrium and ventricle were studied in eight subjects. The pressures were measured via percutaneously introduced catheters, and cardiac output by the Fick method.[8]

Forearm blood flow was measured by venous occlusion plethysmography in the eight subjects already mentioned. In eight additional subjects, forearm and calf blood flow were measured simultaneously by occlusion plethysmography. In these subjects, an intra-arterial PGI₂ infusion into the brachial artery was added so as to make it possible to study the blood flow effect of a higher local concentration without untoward system effects.

Coronary sinus blood flow and myocardial oxygen extraction was measured by a thermodilution catheter, introduced percutaneously via an arm vein in six subjects.

Splanchnic blood flow was measured in six subjects, utilizing constant rate IV infusion of indocyanin green (Cardiogreen), with blood sampling for dye and oxygen analysis from percutaneous catheters in the brachial artery and the hepatic vein.

In all series, measurements were made with the subject in the supine position before PGI₂ infusion (basal) and during 20-minute consecutive periods of PGI₂ infusion at 160, 500, and 1000 ng/min (corresponding to 2 ng, 7 ng, and 13 ng $\times$ min^{-1} $\times$ kg^{-1} body weight). In addition, forearm blood flow was also studied during intra-arterial infusion, and cardiac output and forearm blood flow during intravenous infusion, of PGE₁ and PGF₂ₐ.[9]

The studies were approved by the Ethical Committee of the Karolinska Institute.

Results

The highest PGI₂ dose increased cardiac output by about 80% (Fig 10–1) and decreased mean arterial pressure slightly, which means

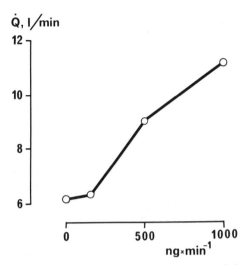

Fig 10–1.—Cardiac output before and at the end of each of three consecutive 20-minute periods of IV prostacyclin infusion.

that the total systemic vascular resistance decreased by 50% (Fig 10–2). The pulmonary artery pressure increased very slightly.

The increase in cardiac output was a result of increases in both stroke volume and heart rate of similar magnitudes (Fig 10–3).

At the same time as the cardiac output increased significantly by 80%, forearm blood flow and calf blood flow showed statistically insignificant increases of 20% to 30% (Fig 10–4). However, with intra-arterial infusion into the brachial artery, which made it possible to produce higher local concentration of PGI_2 without intolerable systemic effects, it was possible to increase forearm blood flow significantly (Fig 10–5). Coronary blood flow did not change at all until at the highest dose level when an insignificant increase of 10% was recorded (Fig 10–6). Coronary sinus O_2 saturation remained unaltered, which means that coronary blood flow varied directly with myocardial oxygen uptake (Fig 10–7), suggesting that the flow increase at the highest dose was the result of an increased myocardial oxygen utilization and not of a direct vasodilating influence of PGI_2. The factor responsible for the increased myocardial oxygen demand was most probably the increased heart rate.

Splanchnic blood flow increased almost threefold, i.e., from 1.5 to slightly more than 4 L/minute (Fig 10–8).

To produce similar increases in cardiac output and decreases in mean arterial pressure by PGE_1, an approximately tenfold greater IV

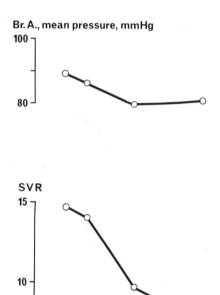

Fig 10–2.—Brachial artery mean pressure and total systemic vascular resistance before and during prostacyclin infusion.

infusion rate was required (Fig 10–9). The tenfold difference in infusion rate required does not necessarily mean a tenfold difference in potency, since PGE_1, but not PGI_2, is efficiently removed in the pulmonary vascular bed (the fractional removal of PGE_1 has been found to be 75% to 90%). However, the most striking difference in effect between PGI_2 and PGE_1 was that the dose of PGE_1, which halved the total systemic vascular resistance, caused a similar decrease in forearm vascular resistance. By contrast, with PGI_2 the decrease in forearm vascular resistance was far smaller than that in total systemic vascular resistance. Thus, unlike PGE_1, PGI_2 has different effects on the vascular resistance of different systemic vascular beds. This is also evidenced by the production of a threefold increase in splanchnic, but only a 10% increase in coronary, blood flow by the same systemic dose of PGI_2.

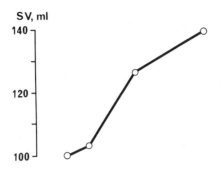

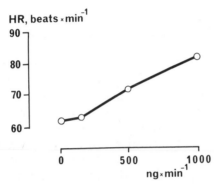

Fig 10–3.—Stroke volume and heart rate before and during prostacyclin infusion.

Discussion

In addition to being a potent inhibitor of platelet aggregation, PGI_2 has been considered a powerful vasodilator. However, its role as vasodilator is based mainly on studies of isolated arterial preparations or animal experiments, and it is well known that a number of prostaglandins have different effects in different vascular beds as well as in different species. The present study shows that PGI_2 is a vasodilator in all systemic vascular beds studied in man, but that its effect differs greatly between different vascular areas, being most pronounced in the splanchnic organs. In this respect it differs qualitatively from PGE_1 and PGE_2, which have similar effects on increasing limb blood flow, cardiac output (present study), splanchnic blood flow, and renal blood flow.[7] If there is a difference at all between different vascular beds in the case of PGE_1, the last-mentioned study suggests that in fact the flow increase is greater in limbs than in the splanchnic vascular bed.

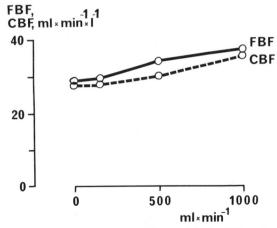

Fig 10–4.—Forearm and calf blood flow before and during IV prostacyclin infusion.

The IV dose which doubled cardiac output in the case of PGI_2, increased and, in the case of PGE_1, decreased the mean pulmonary artery pressure slightly. The increase produced by PGI_2 was smaller than the corresponding increase in pulmonary artery pressure during physical exercise at a load that yields the same increase in cardiac output (together with the cardiac output increase it signifies a significant decrease in pulmonary vascular resistance), suggesting that the direct effect of PGI_2 on the pulmonary vasculature is vasodilatory.

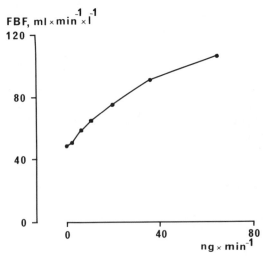

Fig 10–5.—Forearm blood flow before and during IA prostacyclin infusion.

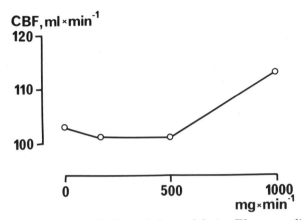

Fig 10–6.—Coronary sinus blood flow before and during IV prostacyclin infusion.

The more pronounced decrease in pulmonary vascular resistance with PGE_1 does not necessarily mean that PGE_1 is a more powerful vasodilator in the pulmonary vasculature. Although the pulmonary and systemic vascular beds were probably exposed to similar concentrations of PGI_2, the removal of PGE_1 in the lungs probably exposed

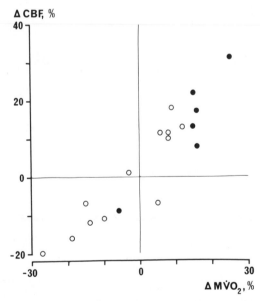

Fig 10–7.—Change in coronary sinus blood flow in relation to simultaneous change in calculated myocardial oxygen uptake (flow × arterial—coronary sinus O_2 difference). Individual data. Filled symbols denote measurements at highest infusion rate.

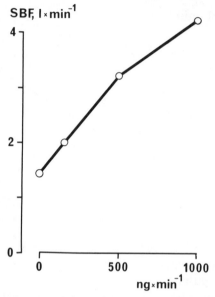

Fig 10–8.—Splanchnic blood flow before and during IV prostacyclin infusion.

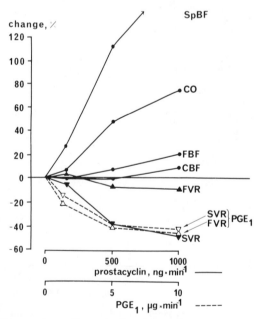

Fig 10–9.—Changes in cardiac output and forearm, coronary, and splanchnic flow during prostacyclin infusion and cardiac output and forearm blood flow during PGE_1 infusion, together with changes in corresponding vascular resistance.

the pulmonary vasculature to far higher concentrations of PGE_1 than were present in the systemic vascular beds.

Of other prostaglandins with effects on vascular tone, it may be mentioned that $PGF_{2\alpha}$ is a systemic vasodilator in some and a vasoconstrictor in other species. In our own studies we found that a constant rate IV infusion of 100 $\mu g/min$ increased mean arterial pressure slightly and cardiac output to the same extent, leaving total systemic vascular resistance unaffected.[9] However, at the same time as the vascular resistance in the average systemic vascular bed was unaffected, forearm vascular resistance was increased significantly. Similarly, the pulmonary vascular resistance was increased. Thus, the finding of different effects in different vascular beds in the case of PGI_2 is itself not unusual among prostaglandins.

Conclusions

PGI_2 decreases total systemic vascular resistance, which in healthy men leads to increased cardiac output with a minor decrease in arterial pressure.

Its vasodilatory potency in the average systemic vascular bed is at least as great as that of PGE_1.

The effect is of short duration.

Unlike PGE_1 the vasodilatory effect of PGI_2 differs greatly between different systemic vascular beds. Of vascular areas receiving a significant fraction of the cardiac output, the splanchnic vascular bed seems to be very sensitive, and heart and skeletal muscle comparatively insensitive, to its vasodilatory stimulus.

ACKNOWLEDGMENTS

This study was supported by the Swedish Medical Research Council (04X-4494). Prostacyclin was kindly provided by Upjohn Company, Kalamazoo, Michigan.

REFERENCES

1. von Euler U.S.: Über die spezifische blutdrucksenkende Substanz des menschlichen Prostata- und Samenblasesekretes. *Klin. Wochenschr.* 14:1182–1183, 1935.
2. Bevegård S., Orö L.: Effect of prostaglandin E_1 on forearm blood flow. *Scand. J. Clin. Lab. Invest.* 23:347–353, 1969.
3. Moncada S., Grylewski R.J., Bunting S., Vane J.R.: An enzyme isolated from arteries transforms prostaglandins endoperoxides to an instable substance that inhibits platelet aggregation. *Nature* 263:663–665, 1976.
4. Bunting S., Gryglewski R.J., Moncada S., Vane J.R.: Arterial walls generate from prostaglandin endoperoxides a substance (prostaglandin X)

which relaxes strips of mesenteric and coeliac arteries and inhibits platelet aggregation. *Prostaglandins* 12:897–913, 1976.

5. Dusting G.J., Moncada S., Vane J.R.: Prostacyclin (PGX) is the endogenous metabolite of arachidonic acid which relaxes coronary arteries. *Prostaglandins* 13:3–15, 1977.

6. Nowak J., Kaijser L., Wennmalm Å.: Cardiac syntheses of prostaglandin from arachidonic acid in man. *Prostaglandins and Medicine* 4:205–214, 1980.

7. Nowak J., Wennmalm Å.: Human forearm and kidney conversion of arachidonic acid to prostaglandins. *Acta Physiol. Scand.* 106:307–312, 1979.

8. Eklund B., Joreteg T., Kaijser L.: Dissimilar effects of prostacyclin on cardiac output and forearm blood flow in healthy men. *Clin. Physiol.* 1:123–130, 1981.

9. Eklund B., Carlson L.A.: Central and peripheral circulatory effects of different prostaglandins given IV to man. *Prostaglandins* 20:333–347, 1980.

The Importance of Renal Prostaglandins in the Maintenance of Renal Blood Flow

MICHAEL J. DUNN AND EDWARD J. ZAMBRASKI

Department of Medicine, Division of Nephrology, Case Western Reserve University and University Hospitals of Cleveland; Department of Physiology, Rutgers University, New Brunswick, New Jersey

Introduction

Renal tissue from animals and man can synthesize all of the known prostaglandins (PGs) and thromboxane A_2 (TXA_2).[1] However, the distribution of the synthetic capacity varies among different portions of the nephron. Table 11–1 summarizes the current information about the sites of PG production within the kidney and the relative abundance of each PG and TX.[2] There is a general belief that PGs synthesized in the cortex primarily alter cortical physiologic and biochemical processes, whereas medullary PGs and TX act locally to modulate medullary events. Table 11–2 lists the major renal actions of the PGs and tabulates the PGs that exert the most potent actions on each individual physiologic process. This review will focus on the importance of renal PGs for the maintenance of renal blood flow (RBF).

PGs and Normal RBF

All PGs and TX have some renal vasoactive properties. PGI_2 and PGE_2 are potent vasodilators and TXA_2 is an intense vasoconstrictor. PGD_2 and PGA_2 are also vasodilatory, whereas $PGF_{2\alpha}$ is weakly va-

TABLE 11–1.—RENAL SITES OF PROSTAGLANDIN SYNTHESIS*

TISSUE[†]	RELATIVE AMOUNTS SYNTHESIZED[‡]
Medullary interstitial cells	$PGE_2 \gg PGF_{2\alpha}$. No PGI_2 or TXA_2
Collecting tubules (papillary)	$PGE_2 \gg PGF_{2\alpha}$
Cortical tubules (proximal and distal)	$PGE_2 > PGF_{2\alpha} > TXA_2$
Cortical arterioles	$PGI_2 > PGF_{2\alpha} > PGE_2$
Glomeruli	$PGE_2 \geq PGF_\alpha > TXA_2 > PGI_2 = PGD_2$

*Adapted from Dunn M.S.: *Kidney Int.* 19:86–102, 1981.
†In vitro studies of isolated portions of the kidney or of cells in culture.
‡These measurements are approximate, especially when made by radiometric thin-layer chromatography. The in vivo synthesis of these products can differ substantially because of cofactors, substrate concentration, and other variables.

TABLE 11–2.—RENAL ACTIONS OF PROSTAGLANDINS*

Renal blood flow
  Vasodilation: PGE_2, PGI_2
  Vasoconstriction: TXA_2, $PGF_{2\alpha}$ (weak)
Glomerular filtration rate†
  Increased: PGE_2, PGI_2
  Decreased: TXA_2
Renin secretion
  Increased: PGI_2, PGE_2, PGD_2
  Decreased: ? TXA_2
Natriuretic: PGE_2, PGI_2, PGD_2?
Water diuretic: PGE_2

*Adapted from Dunn M.S.: *Kidney Int.* 19:86–102, 1981.
†Increments of GFR only occur if vasoconstriction (e.g., resulting from angiotensin II) precedes administration of PGE_2 or PGI_2.

soconstrictive. Infusion of arachidonic acid, the precursor of PG and TX synthesis, vasodilates the renal vasculature in man and in the dog, rabbit, and cat, but not in the rat. Controversy exists as to whether the products of arachidonate cyclo-oxygenation are more vasoconstrictor than vasodilator in the rat.[3, 4]

In the basal or unperturbed state, renal PGs do not exert significant effects on RBF. In experimental animals studied without anesthesia or surgery (i.e., conscious, chronically instrumented dogs), inhibition of PG synthesis by either indomethacin or meclofenamate does not alter RBF.[5, 6] Figure 11–1 depicts the effects of meclofenamate, 2 mg/kg IV, on renal vascular resistance in eight conscious dogs with a chronically implanted electromagnetic flow probe on the left renal artery. Despite reductions of renal venous and urinary

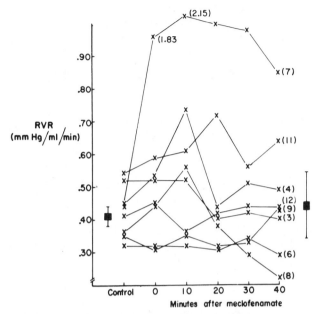

Fig 11–1.—Changes in renal vascular resistance (RVR) observed after meclofenamate treatment (2 mg/kg). Individual animals are identified by number in parentheses. Squares represent means ± SE. (From Zambraski E.J., Dunn M.J.: *Am. J. Physiol.* 236:F552–F558, 1979.)

PGE_2, there was no increment of renal vascular resistance or decrement of RBF except in one dog. Similar results were obtained after indomethacin, 2 mg/kg IV.[6] Nowak and Wennmalm,[7] studying human volunteers, observed a 30% increment in renal vascular resistance after indomethacin 50 mg IV. Infusion of PGE_1 reversed the renal vasoconstriction. However, Muther and Bennett did not find any significant reduction of GFR after the administration of aspirin, 3.5 gm per day for 1 week, to nine normal volunteers.[8] It seems fair to conclude that renal PGs play a negligible role in the control of RBF in normal animals and man unless there is Na depletion (see below).

PGs and Preservation of RBF During Vasoconstriction

Vasoconstriction induced by angiotensin II, vasopressin, or norepinephrine, and renal ischemia after renal artery occlusion or hypotension are potent stimuli of the renal synthesis of vasodilatory PGs. If one blocks fatty acid cyclo-oxygenase, and hence PG production, the vasoconstriction and ischemia become more intense. The release of PGE_2 and PGI_2, in response to angiotensin, vasopressin, or catecholamines, modulates the renal vascular resistance and increases RBF toward normal.[10] We have noted a direct correlation between the compensatory increase of renal PGE_2 synthesis and the recovery of RBF during angiotensin infusion or renal arterial constriction.[6] It seems quite likely that PGI_2 increased similarly, since angiotensin also stimulates renal PGI_2 synthesis.[11] Na-depleted dogs, possibly because of compensatory increases of plasma angiotensin and catecholamines, also develop acute reductions of RBF after inhibition of PG synthesis.[12] Renal PGs exert important vasodilatory actions during acute reductions of cardiac output in dogs, since indomethacin or meclofenamate significantly increase renal vascular resistance after reductions of cardiac output subsequent to inflation of a balloon in the inferior vena cava.[13] Since glomerular filtration rate (GFR) is affected by decrements of RBF, most studies have shown parallel, but less severe, changes of GFR when RBF was reduced after inhibition of PG synthesis.

PGs and Renal Function in Experimental Liver Disease in the Dog

To evaluate the role of PGs in determining kidney function during liver disease, excretion rates of PGE_2, $PGF_{2\alpha}$, and two metabolites of PGI_2 were determined before and after chronic ligation of the common bile duct (CBDL).[14] In 15 dogs, CBDL for 4 to 14 weeks significantly increased serum bilirubin and alkaline phosphatase. At the time of study, seven dogs had ascites and eight were nonascitic. PGE_2 excretion rates, before and after CBDL, were 2.2 ± 0.4 and 3.5 ± 1.0 ng/min, respectively. $PGF_{2\alpha}$ excretion rates increased significantly from 2.4 ± 0.4 ng/min to 4.1 ± 0.8 ng/min after CBDL. Renal PGI_2 synthesis, as assessed by urinary excretion of $6\text{-}KPGF_{1\alpha}$ and 6,15 DK, 13,14 $DHPGF_{1\alpha}$, increased from 1.2 ± 0.2 to 5.3 ± 1.6 and from 1.5 ± 0.2 to 3.5 ± 1.0 ng/min before and after CBDL. To assess the effects of indomethacin, animals were anesthetized and prepared for left kidney studies. Indomethacin (2 mg/kg) caused a 90% reduction in PGE_2 and $PGF_{2\alpha}$ excretion and a 75% decrement of the PGI_2 metabolites in the nonascitic and ascitic animals. In both the ascitic and nonascitic CBDL animals, indomethacin significantly increased mean arterial pressure, decreased renal blood flow by 35%, and decreased glomerular filtration rate by 25% to 40%. Renal vascular resistance almost doubled in the CBDL dogs after indomethacin. Indomethacin had no effect on these parameters in sham-operated animals. These data demonstrated that vasodilatory PGs, especially PGI_2, served an important compensatory role in maintaining renal blood flow and glomerular filtration in CBDL cirrhotic dogs. Similar results have been obtained in several studies of patients with alcoholic cirrhosis and ascites (see below).

Effects of PG Inhibition in Human Disease

Excellent documentation exists about the deleterious effects of indomethacin and other nonsteroidal anti-inflammatory drugs on RBF and GFR in patients with diverse types of diseases. Table 11–3 summarizes some of these reports. Indomethacin, aspirin, and ibuprofen, in conventional doses, reduced GFR by 20% to 50% in patients with parenchymal renal disease, alcoholic liver disease, or congestive heart failure.[15-21] Sodium depletion can also predispose patients to a reduction in GFR after inhibition of PG synthesis. Muther and coworkers measured a 10 to 15 ml/min decrement of GFR in 10 healthy adults receiving 3.5 gm aspirin per day during 10 mEq Na restriction. The decrement of GFR (inulin clearance) correlated directly with the plasma salicylate level.[22] The aforementioned clinical circumstances generally are accompanied by an ineffective or reduced circulating plasma volume with subsequent elevation of plasma angiotensin, catecholamines, and vasopressin. As previously mentioned, these compounds enhance renal PG synthesis (especially PGE_2 and PGI_2), which in turn modulate the renal vasoconstriction.

TABLE 11–3.—EFFECTS OF INHIBITION OF PG SYNTHESIS ON GFR

AUTHOR	DRUG	UNDERLYING DISEASE	% DECREMENT OF GFR
Donker et al.[15]	Indomethacin 150 mg/day	Parenchymal renal disease	20
Arisz et al.[16]	Indomethacin 150 mg/day	Nephrotic syndrome	35
Boyer et al.[17]	Indomethacin 200 mg/day	Alcoholic liver disease	20
Zipser et al.[18]	Indomethacin 200 mg/day	Alcoholic liver disease	50
Walshe and Venuto[19]	Indomethacin 100 mg/day	Severe congestive heart failure	> 75
Berg[20]	Aspirin 750 mg, IV	Chronic renal failure	50
Kimberly et al.[21]	Aspirin 3–6 gm/day	Systemic lupus erythematosus	15–20

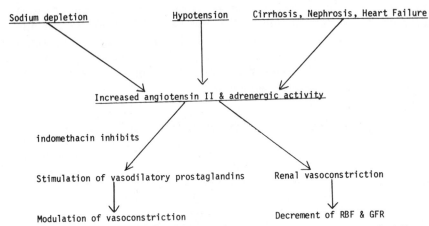

Fig 11–2.—Balance between vasoconstrictor and vasodilator factors in the kidney. Sodium depletion, hypotension, or an ineffective circulatory volume due to cirrhosis, nephrosis, or heart failure exert vasoconstrictor effects on the kidney that are modulated by release of vasodilatory prostaglandins (PGE_2 and PGI_2). If prostaglandin synthesis is inhibited with an anti-inflammatory drug, then renal vasoconstriction is exaggerated, and GFR and RBF decrease significantly. (From Dunn M.J., Zambraski E.J.: *Kidney Int.* 18:609–622, 1980.)

Inhibition of PG production accentuates the renal vasoconstriction with resultant decrements of RBF and GFR. Figure 11–2 summarizes these inter-relationships.

ACKNOWLEDGMENT

This work was supported by NIH grant HL22563.

REFERENCES

1. Dunn M.J., Zambraski E.J.: Renal effects of drugs that inhibit prostaglandin synthesis. *Kidney Int.* 18:609–622, 1980.
2. Dunn M.J.: Prostaglandins and Bartter's syndrome. *Kidney Int.* 19:86–102, 1981.
3. Malik K.V., McGiff J.C.: Modulation by prostaglandins of adrenergic transmission in the isolated perfused rabbit and rat kidney. *Circ. Res.* 36:599, 1975.
4. Gerber J.G., Nies A.S.: The hemodynamic effects of prostaglandins in the rat: Evidence for important species variation in renovascular responses. *Circ. Res.* 44:406, 1979.
5. Terragno N.A., Terragno D.A., McGiff J.C.: Contribution of prostaglandins to the renal circulation in conscious, anesthetized, and laparotomized dogs, *Circ. Res.* 40:590, 1977.
6. Zambraski E.J., Dunn M.J.: Renal prostaglandin E_2 secretion and excretion in conscious dogs. *Am. J. Physiol.* 236:F552–F558, 1979.

7. Nowak J., Wennmalm A.: Influence of indomethacin and of prostaglandin E₁ on total and regional blood flow in man. *Acta. Physiol. Scand.* 102:484–491, 1978.

8. Muther R.S., Bennett W.M.: Effects of aspirin on glomerular filtration rate in normal humans. *Ann. Int. Med.* 92:386–387, 1980.

9. Dunn M.J., Liard J.F., Dray F.: Basal and stimulated rates of renal secretion and excretion of prostaglandins E₂, Fₐ, and 13,14-dihydro-15-keto Fₐ in the dog. *Kidney Int.* 13:136–143, 1978.

10. Dunn M.J.: Renal prostaglandins, in Klahr S., Massry S.: *Contemporary Nephrology.* New York Plenum Publishers, 1981.

11. Shebuski R.J., Aiken J.W.: Angiotensin II stimulation of renal prostaglandin synthesis elevates circulating prostacyclin in the dog. *J. Cardiovasc. Pharmacol.* 2:667–677, 1980.

12. Blasingham M.C., Shade R.E., Share L., Nasjletti A.: The effect of meclofenamate on renal blood flow in the unanesthetized dog: relation to renal prostaglandins and sodium balance. *J. Pharmacol. Exp. Ther.* 214:1–4, 1980.

13. Oliver J.A., Sciacca R.R., Pinto J., Cannon P.J.: Participation of the prostaglandins in the control of renal blood flow during acute reduction of cardiac output in the dog. *J. Clin. Invest.* 67:229–237, 1981.

14. Zambraski E.J., Dunn M.J.: Prostaglandins and renal function after chronic ligation of the common bile duct in dogs. (Submitted for publication.)

15. Donker A.J.M., Arisz L., Brentjens J.R.H., Van Der Hem G.K., Hollemans H.J.G.: The effect of indomethacin on kidney function and plasma renin activity in man. *Nephron* 17:288–196, 1976.

16. Arisz L., Donker A.J.M., Brentjens J.R., Van Der Hem G.K.: The effect of indomethacin on proteinuria and kidney function in the nephrotic syndrome. *Acta Med. Scand.* 199:121–125, 1976.

17. Boyer T.D., Zia P., Reynolds T.: Effect of indomethacin and prostaglandin A₁ on renal function and plasma renin activity in alcoholic liver disease. *Gastroenterology* 77:215–222, 1979.

18. Zipser R.D., Hoefs J.C., Speckart P.F., Zia P.K., Horton R.: Prostaglandins: modulators of renal function and pressor resistance in chronic liver disease. *J. Clin. Endo. Metabol.* 48:895–900, 1979.

19. Walshe J.J., Venuto R.C.: Acute oliguric renal failure induced by indomethacin: possible mechanism. *Ann. Intern. Med.* 91:47–49, 1979.

20. Berg K.J.: Acute effects of acetylsalicyclic acid on renal function in patients with chronic renal insufficiency. *Eur. J. Clin. Pharmacol.* 11:111–116, 1977.

21. Kimberly R.P., Gill J.R., Bowden R.E., Keiser H.R., Plotz P.H.: Elevated urinary prostaglandins and the effects of aspirin on renal function in lupus erythematosus. *Ann. Intern. Med.* 89:336–341, 1978.

22. Muther R.S., Potter D.M., Bennett W.M.: Aspirin-induced depression of glomerular filtration rate in normal humans: role of sodium balance. *Ann. Int. Med.* 94:317–321, 1981.

Clinical Pharmacology of Prostacyclin

GARRET A. FITZGERALD

Division of Clinical Pharmacology
Department of Pharmacology
Vanderbilt University
Nashville, Tennessee

Introduction

The appreciation of the importance of prostacyclin (PGI_2) and thromboxane A_2 (TXA_2) in the regulation of platelet-blood vessel wall interactions[1, 2] has fostered interest in agents that might mimic the antiplatelet and vasodilating properties of endogenous PGI_2 or counter the proaggregant vasoconstrictor effect of TXA_2. Furthermore, the development of techniques that estimated endogenous PGI_2 in human plasma prompted a search for diseases in which "PGI_2 deficiency" might be of etiologic importance.

Measurement of Prostacyclin in Human Biologic Fluids

The earliest attempts at measurement of PGI_2-like activity in human plasma employed bioassay techniques in which venous blood was superfused over organ strips arranged in series in tissue baths.[3] These techniques were replaced by the development of mass spectrometry[4] and subsequently radioimmunoassays[5, 6] for 6-keto-$PGF_{1\alpha}$, the stable inactive hydrolysis product of PGI_2. Bioassay experiments in anesthetized cats and rabbits had suggested that PGI_2 might function as a systemic antiplatelet hormone following release from the lungs into the circulation.[7, 8] This concept appeared consistent with GC-MS measurements of 6-keto-$PGF_{1\alpha}$ in the pulmonary artery and left ventricle of subjects undergoing cardiac catheterization.[9] The transpulmonary difference observed suggested release of about 5 ng/

141

kg/min PGI_2 from the lungs—sufficient to exert an antiplatelet effect. However, the interpretation of these data has been complicated by recent observations suggesting that 6-keto-$PGF_{1\alpha}$ is barely detectable in the plasma of supine human volunteers.[10, 11] The explanation for such disparities between investigators using similar techniques (Table 12–1) is at present unclear, but it does introduce caution into the interpretation of comparative data employing these assays. Besides hydrolysis to 6-keto-$PGF_{1\alpha}$ and subsequent enzymatic conversion to 6,15-diketo-13,14-dihydro-$PGF_{1\alpha}$, PGI_2 may undergo prior dehydrogenation and reduction to 15-keto-13,14-dihydro-PGI_2 (Fig 12–1). The dinor metabolites, which appear in the urine, reflect PGI_2 metabolism by either of these pathways and bypass the possible confounding effect of venous sampling. Development of a mass spectrometric assay for two major PGI_2 metabolites in urine, 2,3-dinor-6-keto-$PGF_{1\alpha}$ and 6,15-diketo-13,14-dihydro-2,3-dinor-$PGF_{1\alpha}$[12] permitted estimation of the rate of entry of endogenous PGI_2 into the circulation.[13] Subjects were infused with vehicle alone or PGI_2 (0.01, 0.04, and 2.0 ng/kg/min) on separate occasions. By regressing the quantities of PGI_2 infused upon the quantities of the metabolites excreted in excess of baseline, the rate of entry of endogenous PGI_2 into the bloodstream was estimated at 0.09 ng/kg/min. This is much less than the threshold dose of exogenous PGI_2 required (2–4 ng/kg/min) for an effect on ADP-induced aggregation.[14] The threshold concentration for PGI_2 in blood required to exert an antiplatelet effect has been estimated as $\geqslant 34$ pg/ml in a study of healthy volunteers[15] and $\geqslant 5$ ng/ml in an investigation of patients with peripheral vascular disease.[16] However, a maximal estimate derived from the urinary data is in the order of 3 to 4 pg/ml endogenous PGI_2 in the plasma of healthy volunteers.[13]

6-Keto-PGE_1 has been recognized as a potentially stable, active metabolite of PGI_2 in man. Such a metabolite might be relevant to the prolonged clinical benefit following PGI_2 infusion claimed for

TABLE 12–1

	6-KETO-$PGF_{1\alpha}$ (pg/ml)	METHODOLOGY
Moncada, Korbut, Bunting, Vane (1979)	1–200	Bioassay
Masotti, Poggessi, Galanti et al. (1979)	5–25000	Superfusion-Bioassay
Hensby, FitzGerald, Friedman et al. (1979)	140	GC-MS
Nugteren, Christ-Hazelhof, Jouvenaz (1980)	$\leqslant 10$	GC-EC
Hirsch, Hills, Campbell et al. (1981)	160	RIA
Rosenkranz, Fischer, Frohlich (1981)	120	GC-MS
Ciabattoni and Patrono (1981)	$\leqslant 10$	RIA

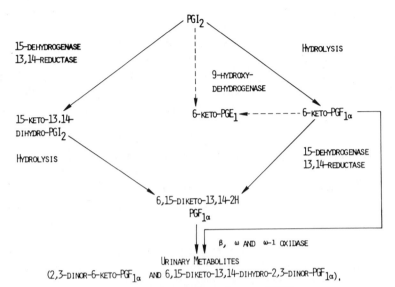

Fig 12–1.—Metabolic pathways of PGI$_2$.

some patients with peripheral vascular disease.[17] Like PGI$_2$, it is a vasodilator, inhibitor of platelet activation, and renin secretagogue.[18, 19] Its synthetic enzyme, 9-hydroxy-prostaglandin dehydrogenase, has been identified in human platelets in vitro.[20] However, we have recently developed a mass spectrometric assay for this compound and identified levels in the order of 10 to 30 pg/ml in resting volunteers.[21] This appeared consistent with the very low estimates of 6-keto-PGF$_{1\alpha}$[10, 11] and endogenous PGI$_2$[13] in human plasma. Furthermore the possibility of a persistent effect of PGI$_2$ due to a long-lived metabolite seems unlikely from the pattern of decay of radioactivity in plasma following a 24-hour infusion of 11-β-(^{3}H)-PGI$_2$ into a healthy volunteer.[22] Radioactivity underwent a triphasic decline in plasma, the $t_{1/2}$ being only 287.5 minutes. Recently 6,15-diketo-13,14-dihydro-2,3-dinor-PGF$_{1\alpha}$ and its ω-oxidized analogue have been identified in human plasma after an infusion of (^{3}H)-labeled and unlabeled PGI$_2$.[23] The additional determination of these longer-lived metabolites might identify an increase in plasma levels of 6-keto-PGF$_{1\alpha}$ which resulted from sampling technique.

Antiplatelet Effects of Prostacyclin Infusion

The chemical synthesis and purification of PGI$_2$ for human use permitted detailed studies in human volunteers. Owing to the extremely short half-life of PGI_2 at 37°C and pH 7.4, the drug was administered in a glycine buffer (pH 10.5) by continuous intravenous infusion. Using single-blind, placebo-controlled conditions, PGI_2 caused a dose-dependent inhibition of ADP-induced platelet aggregation ex vivo.[14] This was accompanied by an increase in plasma cyclic AMP, presumably reflecting the corresponding increase in platelet cyclic AMP.[14] The threshold for this effect lay between 2 and 4 ng/kg/min PGI_2 and it was no longer evident 20 minutes after the infusion was discontinued. Citrated platelet-rich plasma was prepared within 2 minutes in this and a subsequent study,[24] in which similar results were obtained. The inhibitory effect of PGI_2 infusion on ex vivo aggregation,[16, 25, 26] "spontaneous" aggregability[26] and "in vivo" measures of platelet activation, such as β-thromboglobulin and circulating platelet aggregates,[27] has been shown to be similarly transient in patients with peripheral vascular disease and atherosclerotic heart disease. The use of in vivo parameters suggests that the threshold antiplatelet dose of PGI_2 may lie between 1 and 2 ng/kg/min in such patients.[28] A biphasic effect of PGI_2 on platelet aggregation in vitro has been reported,[29] small doses enhancing aggregation. No evidence of such a phenomenon has been established in man although unpublished reports of transient hyperaggregability following a PGI_2 infusion have prompted some investigators to reduce infusions gradually before cessation.

Hemodynamic Effects of Prostacyclin Infusion

Under controlled condition, PGI_2 caused a dose-dependent decline in diastolic pressure and increase in heart rate.[14] Although activation of the baroreflex was expected, the tachycardia ($+25.5 \pm 6.5$ beats/min) seemed disproportionate to the minor diastolic hypotension (-6.3 ± 1.6 mm Hg at PGI_2 8 ng/kg/min vs. control), and plasma concentrations of norepinephrine[14] and epinephrine[30] failed to increase.

However, the interpretation of these data is complex. First, plasma concentrations of catecholamines reflect the resultant of their rate of release into and clearance from the circulation.[31, 32] It is thus possible that the PGI_2 infusion may have altered clearance, perhaps by increasing hepatic blood flow, and consequently obscured a baroreflex-mediated rise in plasma catecholamines. Second, inhibitory presynaptic receptors for prostaglandins have been identified on adrenergic nerves in vitro and may have functioned to offset neuronal release of norepinephrine.[33] However, PGI_2 is a poor agonist in these systems,[34] and the physiologic importance of prejunctional regulatory mechanisms in man has been questioned.[35] The possibility that parasympathetic tone might decrease during PGI_2 infusion in man remains to be explored.

If indirect effects on heart rate were excluded, PGI_2 might be having a direct effect on the heart. Noninvasive evaluation by echocardiography in healthy volunteers demonstrated that a dose-dependent decline in stroke volume accompanied the tachycardia.[36] Thus cardiac output and, by implication, cardiac work underwent little change. Both end-diastolic and end-systolic dimensions underwent a significant reduction during the infusion, suggesting that PGI_2 was acting as both a venodilator and arteriolar dilator in man. Fractional shortening and the velocity of fiber shortening remained unchanged. These effects were evident at doses of PGI_2 (4 to 8 ng/kg/min) that inhibited platelet function and suggested a hemodynamic profile that ought not to be disadvantageous in patients with heart failure or myocardial ischemia. Subsequent administration of PGI_2 to patients with angina and angiographically proven coronary artery disease resulted in a reduction in coronary vascular resistance and mean atrial pacing time to angina. Lactate production during rapid atrial pacing was also reduced.[37]

Humoral Effects of Prostacyclin Infusion

PGI_2 causes a dose-dependent increase in plasma renin activity when administered to healthy volunteers.[14, 30] This reflects an increase in the plasma concentration of active renin, but not of prorenin.[38] Plasma concentrations of angiotensin II and aldosterone also increase during PGI_2 infusion,[30] but sodium and water excretion increase,[38] perhaps due to a direct effect of PGI_2 on the distal renal tubule.[39] Urinary kallikrein excretion is unaltered by intravenous PGI_2.[38] Although a role has been proposed for prostaglandins in the regulation of pituitary hormone release, plasma concentrations of luteinizing and follicle-stimulating hormone are unaltered during PGI_2 infusion in man.[40] Plasma prolactin is similarly unaltered, except in subjects experiencing stressful side effects in whom the hyperprolactinemia may be associated with an increase in plasma cortisol.[40]

Adverse Effects of Prostacyclin Infusion

Subjects usually develop facial flushing at doses in excess of 4 ng/kg/min, which limits the possibility of double-blind studies involving

PGI_2. This is occasionally associated with a throbbing headache, which is reversible on reduction of dose or cessation of the infusion. Nausea and colicky abdominal pain frequently complicate doses in excess of 8 ng/kg/min. Rarely, subjects complain of restlessness during the infusions. Infusions are more readily tolerated if the dose is gradually increased. However, although administration of doses up to 60 ng/kg/min have been reported,[16] doses in excess of 10 ng/kg/min are rarely possible. Moreover, biologic effects are usually not measurable at doses less than 4 ng/kg/min, and so the potential "therapeutic window" for PGI_2 is quite narrow.

Therapeutic Applications of Prostacyclin

Potential therapeutic applications of PGI_2 will be dealt with in greater detail elsewhere in this publication. However, it does seem of great promise in extracorporeal circulations, either alone[41] or in combination with heparin.[42, 43] The role of PGI_2 therapy in other clinical conditions remains to be established. The vasodilator and antiplatelet effects of PGI_2 are desirable in many diseases, and its application has been reported to be favorable in thrombotic thrombocytopenic purpura,[44] persistent fetal circulation,[45] idiopathic pulmonary hypertension,[46] pregnancy hypertension,[47] Raynaud's phenomenon,[48] and angina pectoris.[49] However, controlled clinical trials have yet to be performed in any of these conditions, and so the efficacy of PGI_2 therapy remains to be proven. This caveat is perhaps best exemplified by the place of infusion in the treatment of severe obliterative arterial disease of the extremities. Observational studies have suggested a sustained improvement in blood flow following short-term intra-arterial and intravenous[17, 25, 27] infusions of PGI_2. However, a controlled study has suggested that improvement in blood flow due to bed rest alone may, at least in part, have confounded these results.[26] Orally active stable analogues of PGI_2 are being developed,[50, 51] but have yet to be evaluated in clinical trials.

Conclusion

Although they are probably important in the local regulation of platelet blood vessel wall interactions, neither prostacyclin nor its metabolite 6-keto-PGE_1 is likely to act as circulating antiplatelet hormones under physiologic conditions in man. Synthetic PGI_2 is readily tolerated at doses that exert antiplatelet and vasodilating effects. However, the dose-response curve is steep. Stable orally active analogues of prostacyclin have yet to be evaluated in man. Although of probable value in extracorporeal systems, other potential therapeutic roles remain to be confirmed.

ACKNOWLEDGMENTS

This study was supported by grants from the Wellcome Trust, the Upjohn Company, the Alexander von Humbolt Stiftung, USPHS grant GM 15432, and a Travelling Studentship from the National University of Ireland.

REFERENCES

1. Cohen I.: Platelet structure and function role of prostaglandins. *Ann. Clin. Lab. Sci.* 10:187–194, 1980.
2. Nalbandian R.M., Henry R.L.: Platelet-endothelial cell interactions. *Semin. Thromb. Hemostas.* 5:2, 87, 1978.
3. Masotti G., Puggelesi L., Peggesi G., Galouti G., Trotta F., Neri Serneri G.C.: Prostacyclin production in man, in Lewis P.J., O'Grady J. (eds.): *The Clinical Pharmacology of Prostacyclin.* New York, Raven Press, 1981, pp. 9–20.
4. Hensby C.N., FitzGerald G.A., Friedman L.A., Lewis P.J., Dollery C.T.: Measurement of 6-oxo-PGF$_{1\alpha}$ in human plasma using gas chromatography-mass spectrometry. *Prostaglandins* 18:731–736, 1979.
5. Hirsh P.D., Hills L.D., Campbell W.B., Firth B.G., Willerson J.T.: Release of prostaglandins and thromboxane into the coronary circulation in patients with ischemic heart disease. *N. Engl. J. Med.* 304:685–691, 1981.
6. Hensby C.N., Jogee M., Elder M.G., Myatt L.: A comparison of the quantitative analysis of 6-oxo-PGF$_{1\alpha}$ in biological fluids by gas chromatography mass spectrometry and radioimmunoassay. *Biomed. Mass. Spec.* 8:111–117, 1981.
7. Gryglewski R., Korbut R., Ocetkiewcz A.: Generation of prostacyclin by lungs in vivo and its release into the arterial circulation. *Nature* 273:765–767, 1978.
8. Moncada S., Korbut R., Bunting S., Vane J.R.: Prostacyclin is a circulating hormone. *Nature* 273:767–768, 1978.
9. Hensby C.N., Barnes P., Dollery C.T., Dargie H.S.: Production of 6-oxo-PGF$_{1\alpha}$ by human lung in vivo. *Lancet* 2:1162–1163, 1979.
10. Claeys M., VanHove C., Duchateau A., Herman A.G.: Quantitative determination of 6-oxo-PGF$_{1\alpha}$ in biological fluids by gas chromatography mass spectrometry. *Biomed. Mass. Spec.* 7:11, 12, 544–548, 1980.
11. Patrono C., Ciabattoni G., Peskar B.M., Pugliese F., Peskar B.A.: Is plasma 6-keto-prostaglandin-F$_{1\alpha}$ a reliable index of circulating prostacyclin? *Clin. Res.* 29:276A, 1981. (Abstract)
12. Falardeau P., Oates J.A., Brash A.R.: Quantitative analysis of 2 dinor urinary metabolites of prostaglandin I$_2$. *Analyt. Biochem.* (in press), 1981.
13. FitzGerald G.A., Brash A.R., Falardeau P., Oates J.A.: Estimated rate of prostacyclin secretion in the circulation of normal man. *J. Clin. Invest.* 68:1272–1276, 1981.

14. FitzGerald G.A., Friedman L.A., Miyamori I., O'Grady J., Lewis P.J.: A double-blind placebo controlled evaluation of prostacyclin in man. *Life Sci.* 25:665–672, 1979.
15. Steer M.L., MacIntyre S.E., Levine L., Salzman W.: Is prostacyclin a physiologically important circulating antiplatelet agent? *Nature* 283: 194–195, 1980.
16. Machin S.J., Chamone D.A.F., Defreyn G., Vermylen J.: The effect of clinical prostacyclin infusions in advanced arterial disease on platelet function and plasma 6-keto-PGE$_{1\alpha}$ levels. *Br. J. Haematol.* 47:413–422, 1981.
17. Szczeklik A., Nizankowski R., Skawinski S., Szczeklik J., Gluszko P., Gryglewski R.J.: Successful therapy of advanced arteriosclerosis obliterans with prostacyclin. *Lancet* I:325–326, 1979.
18. Quilley C.P., McGiff J.C., Lee W.H., Sun F.F., Wong P.Y.-K.: 6-Keto-PGE$_1$: a possible metabolite of prostacyclin having platelet antiaggregability effects. *Hypertension* 2:524–528, 1980.
19. Wong P.Y.-K., Malik K.U., Desidero D.M., McGiff J.C., Sun F.F.: Hepatic metabolism of prostacyclin in the rabbit formation of a potent novel inhibitor of platelet aggregation. *Biochem. Biophys. Res. Commun.* 93:486–496, 1980.
20. Wong P.Y.-K., Lee W.H., Chao P.H.-W., Reiss R.F., McGiff J.C.: Metabolism of prostacyclin by 9-hydroxyprostaglandin dehydrogenase in human platelets. *J. Biol. Chem.* 255:9021–9024, 1980.
21. Jackson E.K., Goodman R.P., FitzGerald G.A., Oates J.A., Branch R.A.: Plasma levels of 6-keto-prostaglandin E$_1$ in human subjects: effect of an intravenous prostacyclin infusion. (Submitted for publication.)
22. FitzGerald G.A., Jackson E.K., Brash A.R., Branch R., Oates J.A.: Unpublished data, 1981.
23. Rosenkranz D., Fischer C., Frohlich J.C.: Prostacyclin metabolites in human plasma. *Clin. Pharmacol. Ther.* 29:420–424, 1981.
24. O'Grady J., Warrington S., Moti M.J., Bunting S., Flower R., Fowle A.S.E., Higgs E.A., Moncada S.: Effects of intravenous prostacyclin infusion in healthy volunteers—some pulmonary observations, in Vane J.R., Bergstrom S. (eds.): *Prostacyclin.* New York, Raven Press, 1979.
25. Pardy B.J., Lewis J.D., Eastcott H.G.: Preliminary experience with prostaglandin E$_1$ and I$_2$ in peripheral vascular disease. *Surgery* 826–832, 1980.
26. Hossmann V., Heinen A., Auel H., FitzGerald G.A.: A randomized placebo controlled trial of prostacyclin in peripheral arterial disease of the lower extremeties. *Thromb. Res.* 22:481–490, 1981.
27. Szczeklik A., Gryglewski R.J., Nizankowski R., Skawinski S., Gluszko P., Korbut R.: Prostacyclin therapy in peripheral arterial disease. *Thromb. Res.* 19:191–199, 1980.
28. FitzGerald G.A., Hawiger J., Roberts L.J., Oates J.A.: Unpublished data, 1981.
29. Jorgensen K.A., Dyerberg J., Stoffersen E.: A biphasic effect of prostacyclin on platelet aggregation. *Thromb. Res.* 19:877–881, 1980.
30. Miyamori I., FitzGerald G.A., Lewis P.J.: Prostacyclin stimulates the renin angiotensin aldosterone system in man. *J. Clin. Endocrinol.* 49:943–944, 1979.

31. FitzGerald G.A., Hossmann V., Hamilton C., Davies D., Reid J., Dollery C.T.: Interindividual variation in the kinetics of infused norepinephrine. *Clin. Pharmacol. Ther.* 26:669–675, 1979.

32. FitzGerald G.A., Barnes P., Hamilton C.A., Dollery C.T.: Circulating adrenaline and blood pressure: the metabolic effects and kinetics of infused adrenaline in man. *Eur. J. Clin. Invest.* 10:401–406, 1980.

33. Starke K.: Regulation of noradrenaline release by presynaptic receptor mechanisms. *Rev. Physiol. Biochem. Pharmacol.* 77:1–116, 1977.

34. Hedqvist P.: Actions of prostacyclin (PGI_2) on adrenergic neuroeffector transmission in the rabbit kidney. *Prostaglandins* 17:249–258, 1979.

35. FitzGerald G.A., Watkins J., Dollery C.T.: The regulation of noradrenaline release by peripheral α_2 receptor stimulation. *Clin. Pharmacol. Ther.* 29:160–168, 1981.

36. FitzGerald G.A., Watkins J., Dargie H., Brown M., Lewis P.J.: Cardiac effects of prostacyclin in man, in Lewis P.J., O'Grady J. (eds.): *The Clinical Pharmacology of Prostacyclin.* New York, Raven Press, 1981, pp. 145–152.

37. Bergman G., Atkinson L., Richardson P.J., Daly K., Rothman M., Jackson G., Jewett D.E.: Prostacyclin: haemodynamic and metabolic effects in patients with coronary disease. *Lancet* I:569–572, 1981.

38. FitzGerald G.A., Hossmann V., Konrads J., Hummerich J.: The renin-kallikrein-prostaglandin system: the influence of prostacyclin on prorenin, plasma renin activity and salt excretion in man. *Prostaglandins Med.* 5:445–456, 1981.

39. Gullner H.G., Nicolaou G., Bartter F.C.: Prostacyclin has effects on proximal and distal tubular function in the dog. *Prostaglandins Med.* 6:141–146, 1980.

40. Allolio B., FitzGerald G.A., Hepp F.X., Hossman V., Winkelman A.: Stress related release of prolactin during prostacyclin infusion in man. *Br. J. Clin. Pharmacol.* 10:626–627, 1980.

41. Zusman R.M., Rubin R.H., Cato A.E., Cocchetto D.M., Crow J.W., Tolkoff-Rubin N.: Hemodialysis using prostacyclin instead of heparin as the sole antithrombotic agent. *N. Engl. J. Med.* 304:934–940, 1981.

42. Longmore D.B., Hoyle P.M., Gregory A., Bennett J.G., Smith M.A., Osivand T., Jones W.A.: Prostacyclin administration during cardiopulmonary bypass in man. *Lancet* 2:800–804, 1981.

43. Gimson A.E.S., Hughes R.D., Mellon P.J., Woods H.F., Langley P.G., Canalese J., Williams R., Weston M.J.: Prostacyclin to prevent platelet activation during charcoal haemoperfusion in fulminant hepatic failure. *Lancet* 1:173–175, 1980.

44. FitzGerald G.A., Roberts L.J., Maas R.L., Brash A.R., Stein R., Oates J.A.: Intravenous prostacyclin in thrombotic thrombocytopenic purpura. *Ann. Int. Med.* 95:319–322, 1981.

45. Lock J.E., Olley P.M., Coceani F., Swyer P.R., Rowe R.D.: Use of prostacyclin in persistent fetal circulation. *Lancet* 1:1343–1344, 1979.

46. Watkins W.D., Peterson M.B., Crone R.K., Shannon D.C., Levine L.: Prostacyclin and prostaglandin E_1 for severe idiopathic pulmonary artery hypertension. *Lancet* 1:1083, 1980.

47. Fidler J., Bennett M.J., De Swiet M., Ellis C., Lewis P.J.: Treatment of pregnancy hypertension with prostacyclin. *Lancet* 1:31–32, 1980.

48. Clifford P.C., Martin M.F.R., Sheddon E.J., Kirby J.D., Baird R.N., Dieppe P.A.: Treatment of vasopastic disease with prostaglandin E_1. *Br. Med. J.* 281:1031–1034, 1980.
49. Chierchia S., Crea F., Bernini W., DeCaterina R., Maseri A.: Effects of prostacyclin (PGI_2) continuous infusion in angina at rest. *Circulation* 62(suppl. III): 310, 1980. (Abstract)
50. Hatano Y., Kohli J.D., Goldberg L.I., Fried J., Mehrotra M.M.: Vascular relaxing activity and stability studies of 10,10-difluoro,13,14-dehydro-prostacyclin. *Proc. Natl. Acad. Sci.* 77:6846–6850, 1980.
51. Whittle B.J.R., Moncada S., Whiting F., Vane J.R.: Carbacyclin—a potent stable prostacyclin analogue for the inhibition of platelet aggregation. *Prostaglandins* 19:605–627, 1980.

Conversion of PGI_2 to an Active Metabolite, 6-Keto-PGE_1

PATRICK Y.-K. WONG, ERIC G. SPOKAS,
JOHN C. MCGIFF

Department of Pharmacology
New York Medical College, Valhalla

Since the discovery of prostacyclin (PGI_2) in blood vessels in 1976,[1] it has been assumed to be the principal product of enzymic transformation of the cyclic endoperoxides, PGG_2 and PGH_2, in all vascular elements. Further, prostaglandin (PG) mechanisms within blood vessels are considered to be mediated by prostacyclin;[2] other prostaglandins identified in vascular tissues have been suggested to have relatively unimportant roles or to be artifacts. However, several findings preclude the unqualified acceptance of prostacyclin as the only important vascular prostaglandin: (1) In some blood vessels there is evidence that prostacyclin is not the principal product of enzymic transformation of the cyclic endoperoxides.[3] (2) PGE_2, which is also synthesized in the vascular wall,[4] may be the principal modulator prostaglandin, affecting the vascular actions of vasoactive polypeptides and autonomic nervous activity.[5] (3) Prostacyclin may be transformed by some tissues to a more stable product, 6-keto-PGE_1, having similar biologic potency.[6, 7]

As prostacyclin is unstable under physiologic conditions,[8] its conversion via the 9-hydroxyprostaglandin dehydrogenase (9-OH PGDH) pathway to a stable product, 6-keto-PGE_1, having potent biologic effects, extends the range and duration of those regulatory mechanisms thought to be dependent on prostacyclin. The generation of 6-keto-PGE_1 from PGI_2 may explain the unexpectedly prolonged effects of PGI_2 reported in several studies. In man, inhalation of PGI_2 produced lowering of blood pressure as well as resistance of platelets to the proaggregatory action of ADP for as long as one hour.[9] ADP-induced thrombi formation in the hamster cheek pouch was diminished for 30 minutes after administration of PGI$_2$ was discontinued.[10] Addition of prostacyclin to the incubate of slices of rabbit kidney caused a prolonged release of renin.[11] These studies, when considered together, raise an important question: Are some of the effects now ascribed to prostacyclin dependent upon transformation of PGI$_2$ to 6-keto-PGE$_1$?

Hepatic Metabolism of Prostacyclin

The possibility of the generation of an active metabolite from prostacyclin was first considered during a study of PGI$_2$ metabolism in the isolated perfused liver of the rabbit.[6] Hepatic metabolism of infused {9-³H}-PGI$_2$ was shown by a radiometric method coupled to gas chromatography-mass spectroscopy to be extensive, primarily through β-oxidation and oxidative decarboxylation resulting in the formation of dinor (C$_{18}$) and pentanor (C$_{15}$) metabolites of prostacyclin (Fig 13–1). In the liver, unlike blood vessels,[12] 15-hydroxyprostaglandin dehydrogenase activity was not found. Of the total radioactivity recovered in the liver perfusate, 7% was found to be tritiated water after distillation of the aqueous phase of the perfusate. Recovery of tritiated water indicated the loss of tritium at the 9-position as

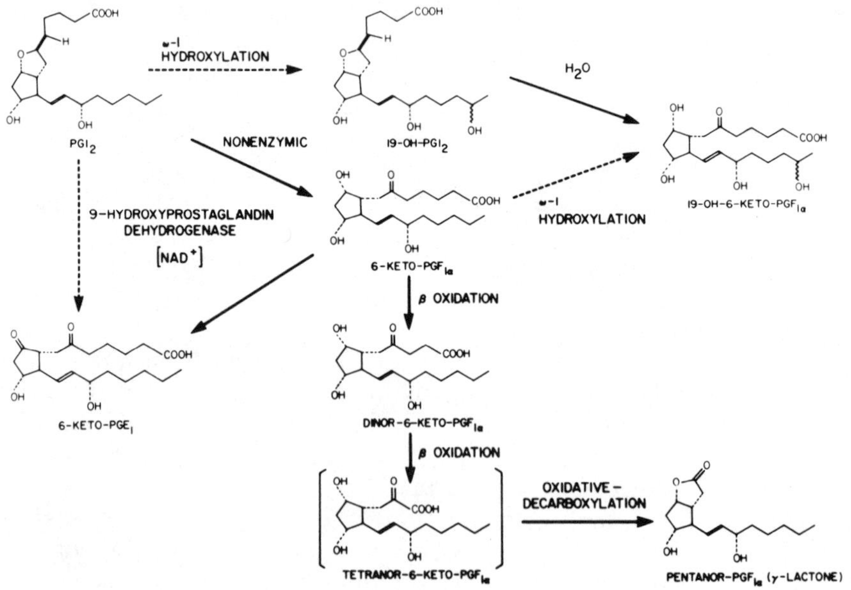

Fig 13–1.—Proposed metabolic pathways of prostacyclin (PGI$_2$) in the rabbit liver. (From Wong P.Y.-K. et al.: *Biochem. Biophys. Res. Commun.* 93:492, 1980.)

{9-³H}-PGI₂ was infused into the liver; this suggested that 6-keto-PGE₁ was a product of PGI₂ under these conditions. Any 6-keto-PGE₁ formed would be unlabeled and, therefore, undetectable by radiometric methods. The formation of this nonradioactive prostaglandin was assessed by scraping the 6-keto-PGE₁ zone from the thin-layer chromatographic plate, eluting the silica gel, suspending the residue in saline, and testing for biologic activity (Fig 13–2). The material in

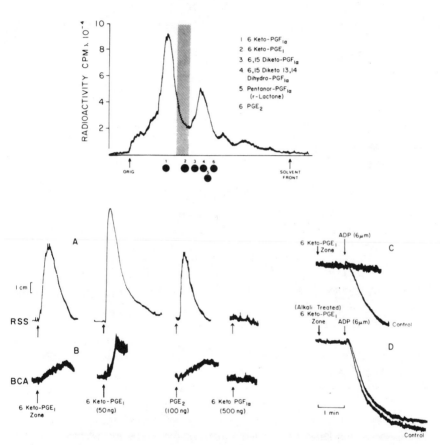

Fig 13–2. — *Upper panel,* radiochromatograph scan of radioactive products extracted from the rabbit liver perfusate after infusion of [9-³H]-PGI₂. Radioactive metabolites were extracted, separated, and identified. *Lower panel,* biologic activity of 6-keto-PGE₁-like substance isolated from TLC. The 6-keto-PGE₁ zone was scraped and eluted from silica gel with chloroform/methanol (1:1, v/v), dried under N₂, and the residue was divided into two parts. One part was suspended in 0.9% saline and tested for 6-keto-PGE₁-like activity on rat stomach strip (RSS) and bovine coronary arteries (BCA) *(A and B).* The other part of the residue was suspended in 50 mM Tris buffer, pH 8.8, and tested for its effect on platelet aggregation *(C and D).*

the 6-keto-PGE$_1$ zone was found to have biologic activity identical to that of authentic 6-keto-PGE$_1$; namely, it contracted the rat stomach strip and bovine coronary artery (Fig 13–2A and B) and inhibited ADP-induced platelet aggregation (Fig 13–2C). Further, alkali treatment, which abolished the platelet antiaggregatory activity of the 6-keto-PGE$_1$ standard, also abolished that of the material recovered from the 6-keto-PGE$_1$ zone (Fig 13–2D). Thus far, the bovine coronary artery is the only tissue that differs qualitatively in its response to 6-keto-PGE$_1$ when compared to PGI$_2$; this tissue is contracted by 6-keto-PGE$_1$ and relaxed by PGI$_2$. The differential response has been exploited in a study on biotransformation of prostacyclin by human platelets.[13]

Platelet Metabolism of Prostacyclin

Although the effects of prostaglandins on platelet function have been well studied,[14] little is known about possible metabolism of prostaglandins by platelets. Compelling evidence has been obtained for enzymic transformation of PGI$_2$ to an active metabolite by platelets. Wong et al. recovered 9-OH PGDH activity primarily from the cytoplasmic fraction of human platelets and purified the enzyme by DEAE-cellulose followed by Sephadex G-200.[15] Gel electrophoresis and isoelectric focusing resulted in a single band of enzyme, having a molecular weight of 60,000 daltons, a pH optimum of 8.5, an isoelectric point of 5.0, and a requirement for NAD$^+$ as cofactor. Purified platelet 9-OH PGDH metabolized the methyl ester of {11$\underline{\ }^3$H}-prostacyclin to a product identified by its mobility on thin-layer plates as {11$\underline{\ }^3$H}-6-keto-PGE$_1$ methyl ester. The methyl ester of prostacyclin was used in this study because it is 10 to 15 times more stable than PGI$_2$, thereby favoring reaction of the purified platelet enzyme with PGI$_2$ methyl ester rather than with the hydrolytic product, 6-keto-PGF$_{1\alpha}$ methyl ester, i.e., significant amounts of unreacted PGI$_2$ methyl ester and the reaction product, 6-keto-PGE$_1$ methyl ester, were recovered (Fig 13–3). PGI$_2$ methyl ester was labeled in the 11-position rather than the 9-position in order to detect 6-keto-PGE$_1$ by radiochromatogram scanning. The 6-keto-PGE$_1$ methyl ester zone of the thin-layer chromatographic plate yielded material that inhibited platelet aggregation induced by ADP, whereas the radioactive peak associated with 6-keto-PGF$_{1\alpha}$ methyl ester did not yield such material (Fig 13–3). As noted previously for 6-keto-PGE$_1$,[6] alkali treatment abolished the platelet antiaggregatory activity of the material obtained from the 6-keto-PGE$_1$ methyl ester zone.

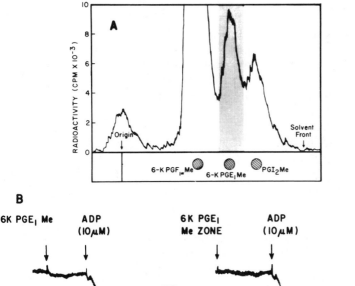

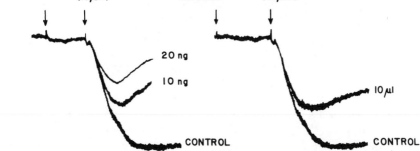

Fig 13–3.—Radiochromatograph scan of the radiometric assay of 9-hydroxyprostaglandin dehydrogenase. *A*, purified platelet enzyme (25 μg) was incubated with [11-^{3}H]-PGI$_2$ Me (Me = Methylester, 500,000 dpm/1.8 μm), NAD$^+$ (4mM), and Tris buffer (pH 8.4, 50 mM, 0.1 mM dithiothreitol) to a volume of 1 ml. After incubation at 37°C for 60 minutes, the reaction was terminated by extraction with precooled ethyl ether (−20°C). The radioactive products extracted were separated by TLC. *B*, the 6-keto-PGE$_1$ Me zone was scraped from the TLC plate, eluted from the silica gel with CHCl$_3$/CH$_3$OH (1:1, v/v), and dried under N$_2$, and the residue was resuspended in Tris buffer (pH 8.4, 50 mM) and tested for its biologic activity on the inhibition of ADP-induced platelet aggregation along with authentic 6-keto-PGE$_1$ Me standard. (From Wong P.Y.-K. et al.: *J. Biol. Chem.* 255:9023, 1980.)

Although the study by Wong et al. was based on the activity of purified 9-OH PGDH of platelets,[15] prostacyclin was shown to gain access to 9-OH PGDH of the intact platelet, a cytosolic enzyme, because in the same study washed human platelets also converted {11$\underline{^3}$H}-PGI$_2$ methyl ester to {11$\underline{^3}$H}-6-keto-PGE$_1$ methyl ester. Unlike prostacyclin, 6-keto-PGF$_{1\alpha}$ was not metabolized by the intact platelet, although the purified platelet enzyme did transform it to 6-

keto-PGE$_1$, an important finding as it provides an explanation for the failure of infused 6-keto-PGF$_{1\alpha}$ to be converted to a biologically active compound.[16] As the purified platelet enzyme can metabolize 6-keto-PGF$_{1\alpha}$, forming 6-keto-PGE$_1$,[15] this finding would appear to be difficult to reconcile with the negligible biologic potency of 6-keto-PGF$_{1\alpha}$ when large amounts are infused intravascularly.[16] An explanation of this seeming discrepancy resides in the inability of 6-keto-PGF$_{1\alpha}$ to bind to platelet-prostaglandin receptors,[17] presumably a prerequisite to metabolism by 9-OH PGDH. In support of the critical role of platelet receptors to prostaglandin-platelet interactions, Schafer et al. have shown that the affinity of PGI$_2$ for the platelet receptor was 1000 times greater than that of 6-keto-PGF$_{1\alpha}$.[17] It is probable, then, that binding by platelets is an obligatory step before prostaglandins are metabolized by the 9-OH PGDH, an enzyme associated with the cytosol. An additional factor that may contribute to the inability of 6-keto-PGF$_{1\alpha}$ to be metabolized by the platelet enzyme relates to the presence of several isomeric forms of 6-keto-PGF$_{1\alpha}$.[18] Thus, the 6-keto-PGF$_{1\alpha}$ formed in vivo may not be in the same isomeric form as the synthetically prepared compound. The possibility that 6-keto-PGE$_1$ may be formed from PGI$_2$ through an unknown intermediate should also be considered.[19]

The possibility of generation of an active metabolite of prostacyclin by blood elements including platelets has been addressed in two recent studies.[13, 20] In the first study, incubation of PGI$_2$ with platelet-rich plasma or platelet-poor plasma resulted after 60 to 150 minutes in the appearance of material in the incubate which contracted the bovine coronary artery, whereas before 30 minutes, only material having prostacyclin-like musculotropic effects was recovered from the incubate.[13] It should be recalled that PGI$_2$ relaxes the bovine coronary artery, whereas 6-keto-PGE$_1$ contracts this blood vessel.[6] This finding was consistent with metabolism of either PGI$_2$ or 6-keto-PGF$_{1\alpha}$ to 6-keto-PGE$_1$ by one or more components of plasma. Additional evidence for platelet metabolism of PGI$_2$ to 6-keto-PGE$_1$-like material was provided by Hoult, Lofts, and Moore.[20] They demonstrated prolongation of platelet antiaggregatory activity and enhancement of the smooth muscle spasmogenic effect after incubating PGI$_2$ in human platelet-rich plasma, but not in platelet-poor plasma. After extraction of incubates for acidic lipids and separation of the acidic lipids by thin-layer chromatography, material was found in the zone of the thin-layer plate corresponding to 6-keto-PGE$_1$ that inhibited platelet aggregation and contracted rat stomach strip. Identification of the metabolite to date rests on characterization of its chromatographic, musculotropic, and platelet antiaggregatory properties, which are indistinguishable from those of authentic 6-keto-PGE$_1$. Sufficient material was not obtained from the liver perfusate to permit unequivocal identification by gas chromatography-mass spectroscopy.[6] Recovery of tritiated water from the liver perfusate provides indirect evidence for production of 6-keto-PGE$_1$ as, in the course of metabolism of PGI$_2$ by 9-OH PGDH, tritium would be lost from the 9-position.

Regulation of Renin Release

The possibility of metabolic transformation of prostacyclin to 6-keto-PGE$_1$ is of great importance to understanding those mechanisms regulating renin release. The relationship of prostaglandins with the renin-angiotensin system are complex, involving modulation of the actions of angiotensins[21, 22] as well as regulation of renin release.[23] Interaction of these systems was first reported in 1970; infusion of angiotensin II increased the concentration of PGE$_2$ in renal venous blood, associated with blunting of the renal vasoconstrictor and antidiuretic actions of angiotensin II.[22] When angiotensin II did not release prostaglandins from the kidney, or when release was inhibited by treatment with indomethacin,[24] the renal vasoconstrictor and antidiuretic effects of the peptide were augmented. It was concluded that release of PGE$_2$ by exogenous angiotensin II modulated the effects of the peptide hormone on renal function. The focus of prostaglandin interactions with the renin-angiotensin system shifted in 1974 when it was reported that administration of arachidonic acid increased renin release.[23] As this effect was prevented by indomethacin, it indicated that transformation of arachidonic acid to a prostaglandin was required. Subsequently, several prostaglandins have been shown to increase renin release. There is evidence that supports the participation of a prostaglandin-dependent component in each of the several signals that affect renin release: tubular, neural, and vascular.[25] For example, stimulation of renin release by a tubular mechanism has been suggested to adjust glomerular filtration rate to the reabsorptive capacity of the individual nephron. This mechanism, referred to as tubuloglomerular feedback, may involve a prostaglandin that induces renin release in response to a signal arising in the renal tubules, such as delivery or reabsorption of sodium and chloride at the macula densa.[26] It is uncertain whether all of the known signals that can release renin must operate through a prostaglandin mechanism. There are studies that do not support this view and suggest that a prostaglandin mechanism serves only to amplify some of these signals.[27] Nonetheless, the possibility exists that a prostaglandin mechanism may be the final common pathway for the multiple signals capable of releasing renin. This mechanism may operate through effects on cyclic nucleotide levels within the cells of the juxtaglomerular apparatus where renin is formed and stored. Increased intracellular levels of cAMP have been linked to stimulation of renin release,[28] and in many tissues, the levels of cyclic AMP are affected by prostaglandins.[29]

The proposal that PGI$_2$ is the arachidonic acid metabolite mediating secretion of renin was based, in part, on in vitro experiments indicating that PGI$_2$ caused the release of renin from rabbit renal cortical slices.[11] Stimulation of renin secretion by PGI$_2$ in the cortical slice preparation was observed over the range of 10^{-7} to 10^{-5}M and was time-dependent, i.e., the response was linear for at least 30 minutes of incubation. This temporal behavior was surprising since PGI$_2$ is rapidly hydrolyzed to 6-keto-PGF$_{1\alpha}$ in aqueous solution at physiologic pH and temperature, the hydrolysis product being inactive in the slice preparation. However, metabolism of prostacyclin to a stable and biologically active product, 6-keto-PGE$_1$, now seems likely in view of the finding that 9-OH PGDH activity is present in the kidney[30] and the demonstration that 6-keto-PGE$_1$ is a potent renin-releasing agent.[31] Formation of 6-keto-PGE$_1$ on oxidation of either prostacyclin or 6-keto-PGF$_{1\alpha}$ has been shown to occur in the rabbit kidney. The highest activity of 9-OH PGDH in the rabbit kidney was found in the cortex and the lowest in the papilla, corresponding to the zonal distribution of renin.[32] Thus, stimulation of renin release previously attributed to PGI$_2$ may have resulted from its conversion to 6-keto-PGE$_1$. A recent study by Yuan et al. has characterized the 9-OH PGDH of rat kidney.[33] The purified enzyme catalyzed NAD$^+$-specific oxidation of 15-keto-13,14-dihydro-PGF$_{2\alpha}$; unlike the enzyme of rabbit kidney,[32] it did not catalyze the oxidation of 6-keto-PGF$_{1\alpha}$. Thus, when interpreting the functional consequences of 9-OH PGDH activity, not only differences among tissues, such as the platelet versus the kidney, but also differences between species, such as rabbit and rat, should be considered.

That 6-keto-PGE$_1$ is a potent renin secretagogue is evident in studies on renin release from the dog kidney in situ[34] and from slices of rabbit renal cortex.[31] Spokas et al. have shown a concentration-dependent relationship for 6-keto-PGE$_1$ when added to the incubate of rabbit renal cortical slices.[31] The threshold concentration of 6-keto-PGE$_1$, which released renin, was lower than that of PGI$_2$. Jackson et al. have compared the relative potencies of infusions of PGI$_2$ and 6-keto-

PGE_1 into the renal artery of the dog on renin secretion rate and renal blood flow.[34] As a renin secretagogue, 6-keto-PGE_1 was five times more potent than PGI_2; as a renal vasodilator agent, 6-keto-PGE_1 was three times more potent. All studies thus far have indicated that the range of cardiovascular effects of PGI_2 and 6-keto-PGE_1 are similar, although some differences may exist in their relative potencies.

We conclude that a biologically active metabolite is generated from prostacyclin in the liver, platelets, and kidney, and perhaps in other tissues. These studies point to the transformation of PGI_2 to a potent and stable material, 6-keto-PGE_1. Further, they raise the possibility that some of the biologic actions of prostacyclin are mediated by 6-keto-PGE_1. Delineation of the spectrum of biologic activity of 6-keto-PGE_1 should contribute to our understanding of prostacyclin-related mechanisms.

REFERENCES

1. Moncada S., Gryglewski R., Bunting S., Vane J.R.: An enzyme isolated from arteries transforms prostaglandin endoperoxides to an unstable substance that inhibits platelet aggregation. *Nature* 263:663–665, 1976.
2. Dusting G.J., Moncada S., Mullane K.M., Vane J.R.: Implications of prostacyclin generation for modulation of vascular tone. *Clin. Sci. Mol. Med.* 55:195s–198s, 1978.
3. Terragno N.A., Terragno A.: Prostaglandin metabolism in the fetal and maternal vasculature. *Fed. Proc.* 38:75–77, 1979.
4. Terragno D.A., Crowshaw K., Terragno N.A., McGiff J.C.: Prostaglandin synthesis by bovine mesenteric arteries and veins. *Circ. Res.* 36:76–80, 1975.
5. Terragno N.A., Terragno D.A., McGiff J.C.: Contribution of prostaglandins to the renal circulation in conscious, anesthetized, and laparotomized dogs. *Circ. Res.* 40:590–595, 1977.
6. Wong P.Y.-K., Malik K.U., Desiderio D.M., McGiff J.C., Sun F.F.: Hepatic metabolism of prostacyclin (PGI_2) in the rabbit: formation of a potent novel inhibitor of platelet aggregation. *Biochem. Biophys. Res. Commun.* 93:486–494, 1980.
7. Quilley C.P., Wong P.Y.-K., McGiff J.C.: Hypotensive and renovascular actions of 6-keto-prostaglandin E_1, a metabolite of prostacyclin. *Eur. J. Pharmacol.* 57:273–276, 1979.
8. Dusting G.J., Moncada S., Vane J.R.: Recirculation of prostacyclin (PGI_2) in the dog. *Br. J. Pharmacol.* 64:315–320, 1978.
9. Szczeklik A., Gryglewski R.J., Nizankowska E., Nizankowski R., Musial J.: Pulmonary and anti-platelet effects of intravenous and inhaled prostacyclin in man. *Prostaglandins* 16:651–659, 1978.
10. Higgs E.A., Higgs G.A., Moncada S., Vane J.R.: Prostacyclin (PGI_2) inhibits the formation of platelet thrombi in arterioles and venules of the hamster cheek pouch. *Br. J. Pharmacol.* 63:535–539, 1978.

11. Whorton A.R., Misono K., Hollifield J., Frolich J.C., Inagami T., Oates J.A.: Prostaglandins and renin release: stimulation of renin release from rabbit renal cortical slices by PGI_2. *Prostaglandins* 14:1095–1104, 1977.

12. Wong P.Y.-K., McGiff J.C.: Detection of 15-hydroxyprostaglandin dehydrogenase in bovine mesenteric blood vessels. *Biochim. Biophys. Acta* 500:436–439, 1977.

13. Gimeno M.F., Sterin-Borda L., Borda E.S., Lazzari M.A., Gimeno A.L.: Human plasma transforms prostacyclin (PGI_2) into a platelet antiaggregatory substance which contracts isolated bovine coronary arteries. *Prostaglandins* 19:907–916, 1980.

14. Moncada S., Vane J.R.: Pharmacology and endogenous roles of prostaglandin endoperoxides, thromboxane A_2, and prostacyclin. *Pharmacol. Rev.* 30:293–331, 1979.

15. Wong P.Y.-K., Lee W.H., Chao P.H.-W., Reiss R.F., McGiff J.C.: Metabolism of prostacyclin by 9-hydroxyprostaglandin dehydrogenase in human platelets. *J. Biol. Chem.* 255:9021–9024, 1980.

16. Miller O.V., Aiken J.W., Shebuski R.J., Gorman R.R.: 6-keto-prostaglandin E_1 is not equipotent to prostacylin (PGI_2) as an antiaggregatory agent. *Prostaglandins* 20:391–400, 1980.

17. Schafer A.I., Cooper B., O'Hara D., Handin R.I.: Identification of platelet receptors for prostaglandin I_2 and D_2 *J. Biol. Chem.* 254:2914–2917, 1979.

18. Flower R.: Discussion in Metabolic Disposition of Prostacyclin, in Vane J.R., Bergstrom S. (eds.): *Prostacyclin.* New York, Raven Press, 1979, pp. 130–131.

19. Quilley C.P., McGiff J.C., Lee W.H., Sun F.F., Wong P.Y.-K.: 6-keto-PGE_1: a possible metabolite of prostacyclin having platelet antiaggregatory effects. *Hypertension* 2:524–528, 1980.

20. Hoult J.R.S., Lofts F.J., Moore P.K.: Stability of prostacyclin in plasma and its transformation by platelets to a stable spasmogenic product. *Br. J. Pharmacol.* 68:218, 1981. (Abstract)

21. McGiff J.C., Crowshaw K., Terragno N.A., Lonigro A.J.: Renal prostaglandins: possible regulators of the renal actions of pressor hormones. *Nature* 227:1255–1257, 1970.

22. McGiff J.C., Crowshaw K., Terragno N.A., Lonigro A.J.: Release of a prostaglandin-like substance into renal venous blood in response to angiotensin II. *Circ. Res.* 27(suppl. 1):121, 1970.

23. Larsson C., Weber P., Ånggård E.: Arachidonic acid increases and indomethacin decreases plasma renin activity in the rabbit. *Eur. J. Pharmacol.* 28:391–394, 1974.

24. Aiken J.W., Vane J.R.: Intrarenal prostaglandin release attenuates the renal vasoconstrictor activity of angiotensin. *J. Pharmacol. Exp. Ther.* 181:678–687, 1973.

25. Weber P.C., Scherer B., Lange H.-H., Held E., Schnermann J.: Renal prostaglandins and renin release: relationship to regulation of electrolyte excretion and blood pressure, in *Proceedings of VIIth International Congress of Nephrology.* Montreal, Canada, June 18–23, 1978. Basel, München, Paris, London, New York, Sydney, S. Karger, 1978, pp. 99–106.

26. Schnermann J., Weber P.C.: A role of renal cortical prostaglandins in the

control of glomerular filtration rate in rat kidneys, in *Advances in Prostaglandins and Thromboxane Research*. New York, Raven Press, 1980, vol. 7, pp. 1047–1055.

27. Oates J.A., Whorton A.R., Gerkens J.F., Branch R.A., Hollifield J.W., Frölich J.C.: The participation of prostaglandins in the control of renin release. *Fed. Proc.* 38:72–74, 1979.

28. Winer N., Chokshi D.S., Walkenhorst W.G.: Effects of cyclic AMP, sympathomimetic amines, and adrenergic receptor antagonists on renin secretion. *Circ. Res.* 29:239–248, 1971.

29. Klein I., Levey G.S.: Effect of prostaglandins on guinea pig myocardial adenyl cyclase. *Metabolism* 20:890–896, 1971.

30. Hoult J.R.S., Moore P.K.: Pathways of prostaglandin $F_{2\alpha}$ metabolism in mammalian kidneys. *Br. J. Pharmacol.* 61:615–626, 1977.

31. Spokas E.G., Ferreri N.R., Wong P.Y.-K., McGiff J.C.: Effect of 6-keto prostaglandin E_1 (6-keto-PGE$_1$) on renin release from rabbit renal cortical slices. *Circulation III*:287, 1980.(Abstract)

32. Wong P.Y.-K., McGiff J.C.: Metabolism of prostacyclin (PGI$_2$) by 9-hydroxy prostaglandin dehydrogenase (9-OH PGDH) in rabbit kidney and liver. Comparison of enzyme distribution and substrate specificity, in *Prostaglandins and the Kidney: International Symposium*. Stuttgart, Germany, July 23–24, 1980. (Abstract No. 8)

33. Yuan B., Tai C.L., Tai H.-H.: 9-Hydroxyprostaglandin dehydrogenase from rat kidney. *J. Biol. Chem.* 255:7439–7443, 1980.

34. Jackson E.K., Herzer W.A., Zimmerman J.B., Branch R.A., Oates J.A., Gerkens J.F.: 6-Keto-prostaglandin E_1 is more potent than prostaglandin I_2 as a renal vasodilator and renin secretagogue. *J. Pharmacol. Exper. Ther.* 216:24–27, 1981.

PART III

PROSTAGLANDINS IN PERIPHERAL VASCULAR DISEASE

Indications for Prostaglandin Treatment of Peripheral Vascular Disease

JAMES W. HOLCROFT AND F. WILLIAM BLAISDELL

Department of Surgery
University of California, Davis

Introduction

The term "peripheral vascular disease" refers to any disease that involves arteries or arterioles exclusive of the coronary circulation.[1] The term, as such, encompasses a large number of diseases that can present themselves in many forms and can be treated in many ways. In order to understand the role of prostaglandins in peripheral vascular disease, it is necessary to understand these variations. The purpose of this chapter is to present an overview of peripheral vascular disease, so that the potential preventive and therapeutic role of prostaglandins can be placed in perspective.

Pathology of Peripheral Vascular Disease

Atherosclerosis is the pathologic process in most patients with peripheral vascular disease. The disease affects the intima primarily in some cases, and the media primarily in other cases. If the disease involves the intima, it is termed "atherosclerotic occlusive disease," as its primary manifestation is obstruction of the arterial lumen. If the disease involves the outer layers of the media, its primary manifestation is arterial dilation (with maintenance of an adequate lumen) and is referred to as "atherosclerotic aneurysmal disease." Prostaglandins probably have no role to play in the aneurysmal form of atherosclerosis, but they probably do, or can, play a role in the occlusive form of the disease.

In the occlusive form of atherosclerosis, the disease can affect the extracranial cerebrovasculature, the mesenteric arteries, the renal arteries, the infrarenal abdominal aorta, the iliac arteries, the femoral arteries, the popliteal artery, the arteries in the calf, and the arteries in the feet. The disease assumes characteristic patterns.[2] These patterns are important, both for the symptoms they produce and for the sources of therapy that are currently available to patients with these disease patterns.

Extracranial cerebrovascular disease most commonly involves the bifurcations of the common carotid arteries. It occasionally involves the origin of the left common carotid artery, the innominate artery, and the origins of the vertebral arteries. Symptoms of vascular insufficiency are produced either by obstruction with resultant inadequate perfusion of the brain, or by embolization to the brain of debris from the atherosclerotic plaque.

The mesenteric arteries are rarely affected by atherosclerotic occlu-

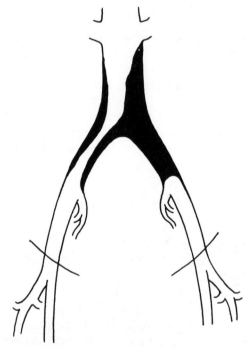

Fig 14–1.—Aortoiliac occlusive disease involves the distal, infrarenal abdominal aorta and spills over into the origins of the common iliac arteries. The disease may progress to occlusion. (From Moore W.S., Blaisdell F.W.: In *Current Problems in Surgery*. Chicago, Year Book Medical Publishers, 1973.)

sive disease. In those few cases in which the mesenteric arteries are involved, the disease is always confined to the origins of the arteries. The disease involves the ventral surface of the aorta in contrast to other forms of atherosclerotic disease in which the disease is usually more extensive on the dorsal surface of the involved vessel. The disease in the mesenteric vessels produces mesenteric ischemia by obstructing flow. To the best of our knowledge, debris from these atherosclerotic plaques rarely embolizes distally.

Atherosclerotic disease in the renal arteries also almost always involves the origins of the vessels. It produces renal ischemia, loss of renal function, and hypertension by obstructing flow. These lesions rarely embolize.

Atherosclerotic occlusive disease of the infrarenal abdominal aorta is usually most extensive at the distal end of the vessel, where it bifurcates into the iliac arteries (Fig 14–1). The disease usually

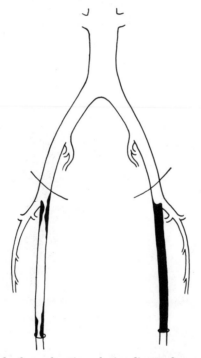

Fig 14–2.—Femoral atherosclerotic occlusive disease frequently begins at the origin of the superficial femoral artery or the distal superficial femoral artery as it courses through Hunter's canal. If either lesion progresses to occlusion, a thrombus will develop throughout the length of the vessel. (From Moore W.S., Blaisdell F.W.: In *Current Problems in Surgery*. Chicago, Year Book Medical Publishers, 1973.)

spills over into the iliac arteries, and this form of the disease is characteristic enough to have earned its own descriptive term, "aortoiliac disease." Symptoms are usually produced by obstruction, but occasionally debris from the atherosclerotic plaque embolizes distally to occlude small arteries in the feet.

Atherosclerotic occlusive disease in the femoral arteries usually begins in the distal superficial femoral artery, just as the vessel passes through Hunter's canal (Fig 14–2). The common femoral artery is the next most commonly involved, the disease progressively occluding the origin of the superficial femoral artery and, slightly less commonly, the origin of the profunda femoris artery (Fig 14–3). The disease in the profunda rarely involves more than the first few centimeters. An exception occurs in diabetics, in whom the disease may extend distally. Again, symptoms are produced by obstruction rather than by embolization.

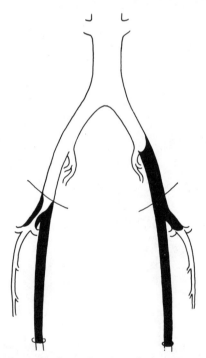

Fig 14–3.—Severe femoral atherosclerotic occlusive disease will involve not only the superficial femoral artery, but also the origins of the profunda femoris artery and, occasionally, the common femoral artery. In most nondiabetics, the profunda disease is confined to the origin, so that collaterals can form to supply the leg through distal branches of the profunda. (From Moore W.S., Blaisdell F.W.: In *Current Problems in Surgery*. Chicago, Year Book Medical Publishers, 1973.)

The popliteal artery can be involved anywhere along its course from the adductor canal to its trifurcation. Symptoms usually result from obstruction.

The trifurcation vessels—the anterior tibial, posterior tibial, and peroneal arteries—are usually involved only at their origins (Fig 14–4). In blacks and diabetics, the disease may extend further down the vessels as they pass through the calf. Symptoms are produced by obstruction.

Atherosclerotic occlusive disease involving the arteries in the feet is confined to diabetics (Fig 14–5). Symptoms are produced by obstruction.

Several other pathologic processes produce peripheral vascular disease besides atherosclerosis. These include diabetic small arterial disease, fibromuscular dysplasia, Buerger's disease, and vasospastic dis-

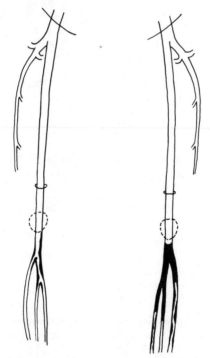

Fig 14–4.—Popliteal atherosclerotic occlusive disease usually involves the origins of the anterior tibial, posterior tibial, and peroneal arteries. In nondiabetics, the disease seldom extends further down the vessels, although the disease in the origin of the arteries can become extensive enough so that the distal popliteal artery becomes occluded. (From Moore W.S., Blaisdell F.W.: In *Current Problems in Surgery.* Chicago, Year Book Medical Publishers, 1973.)

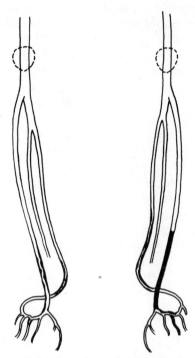

Fig 14–5.—Diabetics can develop atherosclerotic occlusive disease involving the distal arteries in the calf and even the arteries in the foot. (From Moore W.S., Blaisdell F.W.: In *Current Problems in Surgery*. Chicago, Year Book Medical Publishers, 1973.)

orders. All of them, with the exception of fibromuscular dysplasia, produce symptoms by local vascular obstruction rather than by embolization.

Diabetic small vessel disease obstructs arterioles, as opposed to arteries. Diabetics may have atherosclerosis in addition to their small vessel disease, but the small vessel disease, as such, is not atherosclerotic in origin.

Fibromuscular dysplasia is a disease characterized by membrane-like intrusions of the intima and media into the lumen of the vessel. The intrusions obstruct flow and set up eddy currents that allow microthrombi to form and possibly embolize. The disease affects the middle portion of the renal arteries, the distal extracranial portion of the internal carotid arteries, and occasionally, the external iliac arteries.

Buerger's disease (thromboangiitis obliterans) obstructs the arteries of the legs, feet, forearms, and hands. The obstructions are patchy and random. They occur anywhere along the course of the arteries, with skip areas between obstructions. The etiology is unknown, although the disease occurs only in cigarette smokers, who frequently have an extraordinary addiction to tobacco.

Of the vasospastic disorders, Raynaud's disease is the most common. It occurs either by itself or in conjunction with autoimmune diseases, such as scleroderma. The arteries in the hands and feet are most commonly affected, although the arteries in the forearm and leg occasionally go into spasm as well. The etiology is unknown. The arteries are normal pathologically.

Symptoms of Peripheral Vascular Disease

The symptoms of peripheral vascular disease reflect inadequate circulation due to obstruction of an artery or embolization with obstruction distal to the point where the embolus lodges. If obstruction occurs suddenly, the symptoms are worse than if it develops slowly, because slow obstruction allows collaterals to develop.

Acute occlusion of the extracranial cerebrovasculature may be symptomatic or may produce a stroke. Intermittent embolization from an atherosclerotic plaque in the extracranial arteries can cause transient cerebral ischemic attacks or transient blindness—amaurosis fugax. Acute occlusion of the mesenteric vessels usually produces a bowel infarction. Acute occlusion of one renal artery may be asymptomatic or associated with flank pain; occlusion of both produces anuria. Acute occlusion of any of the large arteries that supply the lower extremity will produce any or all of the five "P's"—pulselessness, pallor, pain, paresthesias, and paralysis. The last symptoms indicate the greater degrees of ischemia. Pain, loss of sensation, and, in particular, muscle paralysis indicate impending limb loss. Acute occlusion of the smaller vessels—in the calf or distally—may be asymptomatic or may produce necrosis of the part supplied by the artery. For example, an acute isolated occlusion of the anterior or posterior tibial artery in a patient with otherwise normal vessels will be asymptomatic; an acute occlusion of the distal arteries to the toe usually causes necrosis of at least part of the toe.

Chronic occlusions usually produce fewer symptoms. Slow progression of atherosclerosis of the extracranial cerebrovasculature, which leads to occlusion of one of the extracranial arteries, usually is asymptomatic. Slow occlusion of more than one of the extracranial arteries may produce a stroke.

Slow occlusion of the celiac axis or of the superior or inferior mesenteric artery almost always is asymptomatic. Occlusion of two or more of these vessels produces postprandial abdominal pain—abdominal angina—and weight loss.

Slow occlusion of one renal artery may produce the symptoms of hypertension. Obstruction of both renal arteries produces the symptoms of renal failure.

Isolated, chronic occlusion of the aortoiliac, femoral, or popliteal arteries usually produces only symptoms of claudication, that is, discomfort in muscle groups on exercise when demand for blood flow is the greatest. To produce symptoms of severe ischemia, two or more sequential segments of the arterial tree need to be occluded.[3]

The symptoms of claudication and rest pain distinguish mild ischemia from severe ischemia. Claudication comes from the Latin "claudicare," meaning "to limp." The patient complains of pain, tiredness, or aching in a large muscle group on walking a specified distance. The discomfort disappears within a few minutes with rest; it recurs with walking the same distance again. The muscle group affected is distal to the level of arterial obstruction. Patients with calf claudication have obstruction of the popliteal, femoral, or aortoiliac system. Patients with thigh claudication have obstruction of the femoral or aortoiliac system; patients with buttock claudication have aortoiliac occlusive disease.

Rest pain is pain at rest in the distal part of the foot. It is usually most severe at night, when the patient is lying flat. The pain is worse at night presumably for two reasons: (1) There are fewer sensory distractions at night, so that the patient thinks more about his pain. (2) The foot is at the same level as the heart. The patient does not have the advantage of having a long column of blood pushing blood down into his foot, an advantage he would have during the day when in an erect position. In this last regard, rest pain is sometimes alleviated when the patient sits up and dangles his foot over the side of the bed.

A precise definition of rest pain is important. If the patient truly has rest pain, he will almost certainly come to amputation unless the ischemia can be relieved. Claudication, on the other hand, can usually be tolerated for years. Most patients with claudication as their only sign of ischemia will die of other diseases before their leg becomes jeopardized by the ischemia.

Not all patients with severe ischemia of their legs have rest pain. Diabetics with peripheral neuropathies, in particular, can develop frank gangrene and have no pain. The peripheral neuropathy can complicate the diabetic's care considerably. The patient may not realize the seriousness of his ischemia, and diabetics sometimes do not consult a physician until necrosis affects much of their foot.

Some symptoms of peripheral vascular disease are fairly specific for a particular disease process. Patients with fibromuscular dysplasia of the internal carotid artery may complain of a loud bruit in their ears. Male patients with aortoiliac atherosclerotic occlusive disease may have impotence. Patients with Raynaud's disease can present a characteristic triad of symptoms.

This triad of symptoms typically begins after the patient's extremity is exposed to the cold. The involved extremity becomes extremely pale, then cyanotic, and later, as spasm breaks and perfusion improves, ruborous. The extremity sometimes becomes numb with the onset of symptoms and sometimes painful. Occasionally, the disease becomes so severe that skin necrosis develops.

Signs of Peripheral Vascular Disease

The signs, like the symptoms of peripheral vascular disease, arise from inadequate blood supply to specific tissues.

The signs of cerebrovascular insufficiency are those neurologic abnormalities associated with the area of the eye or brain made ischemic by the disease. Patients with emboli to the retinal artery can have cholesterol plaques in branches of that artery and these can be seen by the opthalmoscope; they can also be partially blind as a result of the embolus. Severe ischemia of the brain can progress to a stroke, with loss of function related to the area of the brain involved. However, many patients with extracranial cerebrovascular disease have intermittent ischemia with transient brain dysfunction; these patients have no permanent neurologic signs.

Chronic mesenteric vascular insufficiency is characterized by signs of chronic weight loss. The patient may also have an abdominal bruit. Acute mesenteric occlusion causes an acute abdomen and subsequent peritonitis and death if not operated upon promptly.

In most cases, the only sign of unilateral chronic renal arterial obstruction is hypertension. Bilateral obstruction can cause signs of chronic renal failure.

Atherosclerotic occlusive disease of any of the arteries going to the lower extremities is characterized by signs ranging from a slight diminishment of the pulses to ischemic necrosis of the lower half of the body. The physical exam is usually all that is necessary to assess the severity of the obstructive process.

The pulses are usually diminished distal to the point of obstruction. However, some patients with less severe disease have normal pulses. In some of these patients, the proximal obstructive process can be demonstrated by asking the patient to exercise to the point at which symptoms develop. On cessation of the exercise, the pulses distal to the obstruction may become weak or absent.[4, 5] This is because the exercise induces peripheral vasodilation with an increased blood flow which the proximally obstructed artery cannot deliver. As a result, a pressure gradient develops across the proximal obstructive lesion, leading to a lower pressure distally.

Proximal obstructive disease produces turbulence in many patients, which can be detected as a bruit over the involved artery distally. Bruits are most easily heard over the femoral arteries in the groin, and occasionally can be heard over the popliteal artery in the popliteal fossa. They are rarely heard distally over the smaller arteries.

Ischemia of the feet is most evident with elevation of the lower extremities 30 to 45 degrees with the patient lying in bed. The ischemic feet become pale or cadaveric, with the paleness most pronounced in the toes.

With the legs and feet still elevated, the patient should then be asked to flex and extend his feet until he develops claudication or for one minute, whichever is shorter. This will empty the veins and also render the marginal limbs pale if significant proximal obstruction exists.

The patient should then be asked to sit up and dangle his feet over the side of the bed in a dependent position. In patients with normal circulation, the veins fill promptly; in patients with inadequate circulation, the veins fill slowly.[6]

The color of the skin of the feet should next be observed. Rapid return of color indicates good circulation and vice versa. Slow return of color, with the ultimate development of an intense red to purplish

Chronic ischemia can also lead to atrophy of the muscles, skin, and hue to the skin of the foot, is called rubor. It indicates severe ischemia. This can be differentiated from the redness of inflammation, since it is cold redness and is due to stasis of blood in a vasculature dilated by the accumulation of waste products of metabolism.

skin appendages of the lower extremities. These signs include calf atrophy; smooth, shiny skin; thickened toenails; loss of sweat glands; and loss of hair. Minor traumatic lesions heal slowly if at all.

As the ischemia worsens, the skin breaks down with the formation of ischemic ulcers or frank gangrene. This usually occurs on the tips of the toes or on pressure points on the dorsum of the toes or distal foot.

The ulcers may involve only the skin and subcutaneous fat; they may extend down to and beneath the fascia (Fig 14–6). The ulcers are sometimes covered by an eschar of dead skin, which conceals the seriousness of the underlying ischemic necrosis. This eschar is formed by desiccation of the dead tissue, and the resulting necrosis is termed "dry gangrene" (Fig 14–7).

Wet gangrene is formed when ischemic tissue becomes infected. The tissue becomes wet and swollen. The other signs of inflammation—for example, erythema, warmth, and pus formation—do not develop because the circulation is so impaired that the tissue cannot mount a full inflammatory response. Diabetics, particularly those with advanced vascular disease, are vulnerable to infection of their ischemic tissue and the development of wet gangrene.

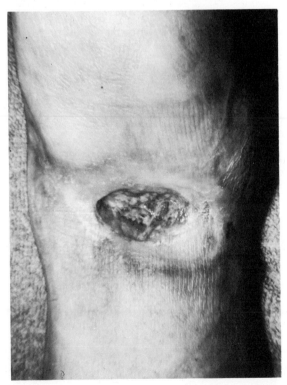

Fig 14–6.—Ischemic ulcer in a patient with severe atherosclerotic occlusive disease. These lesions rarely heal in the absence of improvement of circulation.

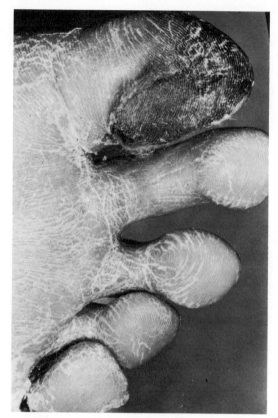

Fig 14–7.—Dry gangrene of the great toe.

Laboratory Evaluation of Peripheral Vascular Disease

Arteriography is the mainstay for diagnosing peripheral vascular disease. It delineates the type of disease and defines the location, extent, and severity of obstructing lesions, and usually easily demonstrates the lesions of atherosclerotic occlusive disease of the large arteries. Fibromuscular dysplasia shows a characteristic arteriographic pattern of beading of the midportion of the renal arteries, the extracranial internal carotid arteries, or the external iliac arteries. Buerger's disease shows segmentally occluded arteries in the legs, feet, forearms, and hands. Vasospastic disorders show spasm of the arteries distal to the knees or elbows if the arteriogram is obtained at the time the patient is having symptoms.

Treatment of Peripheral Vascular Disease

Peripheral vascular disease can be treated with large vessel arterial reconstruction, percutaneous transluminal balloon dilation, sympathectomy, and amputation. Nonoperative treatment includes skin care, exercising to the point of tolerance, cessation of cigarette smoking, and avoidance of cold in patients with Raynaud's disease. Vasodilating agents are of no benefit.

Atherosclerotic occlusive disease of the extracranial, mesenteric, renal, aortoiliac, and femoral arteries can frequently be surgically treated with reconstruction of the involved vessels. The arteries can either be bypassed or their atherosclerotic intima removed by endarterectomy. Atherosclerotic occlusive diseases of some of the larger vessels can also be treated at times with percutaneous transluminal balloon dilation.

Small vessel disease—disease involving the areas distal to the knees and elbows—can seldom be treated with direct surgical or arteriographic techniques. Sympathectomies can help in selected patients, particularly those with vasospastic disorders. Sympathectomy occasionally helps in patients with occlusive diseases if the patient's main problem is impaired skin circulation.

Amputation for peripheral vascular disease need not be the end of useful existence for the patient. The surgeon should maintain a positive attitude when forced to amputate. Most patients with transmetatarsal and below-knee amputations ambulate without crutches, and some younger patients with above-knee amputations can also learn to use a prosthesis. Amputations of the upper extremities are almost never needed for atherosclerotic occlusive disease; they are required at times in patients with Buerger's disease or Raynaud's disease.

Nonoperative treatment does not alter the underlying disease process, but it can prevent the process from worsening and it can allow compensatory mechanisms to exert their effect. The skin of the ischemic extremity must be protected from cuts, bruises, and pressure. A minor break in the skin of a toe can progress to necrosis of the foot. Patients with claudication should exercise to the point of tolerance to stimulate the growth of collaterals. Cessation of cigarette smoking can benefit patients considerably, but seems to be impossible for many. Skin ulcers can be treated with any of a variety of locally applied ointments or solutions, none probably offering much advantage over another. Ischemic ulcers rarely heal unless circulation can be improved.

Potential Role of Prostaglandins

The worst prognosis for limb salvage is in patients with popliteal outflow disease, multiple segmental occlusive disease, Buerger's disease, and severe Raynaud's disease. When patients with these patterns of disease have dependent rubor, rest pain, superficial nonhealing lesions, or peripheral gangrenous lesions of toe tips, the prognosis is poor, and below- or above-knee amputations are often required. In these instances, a relatively small augmentation of blood flow to the skin may be sufficient to relieve rest pain or permit healing of superficial lesions.

The prostaglandins may also prove of value in patients who need augmented skin flow for a limited period of time. Failure of amputations to heal is usually due to inadequate circulation to the skin, as opposed to inadequate circulation to the muscle. Administration of prostaglandins at the time of an amputation might augment skin circulation enough so that the skin flaps of even a distal amputation might heal. Once healed, skin flaps require little blood flow to maintain integrity of intact skin. Thus, even short-term benefit from prostaglandin administration might lead to long-term maintainance of extremity length and function.

Chronic administration of blockers of thromboxane or stimulators of prostacyclin may prevent the development of disease in the first place. These agents could be effective in all of the peripheral vascular disorders, including atherosclerosis, Buerger's disease, and Raynaud's disease.

REFERENCES

1. Rutherford R.B.: *Vascular Surgery.* Philadelphia, W. B. Saunders Co., 1977.
2. Moore W.S., Blaisdell F.W.: Diagnosis and management of peripheral arterial occlusive disease, in Ravitch M. (ed.): *Current Problems in Surgery.* Chicago, Year Book Medical Publishers, 1973.
3. Haimovici H., Steinman C.: Aortoiliac angiographic patterns associated with femoropopliteal occlusive disease: significance in reconstructive arterial surgery. *Surgery* 65:232, 1969.
4. Barner H.B. et al.: Intermittent claudication with pedal pulses. *J.A.M.A.* 204:958, 1968.
5. Keitzer W.F.: Hemodynamic mechanism for pulse changes seen in occlusive vascular disease. *Surgery* 57:163, 1965.
6. Gilfillan R.S., Freeman N.E., Leeds F.H.: A clinical estimation of the blood pressure in the minute vessels of the human skin by the method of elevation and reactive hyperemia. *Circulation* 9:180, 1954.

Prostaglandins and Atherosclerosis

RYSZARD J. GRYGLEWSKI AND ANDREW SZCZEKLIK

N. Copernicus Academy of Medicine
Institute of Pharmacology
Institute of Internal Medicine
Krakow, Poland

Antiaggregatory Prostanoids

Several products of cyclo-oxygenation of polyunsaturated fatty acids (prostanoids) stimulate platelet adenylate cyclase and increase cAMP level in platelets; therefore, they inhibit release reaction, suppress platelet contraction and aggregation, and dissipate white platelet thrombi.

These prostanoids are considered to be tissue hormones (autacoids), and their action is confined to the sites of their generation, i.e., to vascular endothelium and platelet aggregates, although under special circumstances, blood level of antiaggregatory prostanoids may rise to an extent that affects all circulating platelets.

Potent antiaggregatory prostanoids (AP) are generated from arachidonic acid (20:4ω6). The most potent among them is prostacyclin,[1-3] a nonprostaglandin prostanoid whose name was unluckily abbreviated to PGI_2. Recently, it has been proposed that chemically liable PGI_2 is enzymatically converted to 6-keto-prostaglandin E_1 (6-keto-PGE_1).[4, 5] This latter one is chemically stable and biologically active, an antiaggregatory agent. Another AP that derives from arachidonic acid is prostaglandin D_2 (PGD_2).[6] Dihomo-gamma-linoleic acid (20:3ω6) is the substrate for synthesis of prostaglandin E_1 (PGE_1), which is a weaker AP than the three already mentioned.[7] Chemical synthesis leads to another monoenoic AP, that is, 5,6 dihydroprostacyclin (PGI_1).[8] Finally, in vitro eicosapentaenoic acid (20:5ω3) via PGH_3 is enzymatically transformed to two potent APs, which are Δ 17 prostacyclin (PGI_3) and prostaglandin D_3 (PGD_3).[9, 10]

In summary, among monoenoic prostanoids antiaggregatory activity is confined to synthetic PGI_1 and biosynthetic PGE_1 as well as to 6-keto-PGE_1 which originates from dienoic PGI_2. PGI_2 and PGD_2 are dienoic, whereas PGI_3 and PGD_3 are trienoic AP.

At present, the most important of them biologically seems to be PGI_2.

Intravascular activation of platelets has been claimed to be associated with the development of atherosclerosis,[11–13] coronary disease,[14] and thromboembolic disorders.[15] It has been repeatedly suggested that a balance between endogenous generation of vascular PGI_2 and thromboxane A_2 (TXA_2) in platelets may play an essential role in maintaining intravascular homeostasis.[2, 16] In experimental atherosclerosis, a synthetic capacity of PGI_2 in arteries and other tissues is diminished.[13, 17, 18] On the other hand, PGI_2 or PGE_1 were claimed to be beneficial in treatment of peripheral vascular disease,[19, 20] spontaneous angina,[21] myocardial ischemia in dogs,[22] central retinal vein occlusion,[23] pulmonary embolism in dogs,[24] and in cardiopulmonary bypass.[25] In future, this therapeutic approach may be supplemented by activation of physiologic mechanisms that trigger the generation and release of endogenous AP.[26–28]

In one of the pioneering papers on the discovery of prostacyclin[2] we have described that 15-hydroperoxyeicosatetraenoic acid (15-HPETE, 15-HPAA, IC_{50} = 1.5 μM) and tranylcypromine (IC_{50} = 600 μM) are inhibitors of prostacyclin synthetase in porcine aortic microsomes. 15-HPETE inhibits prostacyclin generation also in rabbit arterial slices[29] and in cultured human endothelial cells.[30] 15-HPETE shares its destructive action on prostacyclin synthetase with a vast number of other lipid peroxides.[31] It has been proposed that 15-HPETE suppresses the formation of prostacyclin (PGI_2) as a consequence of the peroxidatic reduction of this hydroperoxide and the release of O_z.[32]

The foregoing in vitro findings prompted us to put forward a hypothesis that an increase in lipid peroxidation promotes the development of atherosclerosis owing to the selective removal of prostacyclin from the body[13, 17] and subsequent activation of blood platelets.[12] We believe that prostacyclin is a natural antiatherosclerotic hormone.[33]

Indeed, feeding rabbits a diet high in oleic acid and in cholesterol leads to a dramatic suppression of prostacyclin generation by aorta, mesenteric arteries, heart,[13, 17] lungs, and kidneys.[18] This suppression is observed as early as one week after feeding the rabbits an atherogenic diet.[34] The selective blockade of prostacyclin generation by lipid peroxides, which are formed during hyperlipidemia, may divert arachidonic acid metabolism from prostacyclin to prostaglandins in arteries[35] and kidney[18] and to thromboxane A_2 in platelets.[12] This last phenomenon has been also observed in atherosclerotic patients.[36, 37]

Until now, we have not been able to produce direct evidence that human atherosclerosis is causally associated with an increased lipid peroxidation. Nonetheless, lipid peroxides have been found in human atherosclerotic arteries,[38] in ceroid atheromatic plaques,[39] and in retina during ocular siderosis.[40] Human atheromatic plaques hardly generate prostacyclin.[41] Low-density lipoproteins were reported to inhibit the generation of an antiaggregatory principle by cultured human endothelial cells[42] and to damage them,[43] whereas high-density lipoproteins were found to prevent the deleterious action of low-density lipoproteins.

We have recently found that serum lipid peroxide levels rise in common types of hyperlipoproteinemias from 2.5 ± 0.1 to 3.8 ± 0.3 nmoles malondialdehyde ml^{-1}.[44] The sum of lipid peroxide concentrations in the lipoprotein fractions is several times higher (10.8 ± 3.0 nmoles MDA ml^{-1} in healthy volunteers and 26.0 ± 3.3 nmoles MDA ml^{-1} in hyperlipoproteinemia type V) than the corresponding serum lipid peroxide concentrations. Most of serum lipid peroxides are accumulated in low-density lipoproteins (LDL). In common types of hyperlipoproteinemias, lipid peroxides may also appear in very low-density lipoproteins (VLDL) and in chylomicrons, but never in high-density lipoproteins (HDL). HDL, when mixed with LDL, seem to protect a hydroperoxy moiety in LDL from being detected by the thiobarbituric acid method or by iodometric titration. LDL, but not HDL, inhibit the release of prostacyclin from superfused bovine coronary artery. Administration of vitamin E (300 mg daily for a week) substantially suppresses lipid peroxide levels in LDL and chylomicrons of patients with hyperlipoproteinemias. At present, we have studied the effect of LDL and HDL of patients with coronary heart disease and healthy volunteers on the generation of PGI_2 by rat aortic slices.

Effect of Low-Density Lipoproteins on Prostacyclin Biosynthesis

Serum low-density lipoproteins (LDL) and high-density lipoproteins (HDL) were prepared by gradient ultracentrifugation and dialyzed from 12 healthy subjects and 15 patients with coronary heart disease and hyperlipoproteinemia.[42] In both lipoprotein fractions, cholesterol and lipid peroxides were determined. The effect of these lipoproteins on spontaneous prostacyclin (PGI_2) biosynthesis in rat aortic slices was studied by bioassay and mass fragmentography of 6-keto-$PGF_{1\alpha}$.[44]

Basal release of prostacyclin by the slices was 1.49 ± 0.04 ng/mg wet tissue (n = 258) by bioassay and 0.96 ± 0.09 ng/mg wet tissue (n = 18) by MID (mean ± S. E.) LDL- and HDL-lipid peroxide concentrations are shown in Figures 15–1, 15–2 and 15–3.

Serum lipoproteins were susceptible to peroxidation during the preparation procedure. LDL were more prone to peroxidation than HDL. Lipid peroxides were hardly formed in lipoproteins when calcium ions had been removed by EDTA (0.01%), and butylated hydroxytoluene (BHT) (0.02%) was present at all stages of their preparation (Figs 15–1, 15–2). LDL prepared without the above precautions either from healthy subjects or from patients with coronary heart disease markedly suppressed prostacyclin generation by rat

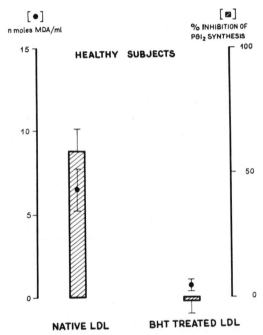

Fig 15–1.—Lipid peroxide content in LDL (dots-nmoles MDA/ml serum) of 12 healthy subjects and percent of inhibition of PGI₂ biosynthesis (columns) in rat aortic slices by LDL prepared by sequential ultracentrifugation without the antioxidant (native LDL) and in the presence of butylated hydroxytoluene (BHT-treated LDL). Rat aortic slices (10 mg/0.1 ml) were preincubated with LDL (0.8 to 1.0 mg protein/ml) at 37 C for 15 minutes and then washed, blotted on filter paper, and incubated with shaking for 3 minutes in 0.1 ml of 0.05 M Tris buffer pH 9.56 at room temperature. PGI₂ or 6-keto-PGF$_{1\alpha}$ were assayed in the supernatant. In control samples, which were preincubated with 0.15 M NaCl, generation of PGI₂, as measured by bioassay, was 1.49 ± 0.04 ng/mg wet tissue (n = 258) or, as measured by mass fragmentography, 0.96 ± 0.09 ng/mg wet tissue (n = 8, mean ± S.E.). Bars represent S.E.

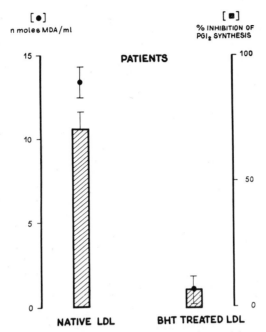

Fig 15-2.—See legend for Figure 15-1. LDL were obtained from 15 patients with coronary heart disease. Seven had myocardial infarction at least three months earlier. Five had severe type of IIA familial hypercholesterolemia; their serum cholesterol ranged from 420 to 545 mg/dl. In the remaining patients, serum cholesterol values were between 250 and 300 mg/dl.

aortic slices (Figs 15–1, 15–2). This inhibition did not depend on LDL-cholesterol, but it did depend on LDL-lipid peroxides (Fig 15–4). In most healthy subjects and patients with coronary heart disease and concomitant hyperlipoproteinemia, LDL deprived of lipid peroxides did not inhibit prostacyclin biosynthesis. However, in one quarter of the patients, those LDL had such inhibitory effect (Fig 15–5). Therefore, in some patients with coronary heart disease there operate mechanisms other than peroxidation of LDL, which might be responsible for the inhibitory activity of this lipoprotein fraction on prostacyclin generation.

HDL prepared by the technique of Nordøy et al. from both controls and patients contained considerably lower amounts of lipid peroxides (2.6 ± 0.6 nmoles MDA ml^{-1}) than LDL.[42] Preparation of HDL in the presence of BHT caused a further decrease in their peroxide content down to 0.5 ± 0.5 nmoles MDA ml^{-1}. Irrespective of the way of preparation of HDL, this lipoprotein fraction did not inhibit significantly

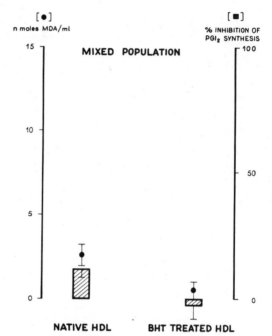

Fig 15–3.—See legend for Figure 15–1. Instead of LDL, HDL of 6 patients with coronary heart disease and 4 healthy subjects were used. Rat aortic slices were preincubated with HDL at a concentration of 0.8 to 1.6 mg protein/ml.

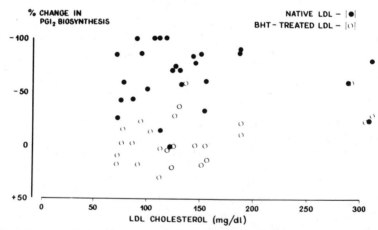

Fig 15–4.—A lack of correlation between cholesterol content in LDL and their inhibitory activity on PGI_2 biosynthesis in rat aortic slices. Closed circles = native LDL; open circles = LDL prepared in the presence of BHT. Inhibitory action of LDL on PGI_2 biosynthesis depends on the presence of lipid peroxides in LDL, but not on LDL cholesterol concentration.

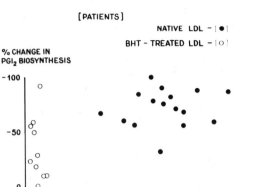

Fig 15–5.—The relation between LDL lipid peroxide content and inhibitory action of LDL on PGI$_2$ biosynthesis in rat aortic slices. For methodologic details see legend for Figure 15–1. LDL were obtained from patients with coronary heart disease and familial type IIA hypercholesterolemia. Closed circles represent data for LDL that were prepared without an antioxidant (native LDL). Open circles refer to LDL that were prepared in the presence of 0.02% of butylated hydroxytoluene (BHT-treated LDL). Note that LDL of some patients though practically deprived of peroxides still inhibit PGI$_2$ biosynthesis.

prostacyclin generation by rat aortic slices. The influence of native HDL on PGI$_2$ synthesis was $-12 \pm 6.1\%$, while that of BHT-treated HDL was $3.4 \pm 6.6\%$ (n = 10, mean $\pm$ S. E.) (Fig 15–3).

In conclusion, LDL-lipids seem to be more susceptible to peroxidation than those of HDL. This peroxidation occurs during fractionation of lipoproteins by the standard gradient ultracentrifugation. However, in the presence of an antioxidant, there still remains a residual amount of lipid peroxides, especially in LDL of patients with coronary heart disease. Therefore, we cannot deny that in vivo spontaneous peroxidation of LDL lipids occurs, although to a small extent. Our finding that LDL prepared by a classic method inhibit PGI$_2$ biosynthesis might be explained as an artifact produced by the preparation technique. This seems to be true in all healthy subjects. However, in some patients with coronary heart disease, even nonperoxidized LDL suppress markedly prostacyclin generation. We therefore believe that mechanisms other than lipid peroxidation might be responsible for inhibition of PGI$_2$ generation by LDL in this subgroup of patients with coronary heart disease.

Irrespective of the mechanism of LDL-induced inhibition of prostacyclin biosynthesis, this biochemical event might be one of the explanations for the proatherogenic properties of LDL. In this respect it should be mentioned that antiatherogenic HDL did not inhibit PGI_2 biosynthesis even when isolated from patients with hyperlipoproteinemia. Our findings may throw a new light on the role of LDL/HDL ratio in development of atherosclerosis.[44]

Mechanisms That Regulate the Release of Antiaggregatory Prostanoids

In human and experimental atherosclerosis, generation of antiaggregatory PGI_2-like activity by arterial walls is diminished. On the other hand, LDL from one quarter of patients with coronary heart disease suppress the synthesis of PGI_2 by aortic slices in vitro. Therefore, study of the mechanisms that regulate the release of endogenous antiaggregatory prostanoids may be of clinical importance.

We have previously reported that biologically active peptides[26, 33, 45, 46] and chemoreceptor stimulants[47, 48] release a PGI_2-like substance into the circulation of anesthetized cats. Recently cholinergic stimuli were shown to produce a similar release of antiaggregatory substances, and this release was potentiated by beta-adrenergic blockade. However, except for the release that was activated by chemoreceptor stimulants, the stability of other "PGI_2-like substances" was higher than that of authentic PGI_2. McGiff's group[4, 5, 49] discovered that biotransformation of PGI_2 may lead to a stable and biologically active 6-oxo-PGE_1. Therefore, we decided that it would be appropriate to refer to "antiaggregatory prostanoids" (AP) rather than to "PGI_2-like substances," especially because of our technique in vivo that did not differentiate between 6-oxo-PGE_1, PGE_1, and PGD_2.

Angiotensin II releases antiaggregatory prostanoids into the circulation, and the lung is the main but not the only target organ for this action of angiotensin II.[33, 46] This finding was confirmed by Mullane and Moncada.[50] Angiotensin II stimulates also the release of PGI_2 from isolated kidney,[51] from perfused lungs,[45] and from perfused mesenteric vascular bed.[45] As previously shown,[33, 46] and now confirmed, only angiotensin II, and not angiotensin I, induces the release of antiaggregatory prostanoids, since captopril inhibits the antiaggregatory prostanoid-releasing effect of angiotensin I. In this respect our results differ from those of Dusting et al.,[52] although we have been also observing that when converting enzyme is active, angiotensin I is somewhat more potent than angiotensin II in releasing antiaggregatory prostanoids into arterial blood. It may well be that the release of antiaggregatory prostanoids from the lungs takes place close to the site of conversion of angiotensin I to angiotensin II. There is little doubt that when releasing antiaggregatory prostanoids, angiotensin II is triggering membrane structures, most probably receptor sites, since its effect is blocked by saralasin and by membrane-active drugs such as lignocaine and chlorpromazine.

Bradykinin was a weaker releaser of antiaggregatory prostanoids than angiotensin II; however, after pretreatment with captopril, bradykinin gained considerable antiaggregatory prostanoid-releasing activity. Captopril by itself did not release antiaggregatory prostanoids. On the contrary, an increase was observed in formation of platelet clumps. This finding might point to the renin/angiotensin system rather than to the kinin system as that responsible for physiologic control of the release of antiaggregatory prostanoids.

It seems that the release of antiaggregatory prostanoids by chemical mediators has little to do with the type of their vascular action. Bradykinin, a vasodilator, and angiotensin II, a vasoconstrictor, are both antiaggregatory prostanoid-releasers.

Unlike the findings of Mullane and Moncada in dogs,[50] we have found that acetylcholine releases antiaggregatory prostanoids into the circulation of anesthetized, heparinized cats. As a matter of fact, metacholine (0.1 to 3.0 μg/kg IV) is the most potent agent in this respect. Even though atropine blocks the aforementioned effect of cholinergic stimulants, we are not sure about the site of action of acetylcholine, since acetylcholine does not activate generation of antiaggregatory prostanoids in perfused lung preparation, and electrical stimulation of peripheral section of vagus nerves is not associated with the release of antiaggregatory prostanoids in anesthetized cats (our unpublished data). We can offer no explanation of this discrepancy. One possibility is that beta-adrenergic tone constitutes a natural counterweight to cholinergically mediated release of antiaggregatory prostanoids. In this respect it is interesting to note that seven beta-adrenergic drugs at the following IV doses (mg/kg)—atenolol (1.0), pindolol (0.3), practolol (5.0), propranolol (0.1), oxprenolol (2.0), sotalol (2.0), and timolol (0.5)—potentiated the antiaggregatory prostanoid-releasing effect of cholinergic mediators and revealed the antiaggregatory prostanoid-releasing effect of prostygmine. It should be kept in mind, however, that the dosage of beta-adrenolytic drugs is important. In high doses some of those drugs (e.g., propranolol) may even inhibit the release of antiaggregatory prostanoids by cholinergic stimuli, probably because of their nonspecific membrane properties. Isoprenaline had a local antiaggregatory effect of its own, which rendered it possible to study its influence on the release of antiaggregatory prostanoids.

At present, it seems that cholinergic mediators stimulate the release of antiaggregatory prostanoids into the circulation while beta-adrenergic tone is counteracting their action.

Perfused lung preparations easily metabolize exogenous arachidonic acid through an oxidative pathway.[53] This is not the case in vivo. Even long-lasting infusions of arachidonic acid at doses up to 100 μg/kg/min into right atrium are of no influence on PGI_2 generation by the lung. Occasionally, arachidonic acid at doses of 200 to 600 μg/kg/min may cause an appearance of antiaggregatory prostanoids in arterial blood corresponding to the concentration of PGI_2 following its intravenous injection at a dose of 1 μg/kg. At best, the conversion rate of arachidonic acid to antiaggregatory prostanoids in the lungs in vivo is 0.5%.[54]

Again pretreatment with beta-adrenergic blocking agents increases 5 to 10 times the conversion rate of arachidonic acid to antiaggregatory prostanoids.

Finally, the release of a PGI_2-like substance from the lungs into the circulation is triggered by respiratory stimulants such as almitrine and doxapram. It is most likely that in the foregoing situation PGI_2 is being released exclusively by a chemoreceptor reflex mechanism, since doxapram and almitrine did not release a PGI_2-like substance from isolated perfused guinea pig lungs (our unpublished data).

In summary, we believe that better understanding of receptor mechanisms that are responsible for secretion of antiaggregatory prostanoids into circulation from lungs and other organs presents an alternative to the therapy with prostacyclin,[19, 20, 23] i.e., the therapy with endogenous antiaggregatory prostanoids. The elucidation of a chemical nature of these prostanoids is a rewarding challenge.

REFERENCES

1. Moncada S., Gryglewski R.J., Bunting S., Vane J.R.: An enzyme isolated from arteries transforms prostaglandin endoperoxides to an unstable substance that inhibits platelet aggregation. *Nature (London)* 263:663–665, 1976.
2. Gryglewski R.J., Bunting S., Moncada S., Flower R.J., Vane J.R.: Arterial walls are protected against deposition of platelet thrombi by a substance (prostaglandin X) which they make from prostaglandin endoperoxides. *Prostaglandins* 12:685–714, 1976.
3. Bunting S., Gryglewski R.J., Moncada S., Vane J.R.: Arterial walls generate from prostaglandin endoperoxides a substance (prostaglandin X)

which relaxes strips of mesenteric and coeliac arteries and inhibits platelet aggregation. *Prostaglandins* 12:897–917, 1976.

4. Wong P.Y.-K., McGiff J.C., Sun F.F., Lee W.H.: 6-Keto prostaglandin E₁ inhibits the aggregation of human platelets. *Eur. J. Pharmacol.* 60:245–248, 1979.

5. Quilley C.P., McGiff J.C., Lee W.H., Sun F.F., Wong P.Y.-K.: 6-keto-PGE₁: A possible metabolite of prostacyclin having platelet antiaggregatory effects. *Hypertension* 2:524–528, 1980.

6. Smith J.B., Silver M.J., Ingerman C.M., Kocsis J.J.: Prostaglandin D₂ inhibits the aggregation of human platelets. *Thromb. Res.* 5:291–299, 1974.

7. Ball G., Brereton G.G., Fulwood M., Ireland D.M., Yates P.: Effect of prostaglandin E₁ alone and in combination with theophylline or aspirin on collagen-induced platelet aggregation and on platelet nucleotides including adenosine 3':5' = cyclic monophosphate. *Biochem. J.* 120:709–718, 1970.

8. Sih J.C., Johnson R.A., Nidy E.G., Graber D.R.: Synthesis of the four isomers of 5-hydroxy-PGI₂. *Prostaglandins* 15:409–421, 1978.

9. Gryglewski R.J., Salmon J.A., Ubatuba F.B., Weatherly B.C., Moncada S., Vane J.R.: Effects of all cis-5,8,11,14,17 eicosapentaenoic acid and PGH₃ on platelet aggregation. *Prostaglandins* 18:453–478, 1979.

10. Smith D.R., Weatherly B.C., Salmon J.A., Ubatuba F.B., Gryglewski R.J., Moncada S.: Preparation and biochemical properties of PGH₃. *Prostaglandins* 18:423–438, 1979.

11. Ross R., Glomset J.A., Karija B., Harker L.: A platelet-dependent serum factor that stimulates the proliferation of arterial smooth muscle cells in vitro. *Proc. Natl. Acad. Sci. USA* 71:1027, 1974.

12. Żmuda A., Dembińska-Kieć A., Chytkowski A., Gryglewski R.J.: Experimental atherosclerosis in rabbits: platelet aggregation, thromboxane A₂ generation and antiaggregatory potency of prostacyclin. *Prostaglandins* 14:1035–1042, 1977.

13. Gryglewski R.J., Dembińska-Kieć A., Żmuda A., Gryglewska T.: Prostacyclin and thromboxane A₂ biosynthesis capacities of heart, arteries and platelets at various stages of experimental atherosclerosis in rabbits. *Atherosclerosis* 31:385–394, 1978.

14. Fleischman A.I., Bierenbaum M.L., Justice D., Stier A., Sullivane A.: In vivo platelet function in acute myocardial infarction, acute cerebrovascular accidents and following surgery. *Thromb. Res.* 6:205, 1975.

15. Vreeken J., Aken W.G.: Spontaneous platelet aggregation of blood platelets as a cause of idiopathic thrombosis and recurrent painful toes and fingers. *Lancet* 2:1394, 1971.

16. Moncada S., Vane J.R.: Pharmacology and endogenous roles of prostaglandin endoperoxides, thromboxane A₂, and prostacyclin. *Pharmacol. Rev.* 30:293–331, 1979.

17. Dembińska-Kieć A., Gryglewska T., Żmuda A., Gryglewski R.J.: Generation of prostacyclin by arteries and by the coronary vascular bed is reduced in experimental atherosclerosis in rabbits. *Prostaglandins* 14:1025–1034, 1977.

18. Dembińska-Kieć A., Rücker W., Schönhöfer P.: Atherosclerosis decreased prostacyclin formation in rabbit lungs and kidneys. *Prostaglandins* 17:831–837, 1979.

19. Szczeklik A., Niżankowski R., Skawiński S., Szczeklik J., Głuszko P., Gryglewski R.J.: Successful therapy of advanced arteriosclerosis obliterans with prostacyclin. *Lancet* 1:1111–1114, 1979.
20. Szczeklik A., Gryglewski R.J., Niżankowski R., Skawiński S., Głuszko P., Korbut R.: Prostacyclin therapy in peripheral arterial disease. *Thromb. Res.* 19:191–199, 1980.
21. Szczeklik A., Szczeklik J., Niżankowski R., Głuszko P.: Prostacyclin for acute coronary insufficiency. *Artery* 8:7–11, 1980.
22. Lefer A.M., Ogletree M.L., Smith J.B., Silver M.J., Nicolaou K.V., Barnette W.E., Gasic G.P.: Prostacyclin: a potentially valuable agent for preserving myocardial tissue in acute myocardial ischemia. *Science* 200:52–54, 1978.
23. Żygulska-Mach H., Kostka-Trąbka E., Nitoń A., Gryglewski R.J.: Prostacyclin in central retinal vein occlusion. *Lancet* 1:1075, 1980.
24. Utsunomiya T., Krausz M.M., Valeri C.R., Shepro D., Hechtman H.B.: Treatment of pulmonary embolism with prostacyclin. *Surgery* 88:25–29, 1980.
25. Plachetka J.R., Salomon N.W., Larson D.F., Copeland J.G.: Platelet loss during experimental cardiopulmonary bypass and its prevention with prostacyclin. *Ann. Thorac. Surg.* 30:58–63, 1980.
26. Gryglewski R.J., Korbut R., Splawiński J.: Endogenous mechanisms which regulate prostacyclin release. *Haemostasis* 8:294–299, 1979.
27. Gryglewski R.J., Radomski M., Swies J., Ocetkiewicz A.: Release of prostacyclin into circulation by chemical mediators. Symposium, Chicago, October 28th–31st, 1978. New York, Raven Press, in preparation.
28. Palonek E., Korbut R., Gryglewski R.J., Gryglewska T.: Mass-spectrometric evidence for spontaneous and angiotensin-induced generation of prostacyclin by perfused cat lungs. *Prostaglandins* 20:993–1006, 1980.
29. Moncada S., Gryglewski R.J., Bunting S., Vane J.R.: A lipid peroxide inhibits the enzyme in blood vessel microsomes that generates from prostaglandin endoperoxides the substance (prostaglandin X) which prevents platelet aggregation. *Prostaglandins* 12:715–735, 1976.
30. Marcus A.J., Weksler B.B., Jaffe E.A.: Enzymatic conversion of prostaglandin endoperoxide H_2 and arachidonic acid to prostacyclin by cultured human endothelial cells. *J. Biol. Chem.* 253:7138–7141, 1978.
31. Salmon J.A., Smith D.R., Flower R.J., Moncada S., Vane J.R.: Further studies on the enzymatic conversion of prostaglandin endoperoxide into prostacyclin by porcine aorta microsomes. *Biochim. Biophys. Acta* 523:250–262, 1978.
32. Kuehl F.A., Jr., Humes J.L., Ham E.A., Egan R.W., Dougherty H.W.: Inflammation: the role of peroxidase-derived products, in Samuelsson B., Ramwell P.W., Paoletti R. (eds.): *Advances in Prostaglandin and Thromboxane Research.* Vol. 6. New York, Raven Press, 1980, pp. 77–86.
33. Gryglewski R.J.: Prostacyclin as a circulatory hormone. *Biochem. Pharmacol.* 28:3161–3166, 1979.
34. Masotti G., Galanti G., Poggesi L., Curcio A., Neri Serneri G.G.: Early changes of the endothelial antithrombotic properties in cholesterol fed rabbits. III. Decreased PGI_2 production by aortic wall. *Thromb. Haemostas.* 42:423, 1979. (Abstract)
35. Berberian P.A., Ziboh V.A., Hsis S.L.: Prostaglandin E_2 biosynthesis:

change in rabbit aorta and skin during experimental atherosclerosis. *J. Lip. Res.* 17:46–52, 1976.

36. Szczeklik A., Gryglewski R.J.: Thromboxane A₂ synthesis in platelets of patients with coronary heart disease, in Carlson L.A., Sirtori C.R., Weber G. (eds.): *Internat. Conf. on Atherosclerosis.* New York, Raven Press, 1978, pp. 597–606.

37. Szczeklik A., Gryglewski R.J., Musiał J., Grodzińska L., Serwońska M., Marcinkiewicz E.: Thromboxane generation and platelet aggregation in survivals of myocardial infarction. *Thromb. Haemostas.* 40:66–74, 1978.

38. Glavind J., Hartman S., Clemensen J., Jessen K.E., Dam H.: Studies on the role of lipid peroxides in human pathology II. The presence of peroxidized lipids in the atherosclerotic aortas. *Acta Pathol. Microbiol. Scand.* 30:1–6, 1952.

39. Hartroft W.S., Prta E.A.: Ceroid. *Am. J. Med. Sci.* 250:324–344, 1965.

40. Hiramitsu T., Majima Y., Hasegawa Y., Hirata K., Yaki K.: Lipid peroxide formation in the retina in ocular siderosis. *Experientia* 32:1324–1327, 1976.

41. Angelo V.M., Mysliwiec M.B., Gaetano G.: Defective fibrinolytic and prostacyclin-like activity in human atheromateous plaques. *Thromb. Haemostas.* 39:535–536, 1978.

42. Nordøy A., Svensson B., Wiebe D., Hoak J.C.: Lipoproteins and the inhibitory effect of human endothelial cells on platelet function. *Circ. Res.* 43:527–533, 1978.

43. Henriksen T.S., Evensen S.A., Carlander B.: Injury to cultured endothelial cells induced by low density lipoproteins: protection by high density lipoproteins. *Scand. J. Clin. Lab. Invest.* 39:369–375, 1979.

44. Szczeklik A., Gryglewski R.J.: Low-density lipoproteins (LDL) are carriers for lipid peroxides and invalidate prostacyclin (PGI₂) biosynthesis in arteries. *Artery*, in press.

45. Grodzińska L., Gryglewski R.J.: Angiotensin-induced release of prostacyclin from perfused organs. *Pharmacol. Res. Commun.* 12:339, 1980.

46. Gryglewski R.J., Spławiński J., Korbut R.: Endogenous mechanisms that regulate prostacyclin release, in Samuelsson B., Ramwell P.W., Paoletti R. (eds.): *Advances in Prostaglandin and Thromboxane Research.* Vol. 7. New York, Raven Press, 1980, pp. 777–787.

47. Gryglewski R.J.: Le poumon producteur de prostacyline. *Ann. Anest. Franc.* 6:613, 1980.

48. Gryglewski R.J.: The lung as a generator of prostacyclin, in *Ciba Foundation Symposium 78, Metabolic Activities of The Lung.* Amsterdam-Oxford-New York, Excerpta Medica, 1980, pp. 147–164.

49. Wong P.Y.-K., Malik K.U., Desiderio D.M., McGiff J.C., Sun F.F.: Hepatic metabolism of prostacyclin (PGI₂) in the rabbit: formation of a potent inhibitor of platelet aggregation. *Biochem. Biophys. Res. Commun.* 93:486, 1980.

50. Mullane K.M., Moncada S.: Prostacyclin release and the modulation of some vasoactive hormones. *Prostaglandins* 20:25, 1980.

51. Silberbauer K., Sinzinger H., Winter M.: Prostacyclin activity in rat kidney stimulated by angiotensin II. *Br. J. Exp. Pathol.* 60:38, 1979.

52. Dusting G.J., Mullins E.M., Doyle A.E.: Angiotensin-induced prostacyclin release may contribute to the hypotensive action of converting en-

zyme inhibitors, in Samuelsson B., Ramwell P.W., Paoletti R. (eds.): *Advances in Prostaglandin and Thromboxane Research.* New York, Raven Press, 1980, pp. 815–819.

53. Barnes P., Dollery C.T., Hensby C.N.: Metabolism of ^{3}H-arachidonic acid in male dog lung in vitro using a perfusion system designed to mimic physiological conditions, in Samuelsson B., Ramwell P.W., Paoletti R. (eds.): *Advances in Prostaglandin and Thromboxane Research.* New York, Raven Press, 1980, pp. 933–936.

54. Nowak J., Radomski R., Kaijser L., Gryglewski R.J.: Conversion of exogenous arachidonic acid to prostaglandins in the pulmonary circulation in vivo. A human and animal study. (In preparation)

Prostaglandins and Vasospasm

BRUCE J. PARDY AND H. H. G. EASTCOTT

St. Mary's Hospital
London, England

Introduction

The vasospastic disorders comprise Raynaud's syndrome, acrocyanosis, livedo reticularis, and persistent cold sensitivity following cold injury. Raynaud's syndrome is the most common of these and principally affects young and middle-aged females, causing inconvenience and in some cases considerable morbidity during the winter months. The severe form of Raynaud's syndrome is termed Raynaud's phenomenon, in which the digital arteries are histologically abnormal secondary to an associated disorder, usually one of the collagenoses. Raynaud's disease is the mild primary form with structurally normal arteries. Simple therapeutic measures are usually effective in the disease, whereas the phenomenon is more resistant and may progress to gangrene necessitating amputation.

Clinical Features

Raynaud's syndrome, first described by Maurice Raynaud in 1862,[1] is characterized by episodic color changes affecting the fingers and, less often, the toes in response to cold and emotional disturbance. Initial pallor is caused by digital arterial and arteriolar constriction, but there may be cyanosis if the microcirculation is filled with sluggishly flowing desaturated blood. Subsequently, hyperemia with flushing occurs as the circulation is restored.

The symptoms of Raynaud's syndrome include sensation of cold, pain, and numbness during, and often between, attacks, and there may be tenderness, stiffness, and clumsiness. The finger pulps become atrophied, but in some cases the fingers are thickened. In Raynaud's phenomenon, there may in addition be fingertip ulceration and focal gangrene, and sepsis in relation to the nails and pulps is frequent.

191

The hand disability is often compounded by the effects of the underlying disorder. In scleroderma, the disorder most commonly associated with Raynaud's phenomenon, the digital skin is thickened and tight, resulting in marked stiffness and, occasionally, fixed flexion deformity. Some of the disorders associated with Raynaud's phenomenon are listed below.

Collagen diseases
  Scleroderma
  Lupus erythematosus
  Rheumatoid arthritis
Buerger's disease (Arteriosclerosis obliterans)
Nerve entrapment
  Thoracic outlet syndrome
Occupational trauma
  Vibrating tools
Malignant disease
Hematologic disorders
  Cryoglobulinemia
  Macroglobulinemia
  Cold agglutinins

Etiology of Raynaud's Syndrome

Hand blood flow is reduced under both basal and cold-provoked conditions,[2-5] but the cause is not clear. Attention has concentrated on functional disturbances of the sympathetic nervous system and digital arteries, and on abnormalities of the circulating blood constituents.

SYMPATHETIC NERVOUS SYSTEM

Apart from structural abnormalities, digital artery caliber depends on physiologic mechanisms controlling vasomotor tone, particularly those concerned with thermoregulation. For this purpose, digital blood flow can vary as much as 100-fold.[2] Vasomotor tone is influenced by the sympathetic nervous system, and by local factors such as serotonin[6] and prostaglandins.[7] Adrenergic sympathetic nerve fibers constrict the digital arteries, which reflexly relax when sympathetic activity ceases. Raynaud[1] and others[8] considered the syndrome to be caused by overactivity of the sympathetic nervous system. However, although the severity of attacks is reduced they still may occur, and the improvement after operation is often only temporary.[9] Thus, factors other than, or in addition to, sympathetic overactivity would appear to be implicated in the etiology.

THE DIGITAL ARTERY

Extensive studies by Lewis indicated the fault in Raynaud's syndrome to be local, that is, an abnormality of digital arterial muscle manifested by excessive vasoconstriction in response to local cooling.[10, 11]

THE BLOOD

Until 1965, sympathetic overactivity and a "local fault" were generally believed to be the two most likely factors in the etiology of Raynaud's syndrome. At that time, on the basis of their finding that blood viscosity and plasma fibrinogen were increased, Pringle and his co-workers suggested that abnormalities of the blood may be important.[12] However, subsequent reports in relation to blood viscosity have been inconsistent. Recent work has shown whole blood viscosity to be normal in both Raynaud's disease and the phenomenon.[13] Blood viscosity corrected for hematocrit at 27 C and low shear rate was reported by early workers to be more reduced in patients than in controls,[14] but this has not been substantiated.[13, 15, 16] Corrected blood viscosity is elevated in Raynaud's phenomenon, probably because plasma fibrinogen is increased.[13] Red cell deformability, another factor affecting blood fluidity, is reduced by cold and acidosis in some Raynaud patients.[17, 18]

Other disturbances of the blood constituents include immunologic abnormalities that may be present in some 80% of patients,[19] elevated circulating immune complex levels,[20] and raised beta-thromboglobulin concentration,[21] suggesting increased platelet activity.

Treatment

Currently available management of Raynaud's phenomenon includes sympathectomy, a variety of drugs, and plasma exchange.

SYMPATHECTOMY

Upper limb sympathectomy is normally not now recommended for Raynaud's phenomenon, except when secondary to digital arteriosclerosis in older males.[9] Complications and side-effects of operation are often unpleasant, and though digital blood flow is markedly increased for a brief period, a return toward presympathectomy levels within two years is not uncommon.[22] The cause for this loss of effect is unknown, but possible mechanisms are increased sensitivity to catecholamines,[23-25] reduced arterial wall amine oxidase content,[26] and failure of arterial wall synthesis of acetyl choline.[27]

DRUGS

Drug treatment includes a variety of vasodilators, oral and intra-arterial reserpine, triiodothyronine, guanethidine, methyldopa, griseofulvin, terbutaline (a beta-adrenergic stimulator), and fibrinolytic agents such as stanozolol, phenformin, and ancrod. Of recent interest are drugs that improve red cell flexibility such as isoxuprine, pentoxifylline, and cinnarizine.

PLASMA EXCHANGE

Plasmapheresis weekly for a month with exchange on each occasion of 2.0 to 2.5 L of plasma for PPF and Haemaccel reduces blood viscosity, plasma fibrinogen, circulating immune complex, and beta-thromboglobulin levels, and increases red cell deformability.[28]

Unsatisfactory features of all of these treatments include their ineffectiveness, side-effects, expense, or complexity.

Prostaglandins

Prostaglandins E_1 and I_2 are vasodilators and inhibitors of platelet aggregation.[29, 30] Both prostaglandins are only briefly active in the circulation. PGI_2 is rapidly hydrated nonenzymatically at pH 7.4 to the inactive 6-Keto-$PGF_{1\alpha}$, and PGI_2 blood concentration is reduced by 50% after passage through the peripheral vascular bed.[31] PGE_1 is 90% removed or inactivated during a single passage through the lungs.[32] Although early reports describing the use of PGE_1 intra-arterially[33] and intravenously[34] in severe lower limb ischemia passed largely unnoticed, considerable interest was stimulated by the recent use of PGI_2.[35] Our preliminary experience with these prostaglandins in lower limb ischemia suggested that they are effective in distal arteriopathy when given intravenously, but not when the proximal axial limb artery is occluded.[36] The incidence of side-effects appears to be higher with PGI_2 than with PGE_1,[36, 37] and this, together with the requirement that PGI_2 be buffered to pH 10.0 during infusion, would seem to favor use of PGE_1 for peripheral vascular disease.

PATIENTS AND METHODS

Four British centers have reported their early experience with prostaglandins in Raynaud's phenomenon.

A combined study from the Rheumatology and Vascular Surgical Departments of the Bristol Royal Infirmary and the Dermatology Department of St. Bartholomew's Hospital, London (hereafter called the Bristol and St. Bartholomew's study), reported the use of a continuous intravenous infusion of PGE_1 for 72 hours in 24 patients with Raynaud's phenomenon (secondary to scleroderma in 18 and to arteriosclerosis in 6), and in 2 patients with Raynaud's disease.[38] Digital amputation had previously been performed in 5 patients, and 8 patients had finger ulceration at the time of presentation.

A further brief report from the same two hospitals (the St. Bartholomew's and Bristol study) described a single-blind crossover study of intravenous 0.9% saline solution and PGE_1 infused for 72 hours in 12 patients with Raynaud's phenomenon secondary to scleroderma.[39] In both studies, PGE_1 was given in a dose of 6 ng/kg/min for the first 24 hours, and then 10 ng/kg/min for the next 48 hours.

We have reported the use of PGE_1 as a continuous intravenous infusion of 10 ng/kg/min for 72 hours in 4 patients at St. Mary's Hospital, and of PGI_2 8 to 15 ng/kg/min by the same route and for the same duration in three patients with Raynaud's phenomenon secondary to polyarteritis nodosa at Northwick Park Hospital, Harrow.[36] Our total experience at St. Mary's Hospital comprises 20 treatments with PGE_1 in 15 patients with Raynaud's phenomenon secondary to scleroderma in eight, Buerger's disease in one, and an unrecognized disorder in five. Nine digits had been amputated in four of the patients. Quadrilateral sympathectomy had been performed in two patients, and upper limb sympathectomy bilaterally in three and unilaterally in four. Eight patients with persistent digital sepsis, focal gangrene, or ulceration received a total of 12 treatments.

RESULTS

Subjective

In the Bristol and St. Bartholomew's study, pain was relieved in 25 of the 26 patients during PGE_1 infusion; 21 were still improved at 2 weeks, and 17 at 6 weeks. In the St. Bartholomew's and Bristol report, pain was relieved more with PGE_1 than with 0.9% saline solution ($P < 0.05$); cold tolerance and the severity of Raynaud's attacks were reduced; and 10 patients preferred PGE_1 to saline solution ($P < 0.001$).

The three patients treated with PGI_2 responded satisfactorily. At St. Mary's, two early patients received an intermittent intravenous infusion of PGE_1 10 ng/kg/min for 10 minutes each hour, and as with other cases of peripheral vascular disease treated in this way, no subjective or objective responses were found.[36] The remaining 18 treatments were given as a continuous infusion. Six patients with pain, but not sepsis or gangrene, were treated on one occasion each, with excellent relief of pain in three, none of whom required further treatment during a mean follow-up period of 11.3 months. One patient had only recently been treated and is uncertain of the result, one was unimproved, and one patient returned home to the Middle East immediately after treatment. One patient with pain and sepsis was improved with PGE_1, but after 7 months required a second infusion for relapse. Another patient with pain and sepsis was also relieved, but there were several recurrences of mild pain during the subsequent 12 months. Treatment of the patient with Buerger's disease and focal digital gangrene was followed by a short period of partial relief and then relapse. Six patients with sepsis, gangrene, or both were treated with PGE_1 followed by immediate debridement of 13 digits and amputation of one mummified thumb under general anesthesia. Pain relief was satisfactory, but recurrence of pain and sepsis necessitated two further infusions of PGE_1 and debridement in one patient, and PGE_1 alone in another patient. The mean interval between the three repeat treatments was 6.6 months.

Objective

HEALING OF SEPSIS, ULCERATION, AND GANGRENE.—Five of eight ischemic ulcers in the Bristol and St. Bartholomew's patients healed within 6 weeks. Finger ulceration in two patients in the St. Bartholomew's and Bristol study healed after PGE_1. At St. Mary's, treatment of the patient with Buerger's disease and focal finger gangrene by PGE_1 without debridement was ineffective. The three treatments without debridement in the two patients with sepsis were associated with healing, but sepsis recurred as previously described. In the six patients having 17 digits debrided and the mummified thumb amputated at the line of demarcation, healing was rapid except in two fingers with persistent sepsis, which came under control with antibiotics, and in the fifth toe of a male patient with scleroderma, amputation being subsequently required.

SKIN TEMPERATURE.—Hand and finger temperatures were analyzed by infrared radiometry in the Bristol and St. Bartholomew's study. Temperature rose from 27.4 ± 0.7 C (mean ± SEM) to 31.3 ± 1.4 C during infusion, was 32.1 ± 1.0 C 24 hours after treatment, and 28.8 ± 0.9 C two weeks later. Thermography was also employed in the St. Bartholomew's and Bristol study, in which temperature rose from 28.7 C (mean ± SEM) to a peak of 30.2 ± 0.2 C on the second day of treatment, and was still 29.6 ± 0.4 two weeks later. There was no rise in temperature during 0.9% saline solution infusion.

Thermistor probes on the pulps of the clinically most affected finger of each hand have been used at St. Mary's, hourly recordings being made before and during the first eight treatments in seven patients in uncontrolled ward conditions. The mean of recordings before treatment during a period of 2 to 12 hours was compared with the mean of recordings made during the last 12 hours of treatment. Finger temperature rose 3.8 ± 2.1 C (mean ± SD).

PULSATILITY INDEX.—Pulsatility index, derived by analysis of Doppler velocity waveforms[40] from the radial artery, fell during treatment with PGE_1 in the Bristol and St. Bartholomew's patients, indicating hand vasodilatation. The index was still low 24 hours after infusion, but had returned to pre-infusion values 2 weeks later.

FINGER PLETHYSMOGRAPHY.—Digital pulse volume recordings from segmental air plethysmographs on the proximal phalanges of two fingers of each hand were analyzed by the Bristol and St. Bartholomew's workers. Pulse volume was elevated 24 hours after starting treatment with PGE_1, and was still elevated 6 weeks later.

DIGITAL COOLING TESTS.—Immersion of the hand encased in a plastic glove in water at 20 C for 1 minute was found by the Bristol and St. Bartholomew's workers to be associated with identical hand and finger temperature responses before and after PGE_1. At St. Mary's, the response of finger systolic pressure (FSP) to local cooling (Medimatic)[41] was measured before and after treatment in a number of patients. A special cuff on the middle phalanx was perfused with water at 200 mm Hg for 5 minutes; cuff pressure was then automatically reduced at 2 mm Hg/second, while the return of blood flow in the finger pulp was detected with a photoplethysmography probe. FSP was measured with the cuff perfusate at 30 C, 15 C, and 10 C. The response to local cooling is indicated by the fall in FSP from that at 30 C to that at 15 C and 10 C. The results have not been fully analyzed, but indicate that while FSP at 30 C is not changed after PGE_1, the effect of cooling, which before treatment usually reduces FSP by more than 30%, is often abolished.

DOPPLER MAPPING.—We have employed mapping of digital artery

segments with detectable blood flow, using 4 and 8 MHz Doppler pencil probes.[42] Each phalanx is regarded as having two digital artery segments, one on either side, with a total of 28 per hand. Again our results have not been analyzed, but the number of segments with detectable flow tends to improve after treatment.

SIDE EFFECTS

PGE_1 infusion into a superficial arm vein caused considerable discomfort within 24 hours, but not if the cannula tip was proximal to the shoulder.[36] Mild headache was not uncommon, and other side-effects seen in our patients were finger swelling, fever, malaise, anorexia, muscle aches, joint pains, gynecologic pain, and diarrhea. Flushing occurred in nine of the Bristol and St. Bartholomew's patients, but we have not seen this complication in any of 40 patients treated for peripheral vascular disease. Postural hypotension was experienced by one Bristol and St. Bartholomew's patient, but has not occurred in our patients who remain in bed.

DISCUSSION

The wide variety of treatments available for Raynaud's phenomenon and the continuing search for new therapies attest to the inadequacies of present-day management. Current interest is being principally directed toward alteration of the flow properties of the blood and to vasodilatation of extremity skin. Clearly, an understanding of the basic fault in Raynaud's phenomenon would narrow the search for an effective therapy, but it is often difficult to know whether an abnormality is cause or effect, changes in plasma fibrinogen and blood viscosity being good examples.

The recorded experience with PGE_1 suggests that it is an effective treatment for pain, sepsis, and focal gangrene in Raynaud's phenomenon, and that extremity skin temperature is elevated during and possibly after treatment, indicating improved blood flow.

Possible mechanisms by which prostaglandin therapy might be expected to improve extremity skin blood flow are (1) a direct action on vascular smooth muscle, (2) inotropic and chronotropic cardiac effects which increase cardiac output,[43] and (3) an effect on thermoregulation with reduced extremity skin vasoconstriction, which will be discussed later. Inhibition of platelet activity is unlikely to be a relevant factor in PGE_1 treatment, for PGE_1 has not been shown to have a detectable effect when given in nonhypotensive dosage,[44] and while PGI_2 is 40 times more potent than PGE_1, there has been no indication that the former is clinically superior in peripheral vascular disease. Also, the life of the platelet is short in relation to the duration of clinical benefit, and there is evidence that a rebound of platelet activity occurs with cessation of prostaglandin infusion.

An initial impediment to the study of PGE_1 was the apparent requirement that because of the nearly complete pulmonary clearance, administration should be by the intra-arterial route. This is technically cumbersome and restricts treatment to one limb at a time. Only with the realization that continuous intravenous infusion in a dose some six times that employed intra-arterially was safe and effective, could patients be studied in suitable numbers. In contrast to PGE_1, few data have been published concerning PGI_2 in peripheral vascular disease, possibly because the frequency and severity of side-effects of this prostaglandin have diverted attention toward PGE_1.

St. Mary's Hospital Trial

We have been examining the effects of sequential 72-hour intravenous infusions of 0.9% saline solution and PGE_1 in a temperature-controlled ward cubicle. During the infusions, we analyzed extremity skin blood flow, this index of prostaglandin activity probably being of clinical relevance as suggested by our preliminary work, which indicated a strong correlation between skin temperature rise and clinical benefit in patients with lower limb distal arteriopathy.[36] Extremity skin temperature and photoplethysmography traces were recorded hourly by day and night using automatic equipment.

The data from this study are not yet available, but some points can be made. Regarding clinical management, we initially under-used antibiotics, and now believe that this therapy should precede prostaglandin treatment if there is any suspicion of nonlocalized sepsis. We have been encouraged by the good results of debridement of septic and necrotic tissue after prostaglandin therapy, and indeed have noticed that pain often is not fully relieved until ischemic tissue has been excised. Healing is usually prompt after debridement, and the evidence that PGE_1 stimulates epidermal growth may be pertinent.[45]

Thermoregulation

During history taking, and from observations in the temperature-controlled ward cubicle, we have been impressed by the generalized rather than local cold sensitivity in the extremeties of our patients.

Peacock noted that reduced hand blood flow at nearly body temperature could not be accounted for solely by a local cold hypersensitivity, and commented that in view of the subjective cold sensitivity in his patients, there "appeared to be impairment of the ability to maintain their general thermal state."[5] For this reason, Peacock gave triiodothyronine to increase body metabolism and heat production.[46] We suggest that disturbance of thermoregulation at hypothalamic level rather than a disturbance of body metabolism may be a significant etiologic factor in Raynaud's syndrome. Inappropriate vasoconstrictor influences of central origin would be exerted on the extremities, normally mediated by the sympathetic nervous system. After sympathectomy, alternative mechanisms could, with time, increasingly transmit the central stimulus. The studies of Lewis in relation to the "local fault" are compatible with a central modulating influence on digital arterial tone.

PGE$_1$ is the most powerful pyretic agent known, when injected into the cerebral ventricles or into the anterior hypothalamus, and the effect is dose-dependent.[47, 48] Should a disturbance of thermoregulation be an etiologic factor in Raynaud's syndrome, the pyrogenic effects of PGE$_1$ could be relevant in promoting extremity blood flow by increased cardiac output and skin blood flow. Manifestations compatible with a pyrogenic action of PGE$_1$ seen in our patients are a feeling of cold during the first night of infusion, an influenza-like syndrome with distaste for smoking, anorexia, malaise, fever, generalized aching pains, and a requirement for fewer bed clothes at home after treatment. Fever has also been reported in neonates having PGE$_1$ infused to maintain ductus patency,[49] and our experience indicates that the febrile syndrome may come to be recognized as the dose-limiting factor in prolonged systemic infusions. One attractive possibility is that an oral stable prostaglandin taken in sufficient dosage to produce a "subclinical fever" might confer prolonged relief of extremity vasoconstriction.

DESIGN OF DEFINITIVE CLINICAL TRIALS

The purpose of future controlled trials must be to show that prostaglandin therapy is effective, particularly in relation to other forms of management, has few side-effects, and is not unduly complex or expensive. However, there is much that must first be known before an appropriate trial can be designed, such as the optimum route of administration, dose, duration and frequency of treatment, and the place of ancillary treatments, such as antibiotics and tissue debridement. This information must be sought from preliminary studies, such as those previously described.

Short term crossover trials of PGE_1 versus an inactive substance will document the effects of PGE_1, but for longer term trials, an inactive substance cannot ethically be employed to treat patients in severe pain, and as will be discussed below, crossover studies with prostaglandins are not feasible. Rather, a sequential study of prostaglandin versus another therapy would seem the most appropriate design.

Indices To Be Analyzed

While clinical improvement is the obvious aim, this index is not always easy to analyze, particularly in Raynaud's phenomenon. For example, analysis of pain, a difficult problem at the best of times, may be made more difficult by patient personality disorders which are common in Raynaud's phenomenon, unreliability in daily completion of pain analysis forms over prolonged periods, confusion of finger joint stiffness or pain with Raynaud pain, the onset of finger swelling with or without joint pain during prostaglandin therapy, the induction of carpal tunnel median nerve entrapment because of hand swelling during prostaglandin infusion, relief of Raynaud pain by analgesic drugs taken for prostaglandin side-effects, and the influence of changing climate. Also, pain associated with sepsis and necrotic tissue may not be relieved without surgical debridement.

The attractiveness of noninvasive objective tests is clear, but the problem is what to measure. The logical choice would seem to be digital blood flow because the response to cold is thought to be caused by constriction of the digital arteries. However, because digital blood flow is relatively difficult to measure, many workers have studied the effect of therapy on hand blood flow, which may not be relevant. It is difficult to measure digital blood flow meaningfully for purposes of comparison on a day-to-day basis because digital blood flow is extremely variable in the individual, and nutritional or capillary blood flow is difficult to distinguish from non-nutritional flow through finger tip arteriovenous shunts. Because of this great variability in digital blood flow, isolated laboratory measurements are valueless for day-to-day comparison, but analysis of the many data points acquired by hourly monitoring over a period of days may be acceptable.

Problems Peculiar to Prostaglandins

Blind crossover trials are difficult to design when the test therapy must be administered intravenously via a central cannula during several days in the hospital, when the test therapy has numerous recognizable side-effects, and when the effect of the test therapy is thought to persist for several months after cessation of treatment.

Problems Peculiar to Raynaud's Phenomenon

The disease state is variable, and the number of patients justifying inpatient treatment for a number of days in any one community is small. Thus, there would appear to be a need for cooperative trials.

In conclusion, definitive trials should probably be of the sequential type, performed on a cooperative basis, comparing the effects of PGE_1 and another therapy on the clinical state and digital blood flow.

REFERENCES

1. Raynaud A.G.M.: De L'Asphyxie Locale et de la Gangrene Symetrique des Extremites. Paris, Rignoux, 1862.
2. Burton A.C.: The range and variability of the blood flow in the human fingers and the vasomotor regulation of body temperature. *Am. J. Physiol.* 127:437–453, 1939.
3. Downey J.A., Frewin D.B.: The effect of cold on blood flow in the hand of patients with Raynaud's phenomenon. *Clin. Sci.* 44:279–289, 1973.
4. Downey J.A., LeRoy E.C., Miller J.M., Darling R.C.: Thermoregulation and Raynaud's phenomenon. *Clin. Sci.* 40:211–219, 1971.
5. Peacock J.H.: The effect of changes in local temperature on the blood flows of the normal hand, primary Raynaud's disease and primary acrocyanosis. *Clin. Sci.* 19:505–512, 1960.
6. Halpern A., Kuhn P.H., Shaftel H.E., Samuels S.S., Shaftel N., Selman D., Birch H.G.: Raynaud's disease, Raynaud's phenomenon, and serotonin. *Angiology* 11:151–167, 1960.
7. Moncada S., Vane J.R.: Prostacyclin formation and effects, in Roberts S.M., Scheinmann F.M. (eds.): *Chemistry, Biochemistry and Pharmacological Activity of Prostanoids.* Oxford, Pergamon Press, 1979.
8. Adson A.W., Brown G.E.: The treatment of Raynaud's disease by resection of the upper thoracic and lumbar sympathetic ganglia and trunks. *Surg. Gynecol. Obstet.* 48:577–603, 1929.
9. Johnston E.N.M., Summerly R., Birnstingl M.: Prognosis in Raynaud's phenomenon after sympathectomy. *Br. Med. J.* 1:962–964, 1965.
10. Lewis T.: Experiments relating to the peripheral mechanism involved in spasmodic arrest of the circulation in the fingers, a variety of Raynaud's disease. *Heart* 15:7–101, 1929.
11. Lewis T., Pickering G.W.: Observations upon maladies in which the blood supply to digits ceases intermittently or permanently, and upon bilateral

gangrene of digits; observations relevant to so-called "Raynaud's disease." *Clin. Sci.* 1:327–66, 1934.

12. Pringle R., Walder D.N., Weaver J.P.A.: Blood viscosity and Raynaud's disease. *Lancet* I:1086–1088, 1965.
13. Ayres M.L., Jarrett P.E.M., Browse N.L.: Blood viscosity, Raynaud's phenomenon and the effect of fibrinolytic enhancement. *Br. J. Surg.* 68:51–54, 1981.
14. Goyle K.B., Dormandy J.A.: Abnormal blood viscosity in Raynaud's phenomenon. *Lancet* I:1317–1318, 1976.
15. Jahnsen T., Nielsen S.L., Skovborg F.: Blood viscosity and local response to cold in primary Raynaud's phenomenon. *Lancet* II:1001–1002, 1977.
16. McGrath M.A., Peek R., Penny R.: Raynaud's disease: reduced hand blood flows with normal blood viscosity. *Aust. NZ. J. Med.* 8:126–131, 1978.
17. Dintenfass L.: Hemorrheological factors in Raynaud's phenomenon. *Angiology* 28:472–81, 1977.
18. Dodds A.J., O'Reilly M.J.G., Yates C.J.P., Cotton L.T., Flute P.T., Dormandy J.A.: Haemorrheological response to plasma exchange in Raynaud's syndrome. *Br. Med. J.* 2:1186–1187, 1979.
19. Porter J.M., Bardana E.J., Baur G.M.B., Wesche D.H., Andrasch R.H., Rosch J.: The clinical significance of Raynaud's syndrome. *Surgery* 80:756–764, 1976.
20. Hamilton W.A.P., Dodds A.J., Hancock M.E.J., Roberts V.C., Vergani D., Cotton L.T.: Circulatory improvement in Raynaud's phenomenon following plasma exchange, in Sieber H.G. (ed.): *Proceedings of the International Symposium on Plasma-Exchange.* Cologne, Diamed. (In Press)
21. Zahavi J., Hamilton W.A.P., O'Reilly M.J.G., Clark S.E., Cotton L.T., Kakkar V.V.: Abnormal platelet function in Raynaud's phenomenon. *Thromb. Haemostas.* 42:146, 1979.
22. Barcroft H., Walker A.J.: Return of tone in blood-vessels of the upper limb after sympathectomy. *Lancet* I:1035–1039, 1949.
23. Duff R.S.: Effect of sympathectomy on the response to adrenaline of the blood vessels of the skin in man. *J. Physiol.* 117:415–430, 1952.
24. Duff R.S.: Effect of adrenaline and noradrenaline on blood vessels of the hand before and after sympathectomy. *J. Physiol.* 129:53–64, 1955.
25. Parks V.J., Skinner S.L., Whelan R.F.: Mechanisms in the return of vascular tone following sympathectomy in man. *Circ. Res.* 9:1026–1034, 1961.
26. Burn J.H., Robinson J.: Effect of denervation on amine oxidase in structures innervated by the sympathetic. *Br. J. Pharmacol.* 7:304–318, 1952.
27. Armin J., Grant R.T., Thompson R.H.S., Tickner A.: An explanation for the heightened vascular reactivity of the denervated rabbit's ear. *J. Physiol.* 121:603–622, 1953.
28. Hamilton W.A.P., White J.M., Cotton L.T.: Plasma exchange in Raynaud's phenomenon. *Lancet II:*475, 1980.
29. Bergström S., Carlson L.A., Weeks J.R.: The prostaglandins: a family of biologically active lipids. *Pharmacol. Rev.* 20:1–48, 1968.
30. Moncada S., Gryglewski R., Bunting S., Vane J.R.: An enzyme isolated from arteries transforms prostaglandin endoperoxides to an unstable substance that inhibits platelet aggregation. *Nature* 263:663–665, 1976.
31. Dusting G.J., Moncada S., Vane J.R.: Disappearance of prostacyclin

(PGI₂) in the circulation of the dog. *Br. J. Pharmacol.* 62:414–415, 1978.
32. Hammond G.L., Cronau L.H., Whittaker D., Gillis C.N.: Fate of prostaglandins E$_1$ and A$_1$ in the human pulmonary circulation. *Surgery* 81:716–722, 1977.
33. Carlson L.A., Eriksson I.: Femoral-artery infusion of prostaglandin E$_1$ in severe peripheral vascular disease. *Lancet* I:155–156, 1973.
34. Carlson L.A., Olsson A.G.: Intravenous prostaglandin E$_1$ in severe peripheral vascular disease. *Lancet* II:810, 1976.
35. Szczeklik A., Nizankowski R., Skawinski S., Szczeklik J., Gluszki P., Gryglewski R.J.: Successful therapy of advanced arteriosclerosis obliterans with prostacyclin. *Lancet* I:1111–1114, 1979.
36. Pardy B.J., Lewis J.D., Eastcott H.H.G.: Preliminary experience with prostaglandins E$_1$ and I$_2$ in peripheral vascular disease. *Surgery* 88:826–832, 1980.
37. Olsson A.G.: Intravenous prostacyclin for ischaemic ulcers in peripheral artery disease. *Lancet* II:1076, 1980.
38. Clifford P.C., Martin M.F.R., Sheddon E.J., Kirby J.D., Baird R.N., Dieppe P.A.: Treatment of vasospastic disease with prostaglandin E$_1$. *Br. Med. J.* 281:1031–1034, 1980.
39. Martin M., Dowd P., Ring F., Dieppe P., Kirby J.: Prostaglandin E$_1$ (PGE$_1$) in the treatment of systemic sclerosis (SS). *Ann. Rheum. Dis.* 39:194, 1980.
40. Gosling R.G., King D.H., Newman D.H.: Ultrasonic angiology, in Harcus A.W., Adamson L. (eds.): *Arteries and Veins.* Edinburgh, Churchill Livingstone, 1975, pp. 61–84.
41. Nielsen S.L.: Raynaud phenomena and finger systolic pressure after cooling. *Scand. J. Clin. Lab. Invest.* 38:765–770, 1978.
42. O'Reilly M.J.G., Dodds A.J., Roberts V.C., Cotton L.T.: Plasma exchange and Raynaud's phenomenon—its assessment by Doppler ultrasound velocimetry. *Br. J. Surg.* 66:712–715, 1979.
43. Priano L.L., Miller T.H., Traber D.L.: Use of prostaglandin E$_1$ in treatment of experimental hypovolemic shock. *Circ. Shock* 1:221–230, 1979.
44. Van den Broeke J.J., Van den Dungen J.J.A.M., Brenken U., Karliczek G.F., Homan van der Heide J.N., Wildevuur Ch.R.H.: Haemodynamic side effects of prostaglandin (PGE$_1$) in patients before and during cardiopulmonary bypass. *Eur. Soc. Surg. Res.* 12(suppl 1):49, 1980.
45. Bentley-Phillips C.B., Paulli-Jorgenson H., Marks R.: The effects of prostaglandins E$_1$ and F$_{2\alpha}$ on epidermal growth. *Arch. Dermatol. Res.* 257:233–237, 1977.
46. Peacock J.H.: The treatment of primary Raynaud's disease of the upper limb. *Lancet* II:65–68, 1960.
47. Feldberg W., Saxena P.N.: Fever produced by prostaglandin E$_1$. *J. Physiol.* 217:547–556, 1971.
48. Milton A.S., Wendlandt S.: Effect on body temperature of prostaglandins of the A, E and F series on injection into the third ventricle of unanesthetized cats and rabbits. *J. Physiol.* 218:325–336, 1971.
49. Coceani F., Olley P.M.: Prostaglandins, their synthesis inhibitors and ductus arteriosus, in Karim S.M.M. (ed.): *Practical Applications of Prostaglandins and Their Synthesis Inhibitors.* Lancaster, MTP Press, 1979, pp. 53–75.

Intravenous Prostaglandin E_1 (PGE$_1$): Its Use in Peripheral Vascular Disease Complications

JOANN L. DATA

Burroughs Wellcome Co.
Research Triangle Park, North Carolina
(formerly Bronson Clinical Investigational Unit
Upjohn Company, Kalamazoo, Michigan)

Introduction

Prostaglandin E_1, one of the naturally occurring prostaglandins with both vasodilatory and platelet antiaggregatory properties, has been reported by various investigators to be a useful adjunct in peripheral vascular disease.[1-10] Because of its rapid pulmonary clearance, PGE$_1$ was tested early intra-arterially with reported success in healing of ulcerations and relief of pain, both in the infused limb and in the contralateral noninfused limb.[1, 9] However, because of the inconvenience and high morbidity from intra-arterial infusions, trials utilizing the intravenous route have been conducted. Unfortunately, subsequent double-blind studies have not convincingly supported the intravenous route as an appropriate therapeutic route.

Controlled studies in peripheral vascular disease are difficult because of the multiplicity of diseases classified as peripheral vascular disease, the variability of a given disease, and the instability of the condition in a given patient. Consequently, in our peripheral vascular disease studies, we chose to evaluate only patients with *stable* peripheral vascular disease and to utilize a treatment plan based on the stability of the vascular system.

Materials and Methods

Over the past three years we have treated 23 patients who have had one or more complications of a variety of different peripheral vascular diseases with intravenous prostaglandin E_1 by three different protocols. Table 17-1 outlines the disease categories of the first 18 patients who were treated by one or both of the first two protocols, and who now have been followed for at least 12 months following PGE_1 infusions. Three patients had primarily larger vessel disease, and the remaining 15 had one of a variety of small vessel diseases. Ten of these patients were diabetic and six of these diabetics had stable or worsening ulcerations of 3 to 6 months' duration.

All patients gave informed consent after hearing explanations of the protocol design and assessments of the risks and benefits. Patients were assigned to one of two protocols:

1. *Protocol A*—the desired protocol whereby the patient was given drug or placebo under single-blind label depending on his vascular status.

2. *Protocol B*—an open-labeled study in which the patient received only prostaglandin E_1 because of sudden deterioration of the existing vascular condition.

Eleven patients plus four of our diabetics with ulcerations were

TABLE 17–1.—PATIENT PROFILE FOR
PROTOCOLS A AND B

PROFILE	NO. OF PATIENTS
Arteriosclerotic vascular disease (nondiabetic)	3
Small vessel disease (diabetic), without ulcerations	2
Small vessel disease (diabetic), with ulcerations	6
Diabetics with wet gangrene	2
Raynaud's disease, with ulceration	1
Raynaud's disease, without ulcerations	1
Scleroderma	2
Total	17

TABLE 17–2.—STUDY DESIGN FOR PROTOCOL A

Admission A	Hx + PE + vascular evaluation + photographs
Admission B	Placebo (diluent for PGE_1 in D_5W or NS)
Admission C	Randomized $PGE_1 - 1$ gm/hr $\times$ 72 vs. placebo
Admission D	Evaluate. Reinfuse according to design (Figs 17–1, 17–2)

treated under protocol A (Table 17–2). Each patient was initially brought in for a three-day detailed evaluation of his clinical and vascular status, including assessment of Doppler pressures and pulse volume recordings, a measure of pulsatile blood flow. Detailed photographs of the ulcerations were also made.

Ten days after discharge, patients were readmitted and, if they had stable vascular status, received placebo (ethanol diluent for E_1 in either NS or D_5W 50cc/hr × 72 hrs). Following re-evaluation of their vascular status, patients were discharged.

Ten days later they were readmitted and, if still stable, were randomized to either drug (1 μg/hr) or placebo therapy. Drug or placebo was infused in D_5W or NS for 72 hours, and this sequence of events continued for as long as necessary to complete this protocol. The details of various possible treatment plans are outlined in Figures 17–1 and 17–2.

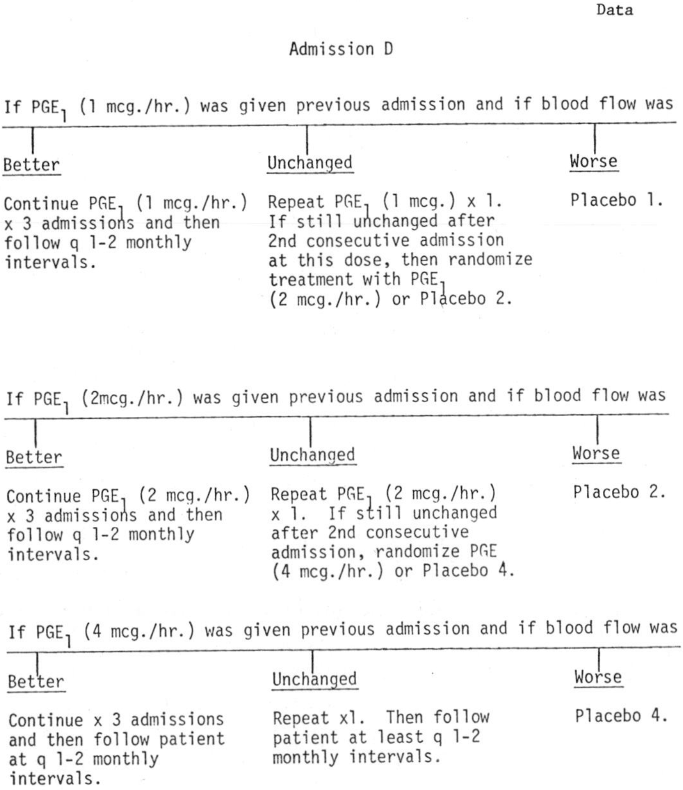

Data

Admission D

If PGE$_1$ (1 mcg./hr.) was given previous admission and if blood flow was

Better	Unchanged	Worse
Continue PGE$_1$ (1 mcg./hr.) x 3 admissions and then follow q 1-2 monthly intervals.	Repeat PGE$_1$ (1 mcg.) x 1. If still unchanged after 2nd consecutive admission at this dose, then randomize treatment with PGE$_1$ (2 mcg./hr.) or Placebo 2.	Placebo 1.

If PGE$_1$ (2mcg./hr.) was given previous admission and if blood flow was

Better	Unchanged	Worse
Continue PGE$_1$ (2 mcg./hr.) x 3 admissions and then follow q 1-2 monthly intervals.	Repeat PGE$_1$ (2 mcg./hr.) x 1. If still unchanged after 2nd consecutive admission, randomize PGE (4 mcg./hr.) or Placebo 4.	Placebo 2.

If PGE$_1$ (4 mcg./hr.) was given previous admission and if blood flow was

Better	Unchanged	Worse
Continue x 3 admissions and then follow patient at q 1-2 monthly intervals.	Repeat x1. Then follow patient at least q 1-2 monthly intervals.	Placebo 4.

Fig 17–1.—Flow diagram for patients randomized to PGE$_1$ on Admission C, Protocol A, and to PGE$_1$ at subsequent randomizations.

Data

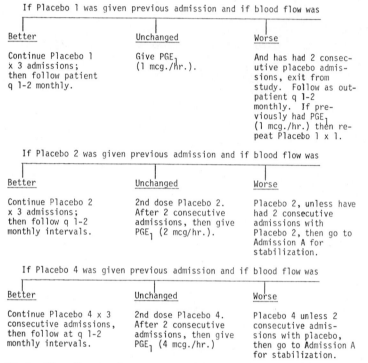

Admission D

If Placebo 1 was given previous admission and if blood flow was

Better	Unchanged	Worse
Continue Placebo 1 x 3 admissions; then follow patient q 1-2 monthly.	Give PGE₁ (1 mcg./hr.).	And has had 2 consecutive placebo admissions, exit from study. Follow as outpatient q 1-2 monthly. If previously had PGE₁ (1 mcg./hr.) then repeat Placebo 1 x 1.

If Placebo 2 was given previous admission and if blood flow was

Better	Unchanged	Worse
Continue Placebo 2 x 3 admissions; then follow q 1-2 monthly intervals.	2nd dose Placebo 2. After 2 consecutive admissions, then give PGE₁ (2 mcg/hr.).	Placebo 2, unless have had 2 consecutive admissions with Placebo 2, then go to Admission A for stabilization.

If Placebo 4 was given previous admission and if blood flow was

Better	Unchanged	Worse
Continue Placebo 4 x 3 consecutive admissions, then follow at q 1-2 monthly intervals.	2nd dose Placebo 4. After 2 consecutive admissions, then give PGE₁ (4 mcg./hr.)	Placebo 4 unless 2 consecutive admissions with placebo, then go to Admission A for stabilization.

Fig 17–2.—Flow diagram for patients randomized to placebo on Admission C, Protocol A, and to placebo therapy at subsequent randomizations.

If initially the patient received PGE_1 and on admission D was stable, he received a second treatment of PGE_1 and then was rerandomized to PGE_1 2μg/hr or placebo 2 (Fig 17–1). Likewise a decision as to the vascular status was made on each admission. The maximum number of allowable infusions at each dose rate was four.

Similarly, if a patient received placebo initially and remained stable (Fig 17–2), he would then move to the PGE_1 infusion regimen just presented. If his condition had worsened, he would receive a second placebo infusion with his vascular surgeon in attendance and if better would continue to receive placebo. No patient in the study demonstrated a placebo improvement, most remaining stable during the administration.

Patients on protocol B (Table 17–3) had similar admissions, and

TABLE 17-3.—Study Design for Protocol B

Admission A & B	Same as Protocol A
Admission C	PGE₁ according to flow diagram in Fig 17-1

TABLE 17-4.—Study Design for Protocol C

Admission A	Hx + PE + vascular evaluation + photographs
Admission B	If stable, randomized to PGE_1 or placebo
Day 2	0 hr—5 µg PGE_1 or placebo equivalent (P)
	2 hr—10 µg PGE_1 or P
	4 hr—15 µg PGE_1 or P each over 5 min
	6 hr—20 µg PGE_1 or P
	8, 10, 12 hr—20 µg PGE_1 or P
Days 3, 4	24, 26, 28, 30, 32, 34, 36, 48, 50, 52, 54, 56, 58, 60 hr—20 µg PGE_1 or P
Admission C	3 weeks after Admission B; 20 µg PGE_1 or P at times in Admission B
Admission D	3 weeks after Admission C; evaluate ulcer, repeat vascular exam and photographs; break code

because of a worsening vascular condition, threatening amputation, they were given PGE_1 under open label in the same dose rates as outlined in protocol A.

As these first two studies suggested that PGE_1 was most likely to benefit patients with ulcerations as the primary manifestation of peripheral vascular disease, a third protocol was conducted to look at that subgroup of patients. Also suggested was the need to give more drug in a shorter period of time, intermittently to minimize venous irritation. We thus modified an intravenous infusion program that had been reported to be well tolerated in Swedish studies. Patients were randomized to either PGE_1 or placebo (ethanol vehicle of PGE_1 in normal saline) after assurance of stabilization of their vascular condition. In a double-blind fashion, patients received either drug or placebo by the schedule outlined in Table 17-4. On day 1, 5µg of PGE_1 or the equivalent volume of placebo was given intravenously over 5 minutes. Two hours later he received 10µg of PGE_1 or equivalent placebo; at hour four, 15µg; and at hour 6, 20µg; each infusion lasting 5 minutes. All subsequent infusions (7 per day for 3 days) were 20µg of PGE_1 or equivalent volume of placebo. Dosage increments were made only if the previous dose was tolerated. Patients were discharged on day 5 and returned in 3 weeks for a second series of double-blind infusions. One month later the effect on ulcer healing was noted, and the code was broken. If the patient had received placebo or if incomplete healing was seen on PGE_1, follow-up infusions were given at monthly intervals to achieve ulcer healing.

Case Histories

A brief clinical description of two of our diabetics with ulcerations provides an outline of how protocols A and B were conducted.

Subject #6A, a 70-year-old diabetic woman who was taking oral hypoglycemic medication, had failed to heal two ulcerations on the lateral aspect of the right foot for more than six months following a femoral-popliteal bypass. She was randomized to PGE_1 initially and received a total of four infusions of 1μg/hr PGE_1, followed by four of 2μg/hr for 50 to 60 hours each, never tolerating the full 72-hour course because of erythema and tenderness at the infusion site. Following these infusions her ulcerations had improved, although they were not healed, and she was examined at monthly intervals for four months until her lesions showed no further improvement. She was then readmitted for four infusions at 4μg/hr. Figure 17–3 demonstrates her ulcerations before and after therapy. Over the course of one year she received a total of 1.8 mg of PGE_1. Ten months postinfusion, her condition continues to be improved.

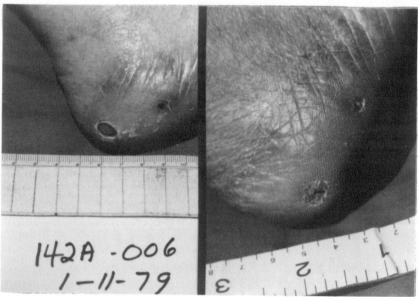

Fig 17–3.—Subject 6A before PGE_1 *(left)* and after multiple 72-hour infusions *(right)*. Total amount of PGE_1 administered—1.8 mg over nine months.

Subject #3B, a 67-year-old diabetic woman facing amputation of her right leg for a painful ulceration of the heel, as well as ulcerations between several of the toes, volunteered and began participation in protocol A. Because of rapid deterioration on placebo she was switched to PGE_1. Good results were seen following 1.9 mg over the six-month protocol, though she did not have complete resolution. Maximum allowable drug had been given, so that she was observed closely over the next year. Her ulcer continued to heal despite discontinuance of the drug. Figure 17–4 shows her heel ulceration before and six months after therapy.

Results

In protocols A and B the major beneficial effects were seen in patients with ulcerations. Four of the six diabetics with ulcerations had complete healing of their ulcerations, as did one patient with Raynaud's disease who had ulcerations of the fingertips. One of the two patients with scleroderma had partial healing of ulcerated areas; the other developed sepsis necessitating discontinuance of PGE_1 infusions. Neither of the two patients with wet gangrene was benefitted. Minimal improvement was seen in claudication symptoms of the re-

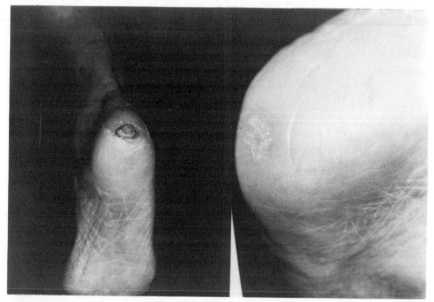

Fig 17–4.—Subject 3B before PGE_1 *(left)* and after multiple 72-hour infusions *(right)*. Total amount of PGE_1 administered—1.9 mg over six months.

maining subjects. The major side-effect seen with this mode of peripheral continued intravenous infusion of PGE$_1$ was venous irritation.

The eight patients with ulceration who participated in this later protocol, two of whom had been subjects in protocol A and B, had the following results. Of the four placebo patients, two demonstrated improvement, no change was seen in a third, and the condition of the fourth worsened. Subsequently PGE$_1$ provided healing of one ulceration and marked improvement of two others. The fourth patient, for conflicting medical reasons, received no PGE$_1$. In the PGE$_1$-treated group, one ulceration was healed, two improved, and one worsened, the latter being a patient previously treated under protocol B.

With this third protocol, transient tachycardia was occasionally observed at the 20-μg dose. Venous erythema was noted, but was transient and did not require premature cessation of infusions. Patients were more mobile in the third study, but needle replacement (a heparin lock) was an occasional problem.

Conclusion

All studies suggested that PGE$_1$ does promote ulcer healing. Also apparent is the "large placebo effect" in this disease, probably related to improved medical treatment in a hospital setting.

Further studies at higher doses, to maximize possible beneficial effects from a rapidly cleared drug, and with shorter hospitalization, to minimize the placebo effect, will be necessary to verify the efficacy of prostaglandin E$_1$ intravenously as a treatment for peripheral vascular disease ulcerations. Such studies are currently being conducted.

REFERENCES

1. Carlson L.A., Eriksson I.: Femoral artery infusions of prostaglandin E$_1$ in severe peripheral vascular disease. *Lancet* I:155, 1973.
2. Carlson, L.A., Olsson A.G.: In Karim S.M. (ed.): *Practical Applications of Prostaglandins and Their Synthesis Inhibitors.* Baltimore, University Park Press, 1979, pp. 39–51.
3. Nielson P.E., Nielson S.L., Holstein P., Hansen E.H., Lassen N.A.: Intraarterial infusion of prostaglandin E$_1$ in normal subjects and patients with peripheral arterial disease. *Scand. J. Clin. Lab. Invest.* 36:633–640, 1976.
4. Nielson P.E., Holstein P., Nielson S.L.: Prostaglandin E$_1$, for impending gangrene. *Lancet* I:192, 1977.
5. Gruss J.D., Kawai S., Karadedos C., Bartels D.: Erste Erfahrungen mit der intraarteriellen Langzeitperfusion von Prostaglandin E$_1$ bei fortgeschritt ener arterieller Verschlusskrankheit der Unteren Extremitaeten

im Stadium IV. (summary English). *Deut. Med. Wochkenschr.* 103:1624–1625, 1978.

6. Sethi G.K., Scott S.M., Takano T.: Effect of intraarterial infusion of PGE₁ in patients with severe ischemia of lower extremity. *J. Card. Surg.* 21:185–192, 1980.

7. Sakaguchi S., Kushaba A., Mishima Y., Kamiya K., Nishimura A., Furukawa K., Shionoya S., Kawashma M., Kaisumura T., Sakuma A.: A multi-clinical double blind study with PGE₁ (α-cyclodextrin clathrate) in patients with ischemic ulcer of the extremities. *VASA* 7:263–266, 1978.

8. Pardy B.J., Lewis J.D., Eastcott H.H.G.: Preliminary Experience with Prostaglandins E₁ and I₂ in Peripheral Vascular Disease. Presented Society of Vascular Surgery 34th Annual Meeting. Chicago, 1980. (Abstract)

9. Carlson L.A., Jogestrand T., Kaijser L., Olsson A.G.: Clinical experience with prostaglandin E₁ in severe peripheral arterial disease. *Lakartidningen* 74:2629–2633, 1977. (Translated from Swedish)

10. Clifford P.C., Martin M.F.R., Sheddon E.J., Kirby J.D., Baird R.N., Dieppe P.A.: The treatment of vasospastic disease with prostaglandin E₁. *Br. Med. J.* 281:1031–1034, 1980.

Intravenous Infusions of Prostaglandins E_1 and I_2 for the Treatment of Small Artery Ischemia and Peripheral Vasospasm

P. A. DIEPPE, P. C. CLIFFORD, M. F. R. MARTIN,
J. T. WHICHER, R. N. BAIRD

Departments of Medicine and Surgery
Bristol (England) Royal Infirmary

Introduction

Peripheral vascular diseases may cause vasospasm, severe pain, ulceration, and gangrene of the hands and feet. Intermittent attacks of digital vasospasm (Raynaud's phenomenon) are common, and often disabling; they may occur with or without other clinical signs of ischemia, and in the presence or absence of obvious arterial disease.[1, 2]

A variety of treatments have been used for peripheral ischemia and vasospasm; these include sympathectomy, oral vasodilator drugs, low-molecular-weight dextran infusions, intra-arterial reserpine, fibrinolytic therapy, anabolic steroids, plasmapheresis, and prostaglandins. The fact that so many treatments have been tried testifies to the inability of most of them to produce lasting benefit.[1, 2]

Over the last three years, several patients have been treated with intravenous infusions of prostaglandin E_1 (PGE_1) or prostacyclin (PGI_2) at the Bristol Royal Infirmary, England. In conjunction with workers at St. Bartholomew's Hospital, London, we have attempted to carry out a logical sequence of treatment protocols to evaluate the efficacy of these agents, and to investigate their mode of action. Many of the results have been published elsewhere.[3–8] This paper summarizes the experience gained with these infusions at Bristol, and attempts to draw some conclusions about the efficacy of this therapy.

Materials and Methods

PGE$_1$ (Alprostadil, Upjohn Ltd.) and PGI$_2$ (Burroughs Wellcome Ltd.) were given by intravenous infusions through central venous catheters situated in the subclavian vein. PGE$_1$ was given in an initial dose of 6 ng/kg/min, increasing to 10 to 12 ng/kg/min in most patients, and up to 25 ng/kg/min in a few. The initial dose of PGI$_2$ was 2.5 ng/kg/min, increasing to a maximum of 10 ng/kg/min. The doses were titrated according to side-effects and subjective responses. All infusions were given in normal saline and continued for 72 hours.

Subjective assessments included pain score (10 cm visual analogue scale) and patient opinion of changes in warmth and cold tolerance (better, same, or worse). The frequency and duration of Raynaud's attacks were recorded, and the physician's overall rating of response was noted. A note was also made of the site and size of any areas of ischemic ulceration and gangrene. Patients were asked to record any side-effects.

Regular recordings were made of pulse, blood pressure, and temperature. Peripheral blood flow was assessed by three independent, objective methods: (1) Doppler studies were made of peripheral arteries at the wrist, groin, and ankle, and the pulsatility index (PI) was derived from analysis of the waveforms. (2) Digital pulse volume recordings (PVR) were made with a plethysmograph attached to the index and middle fingers, and mean PVR calculated from 5 consecutive recordings. (3) Infra-red temperature recordings of the hands were made using a Bofors thermographic camera or Heinmann radiometer. All objective recordings were made after 30 minutes equilibration in a temperature-controlled room; the techniques have been described fully elsewhere,[9-14] and discussed in previous communications on prostaglandin therapy.[3-6]

Venous blood samples were taken to monitor hematologic and biochemical responses. In addition to a full blood count and standard 12-channel biochemical screen, the serum level of C-reactive protein (CRP) and other acute phase proteins was measured by radioimmunoassay.

Patient Groups and Results

Three different treatment protocols have been completed on separate groups of patients.

COMPARISON OF PGE₁ AND NORMAL SALINE INFUSIONS

Twelve patients with systemic sclerosis, severe peripheral ischemia, and vasospasm entered a single-blind, blind-observer, crossover trial comparing saline infusions with PGE₁ in normal saline.[3] The treatments were randomized, and separated by four or five weeks. Analysis of subjective and objective data showed that PGE₁ resulted in a significant decrease in pain, attacks of vasospasm, and a significant rise in hand temperature measured thermographically.

The published data showed that PGE₁ was of greater benefit than placebo;[3, 15] and we therefore decided that no subsequent placebo-controlled trials would be carried out in our unit.

EXPERIENCE WITH PROSTACYCLIN (PGI₂)

Ten patients with systemic sclerosis were treated with PGI₂ infusions. Side-effects were common, and the majority only tolerated doses in the low part of the quoted range (2.5 to 5 ng/kg/min). Transient joint claudication was a distinctive side-effect occurring in seven patients at the start of the infusion. Other problems included hypotension,[6] headache,[8] and abdominal symptoms.[8] Eight patients reported marked subjective improvement in ischemic problems, and in six, radiometry demonstrated a sustained rise in hand temperature. The beneficial response lasted for about six weeks.[6]

The incidence and severity of unpleasant side-effect experienced during these infusions was much greater than that occurring with the use of PGE₁. In view of this we have not continued to treat these patients with PGI₂, but have gained further experience with PGE₁ instead.

PROSTAGLANDIN E₁ INFUSIONS

A total of 53 patients have now been treated with PGE₁ infusions— 37 women and 16 men (mean age 57 years, range 17 to 80). Criteria for patient selection included: (1) predominant small vessel disease, (2) severe ischemic pain and/or vasospasm, and (3) digital ischemic ulcers or gangrene. Thirty-three had a connective tissue disease (systemic sclerosis 26, lupus erythematosus 2, rheumatoid vasculitis 2, and "overlapping syndrome" 3) and 20 had small-artery ischemia of another cause (e.g., small artery arteriosclerosis 12, primary Raynaud's syndrome 4, "Trash" foot syndrome 2, and Buerger's disease 2). Treatment was given only if there were severe symptoms, with or without digital ulceration or gangrene.

Most patients reported a marked reduction of rest pain within 24 hours of starting the infusion, and the majority of those with vasospasm had fewer and less severe attacks in the immediate postinfusion period. Thirteen patients had ulcers prior to treatment; eight of these had healed two months later and 2 others had improved. The duration of the subjective response varied from one week to six months, with a mean of six weeks.

Changes in objective measurements are shown in Table 18–1. Data from the various tests were available on different numbers of patients. The Doppler studies showed no change in pulse transit time, but the pulsatility index (PI) fell during the infusion, indicating vasodilation, and had returned to preinfusion levels by two weeks. Oral thermometer recordings showed a rise in body temperature during the infusion in 56% of patients; this was maximal on the third day, and the mean increase was 1.3°C. Fever subsided quickly once treatment was stopped. The pulse volume and temperature recordings indicated a more sustained rise in peripheral blood flow, maintained six weeks after treatment.

There was no significant change in any of the hematologic or biochemical indices except for the peripheral blood leucocyte count, and the acute phase protein levels. Most patients had a mild leukocytosis, maximal on the second or third day of treatment (mean increase: 2.15×10^9 cells/dl). An initial analysis of CRP levels suggested that about half the patients had shown an increase during the infusion; however, it became apparent that all except those with systemic sclerosis had increased their levels of CRP and other acute phase pro-

TABLE 18–1.—RESULTS OF TREATMENT WITH PGE₁

	PREINFUSION	48 HRS ON PGE₁	6 WEEKS LATER
Number of patients reporting overall improvement (n = 53)	—	83%	56%
Pain (10-cm Visual Analogue Scale) (n = 26)	7.1 cm	4.6 cm*	5.0 cm*
Radial PI (n = 14)	8.8 ± 0.6	4.6 ± 0.5*	6.9 ± 1.0
PVR (mm) (n = 20)	7.1 ± 1.1	21.6 ± 2.7*	14.2 ± 2.9*
Digital temperature (°C) (n = 46)	27.2 ± 0.2	30.3 ± 0.3*	29.5 ± 0.6*

Mean ± standard error.
*$p < 0.01$, using Student's "t" test.

teins. The lack of response in patients with systemic sclerosis has been documented elsewhere.[7]

No serious side-effects were encountered, but there were several minor ones. Pain and inflammation at the catheter tip occurred (5.6%) if the tip was not situated proximal to the shoulder. Headaches were common (62%), and particularly severe in those with a history of migraine. Peripheral edema was often quite severe (66%), and like the febrile responses (77%), took several days to subside. Hypotensive symptoms (15%), as well as nausea and other gastrointestinal symptoms (34%), were noted.

Discussion

Any therapeutic agent used for peripheral ischemia should be safe and simple to administer, and capable of producing prolonged relief of symptoms and improvement in blood flow. If a new agent is introduced, it needs to be established that it has more than a placebo response, and that it has advantages over existing treatments available.

PGE_1 and PGI_2 are potent vasodilators and inhibitors of platelet aggregation, and might be expected to produce at least a transient increase in blood flow to ischemic limbs. We have therefore attempted to evaluate the potential of these prostaglandins in the treatment of peripheral ischemia and vasospasm.

The doses used were chosen empirically on the basis of earlier reports from other groups.[16-18] Our first few infusions, using short IV lines, resulted in severe pain and inflammation at the catheter tip, but this was overcome by using long lines inserted in the subclavian vein, and a 72-hour constant infusion by this route was a simple and satisfactory way of administering the drugs. Greater flexibility with the doses, the duration of treatment, and type of catheter used would be an advantage, but this was sacrificed in our trials for greater comparability between infusions of the different agents, and between different patients.

Assessment of the responses to many available treatments has been hampered by a lack of controlled clinical trials or of any reliable way of measuring peripheral blood flow. Placebo responses in subjective sensations such as pain, as well as in the severity of vasospasm, might be expected, and we believe that it is essential to obtain controlled data. The initial cross-over trial of PGE_1 against saline (placebo)[3, 15] established to our satisfaction that PGE_1 is significantly better than placebo, but more comparative trials against standard therapy are needed to find out whether the prostaglandins are more beneficial than existing treatments.

The controlled trial also indicated that the objective methods used to assess peripheral blood flow were not altered by saline infusions, and this was confirmed by assessing a few more patients on a saline "run-in" infusion, prior to starting PGE_1.[4] The Doppler studies indicated intense vasodilation during infusions, helping to confirm that the doses used were sufficient to produce a general systemic effect on the circulation after passage through the lungs (which can destroy large quantities of PGE_1[19]). This vasodilation came on within minutes of starting treatment and was accompanied by flushing, a warm feeling, fever, and peripheral edema in the majority. Significant hypotension or tachycardia occurred in a minority.

The PVR and thermographic measurements suggested that infusions of PGE_1 can result in a significant improvement in peripheral blood flow which will last for several weeks after the prostaglandin infusions, when vasodilation has long since disappeared. These objective data correlated well with subjective responses, which lasted for about 6 weeks, and with ulcer healing, which was apparently accelerated in the weeks following treatment.

Most infusions were given during the winter months, when symptoms and signs of ischemia were most severe. The benefit helped carry some patients through the winter, but others still came to surgery some weeks later, and nearly all had little or no evidence of lasting improvement when the next winter came along. Improvement, therefore, lasted for only a matter of weeks.

Not all patients responded, and there were clear differences in the amount of improvement experienced on the "fixed" dose regime used. Patients with severe end-stage scleroderma responded poorly, whereas those with Buerger's disease did remarkably well. Further work is being done to try and establish which patient groups are best suited to this type of treatment.

PGE_1 and PGI_2 apparently produced similar beneficial responses, both subjectively and objectively.[4,6] However, side-effects were more frequent and more severe with PGI_2 in patients with systemic sclerosis. Whether this was due to the type of disease treated, the dose used, or some other factor remains to be seen. Further comparative work between E_1 and I_2, as well as with prostaglandins and other therapy, are clearly needed.

The mechanisms whereby the prostaglandins can produce improvement in blood flow, lasting several weeks, is not clear. In addition to a demonstrable effect on platelets,[6] our co-workers in London have shown that PGI_2 alters lymphocyte responses[8] during therapeutic infusions; thus immunologic as well as vascular alterations may be operative, and further work on the mechanism of action is under way.

The other observation of note recorded in this paper and elsewhere[7] is the acute phase reponse to PGE_1 in man. The acute phase proteins are a heterogenous group of glycoproteins having various moderator roles to play in inflammation. They are produced in the hepatocyte in response to peripheral stimuli.[20] It has previously been shown that prostaglandins stimulate increased acute phase protein production by the rabbit liver,[21] but this has not previously been reported in man. Of great interest is the lack of response in systemic sclerosis. It suggests that prostaglandin infusions may have uncovered a basic cellular defect in this idiopathic disease, and this area of investigation is being pursued vigorously in Bristol. Further work on the mode of action of, and biochemical responses to, prostaglandins may aid our understanding of some vascular diseases, as well as providing a potential new treatment.

Conclusions

We have attempted to obtain data to establish the place of intravenous prostaglandin infusions in the treatment of peripheral vascular disease and vasospasm. The work is incomplete, but a few tentative conclusions can be made.

1. Continuous 72-hour IV infusions are a safe, simple way of administering PGE_1 or PGI_2. Both drugs produce an immediate generalized vasodilation. The infusions result in numerous minor side-effects, more common and severe with I_2 than with E_1 in the doses used.

2. Subjective responses and objective measurements of peripheral blood flow suggest that therapy is followed by improved peripheral blood flow, lasting for a few weeks only. No long-term benefit was obtained.

3. Prostaglandin infusions induce fever, a leukocytosis, alterations in lymphocytes, and acute-phase protein production. These changes may be relevant to their mechanism of action, and may provide important new clues to the variability of response in different ischemic diseases, and to the etiology of some of the conditions mentioned.

The need now is for more controlled, comparative data between prostaglandins and other therapy; for work using more flexible doses and attempting to prolong the beneficial effects; and further investigation of the mode of action of prostaglandins in man.

The transient benefits produced in our patients suggest that PGE_1

may be useful in a "crisis" in peripheral ischemic diseases, and perhaps as a preoperative therapy to aid surgical healing.

ACKNOWLEDGMENTS

We would like to acknowledge the financial support of the British Heart Foundation (P.C.C.) and the Arthritis and Rheumatism Council (P.A.D.).

REFERENCES

1. Coffman J.D., Davies W.T.: Vasospastic diseases; a review. *Progr. Cardiovasc. Dis.* 18:123–146, 1975.
2. Porter J.M., Snider R.L., Bardana E.J., Rosch J., Erdmiller L.R.: The diagnosis and treatment of Raynaud's phenomenon. *Surgery* 77:11–23, 1975.
3. Martin M.F.R., Dowd P.M., Ring E.F.J., Cooke E.D., Dieppe P.A., Kirby J.D.T.: Prostaglandin E_1 in the treatment of systemic sclerosis. *Ann. Rheum. Dis.* 39:44, 1980.
4. Clifford P.C., Martin M.F.R., Sheddon E.J., Kirby J.D., Baird R.N., Dieppe P.A.: Treatment of vasospastic disease with prostaglandin E_1. *Br. Med. J.* 281:1031–1034, 1980.
5. Clifford P.C., Martin M.F.R., Dieppe P.A., Sheddon E.J., Baird R.N.: Prostaglandin E_1 infusion for small vessel ischaemia. *Br. J. Surg.* (In press).
6. Dowd P.M., Martin M.F.R., Cooke E.D., Bowcock S.A., Jones R., Dieppe P.A., Kirby J.D.T.: Therapy of Raynaud's phenomenon by intravenous infusion of prostacyclin (PGI_2). *Br. J. Dermatol.* 106:81–89, 1982.
7. Whicher J.T., Martin M.F.R., Dieppe P.A.: Absence of prostaglandin stimulated increase in acute phase proteins in systemic sclerosis. *Lancet* II:1187–1188, 1980.
8. Kirby J.D.T., Linia D.R.A., Dowd P.M., Kilfeather S., Turner P.: Prostacyclin increases cyclic-nucleotide responsiveness of lymphocytes from patients with systemic sclerosis. *Lancet* II:453–454, 1980.
9. Baird R.N., Bird D.R., Clifford P.C., Lusby R.J., Skidmore R., Woodcock J.P.: Upstream stenosis: its diagnosis by Doppler signals from the femoral artery. *Arch. Surg.* 115:1316–1322, 1980.
10. Gosling R.G., King D.H., Newman D.H.: In Harcus A.W., Adamson L. (eds.): *Arteries and Veins*. Edinburgh, Churchill Livingstone, 1975, pp. 61–84.
11. Darling R.C., Raines J.K., Brener B.J., Austen W.C.: Quantitative segmental pulse volume recorder: a clinical tool. *Surgery* 72:873–877, 1972.
12. Zweifler A.J., Cushing B.A., Conway J.: The relationship between pulse volume and blood flow in the finger. *Angiology* 18:591–598, 1967.
13. Cosh J.A., Ring E.F.J.: Skin temperature measurement by radiometry. *Br. Med. J.* 4:448, 1968.
14. Collins A.J., Ring E.F.J., Cosh J.A., Bacon P.A.: Quantitation of thermography in arthritis using multi-isothermal analysis: 1. The thermographic index. *Ann. Rheum. Dis.* 33:113–115, 1974.
15. Martin M.F.R., Dowd P.M., Ring E.F.J., Cooke E.D., Dieppe P.A., Kirby

J.D.T.: Prostaglandin E₁ infusions for vascular insufficiency in progressive systemic sclerosis. *Ann. Rheum. Dis.* 40:350–354, 1981.

16. Carlson L.A., Olsson A.: Intravenous prostaglandin E₁ in severe peripheral vascular disease. *Lancet* II:810, 1976.

17. Sakaguchi S., Kusaba A., Mishima Y.: A multi-clinical double blind study with prostaglandin E₁ (alpha cyclodextrin clathrate) in patients with ischaemic ulcer of the extremities. *Vasa* 7:263–266, 1978.

18. Szczeklik A., Nizankowski R., Skawinski S., Szczeklik J., Cluszko P., Gryglewski R.J.: Successful therapy of advanced arteriosclerosis obliterans with prostacyclin. *Lancet* I:1111–1114, 1979.

19. Golub M., Zia P., Matsuno M., Horton R.: Metabolism of Prostaglandin A₁ and E₁ in man. *J. Clin. Invest.* 56:1404–1410, 1975.

20. Engler R.: In Peters H., Wright P.H. (eds.): Plasma Protein Pathology. Oxford, Pergammon Press, 1979, pp. 13–21.

21. Shim B.P.: Increase in serum haptoglobin stimulated by prostaglandins. *Nature* 259:326–327, 1976.

Double-Blind Controlled Study of the Effect of Prostaglandin E_1 on Healing of Ischemic Ulcers of the Lower Limb

ANDERS G. OLSSON, GUNNEL ERIKSSON,
ANDERS ERIK EKLUND

*King Gustaf V Research Institute and Department of
Medicine, Karolinska Hospital; Departments of
Dermatology and Surgery, Danderyd Hospital,
Stockholm, Sweden*

Introduction

We have previously noted beneficial effects of intra-arterial infusions,[1] intravenous infusions,[2] and intravenous injections[3] of prostaglandin E_1 (PGE_1) on ulcer healing in patients with end-stage arteriosclerosis of the lower limbs. These observations have so far not been confirmed in controlled studies. This is a report on a controlled study on the effect of PGE_1 on ischemic ulcer healing. PGE_1 was given intravenously in intermittent injections in order to avoid the infusion of large amounts of fluid. Ulcer shape was documented by serial stereophotos, which permitted precise measurement of ulcer area and volume.

Material and Methods

SUBJECTS

All 22 patients who took part in the study had arteriosclerosis with ischemic ulcers due to severe restrictions of the arterial blood flow to the limb. No reconstructive surgery was possible, and amputation

225

was considered imminent. Mean age was 74 years (range 35 to 89 years); 11 were females; and 7 were diabetics. None of the patients had overt cardiac decompensation. Mean ulcer duration before treatment was eight months.

None of the patients had beta-hemolytic streptococci growing in the ulcers. Local treatment of the ulcers during the course of the study consisted of saline dressings within the ulcer and an unidentified cream applied to the surrounding skin.

DESIGN OF STUDY

The study had a double-blind design. Each patient was randomly allocated to treatment group or placebo group. Patients were hospitalized for one week for the treatment. In the treatment group, patients received PGE_1 in the dose of 20 μg diluted into 5 ml of saline every other hour, seven times daily, for three days.[3] In the placebo group, the same volume of saline was given in the same manner. The treatment was repeated five weeks later.

Change in ulcer shape was observed by serial stereophotos taken before and at frequent occasions during and after treatment for one month after the second treatment.[4]

Patients in the placebo group were treated with PGE_1 one month after the second blind treatment if their ulcer had not healed.

Statistical analysis was performed according to Snedecor.[5] The study was approved by the ethical committee of the Karolinska Hospital.

Results

DOUBLE-BLIND CONTROLLED STUDY

Two subjects (both placebo group) were dropped from the study— one because of overt cardiac decompensation and the other because of pneumonia.

The dose of PGE_1 used did not produce any subjective or objective side-effects, and the study remained blind throughout its course. The mean initial ulcer dimensions and the mean daily ulcer area and volume change are given in Table 19–1. In the treatment group, both mean ulcer area and volume decreased numerically but insignificantly. In the placebo group, mean ulcer dimension increased insignificantly. No significant difference existed between treatment and placebo groups.

TABLE 19–1.—MEAN INITIAL ULCER DIMENSIONS,
AND MEAN DAILY CHANGE OVER THE PERIOD OF
OBSERVATION AFTER PGE_1 AND PLACEBO

	PLACEBO	p	PGE_1
Ulcer area			
n	10	—	12
Initial, mm^2 Mean ± SEM	615 ± 153	>0.05	856 ± 368
Change, mm^2/day Mean ± SEM	+1.8 ± 4.6	>0.05	−1.8 ± 3.5
Ulcer volume			
Initial, mm^3 Mean ± SEM	1165 ± 534	>0.05	2144 ± 1478
Change, mm^3/day Mean ± SEM	+6.8 ± 6.9	>0.05	−9.5 ± 17.0

In Figure 19–1 it can be seen that in the placebo group 4 of the 10 subjects responded to the treatment with healing. The corresponding figure in the treatment group was of the same order of magnitude. It can also be seen that the overall decrease in ulcer area and volume

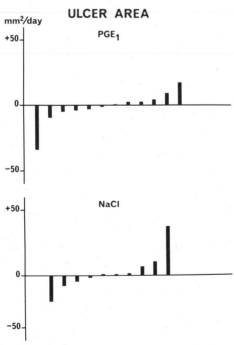

Fig 19–1.—Individual changes in ulcer area two months after the first treatment with PGE_1 and placebo (NaCl) (− = ulcer decrease; + = ulcer increase).

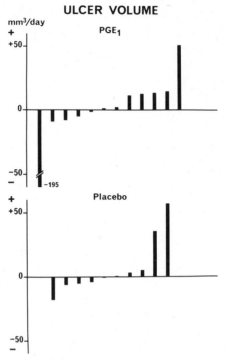

Fig 19-2.—Individual changes in ulcer volume after treatment with PGE₁ and placebo (NaCl).

in the PGE_1 group was mainly due to an extreme healing response in one patient (a diabetic) (Fig 19–2).

A more detailed look at the curves of ulcer shape revealed that many patients responded with a temporary decrease of ulcer measurements after treatment with PGE_1, but not after placebo. This is exemplified by Figure 19–3, which shows the results in a patient who was treated blindly with PGE_1 twice and then openly once. Following each treatment the ulcer size decreased for some weeks. Subsequently it increased, however, and the overall change was an increase in ulcer area and volume. Because of the apparent temporary benefit of PGE_1, we compared the maximal decrease (or minimal increase) daily for each treatment occasion (usually 2 per patient) between the treatment and placebo groups. The results are given in Table 19–2. It can be seen that placebo treatment did not result in any significant reduction in the ulcer size, measured by area or volume, whereas treatment with PGE_1 resulted in significant decreases in both parameters.

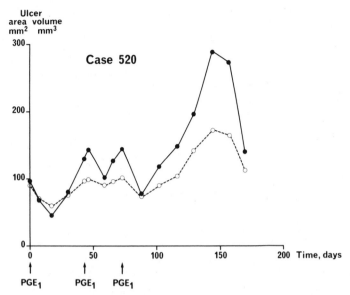

Fig 19–3.—Changes in ulcer area and volume in a patient treated blindly (first two occasions) and openly (third occasion) with PGE₁ in dose of 20 μg every second hour for three days. While the overall change was an increase each PGE₁ treatment resulted in a temporary ulcer decrease (○ = ulcer area; ● = ulcer volume).

OPEN STUDY

Five patients in the placebo group were treated openly with PGE₁ after failure with placebo therapy. When the results observed with these five patients were added to those obtained with the PGE₁ treatment group, the healing effect of PGE₁ became even more apparent (Table 19–2).

Discussion

The overall results of the present study did not show any statistically significant, better healing effect of PGE₁ over placebo when PGE₁ was given as intermittent injections in small doses that avoided side-effects. However, a significant short-term decrease in ulcer size was found in the PGE₁-treated group. The lack of a long-term effect of PGE₁ is, in spite of previous reports, of benefit in patients with ischemic ulcers of the lower limbs.[1-3] There are several possible reasons for this finding.

1. The natural history of this disease is quite variable. Almost half

TABLE 19-2.—MEAN ULCER DIMENSIONS BEFORE EACH
TREATMENT AND AFTER ONE DAY OF MAXIMAL EFFECT (MAXIMAL
DECREASE OR MINIMAL INCREASE) OF EACH TREATMENT OCCASION
IN THE DIFFERENT GROUPS

	PLACEBO	PGE_1	+ PGE_1 AFTER PLACEBO
Ulcer area mm^2 ± SEM			
n	16	20	28
Before	680 ± 162	1248 ± 207	988 ± 222
After	679 ± 163	1236 ± 205	978 ± 220
t	0.3166	2.2090	2.8719
p	NS	<0.05	<0.01
Ulcer volume mm^3 ± SEM			
Before	1214 ± 383	2136 ± 1002	2185 ± 748
After	1201 ± 381	2102 ± 990	2136 ± 736
t	0.5875	2.4305	2.0772
p	NS	<0.05	<0.05

the patients who received placebo showed some healing. In order to
demonstrate a statistically significant beneficial effect of a specific
treatment, a larger number of patients would have to be studied.

2. PGE_1 was given for too short a time. In the design used for the

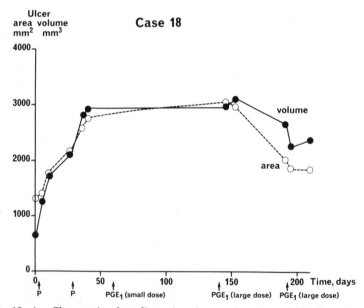

Fig 19-4.—Changes in ulcer dimensions in a patient treated blindly with saline
(two occasions) and then with PGE_1 in a dose of 20 µg twice daily and then in a dose
of 0.5 µg/minute in continuous infusion.

present study, PGE$_1$ was given for three days on two occasions one month apart. If PGE$_1$ were given continuously for several weeks or months, a permanent decrease of ulcer shape and complete healing might occur in more patients.

3. PGE$_1$ was given in too small a dose. Figure 19–4 shows the ulcer development in a patient allocated to the placebo group. During placebo treatment her ulcer increased steadily. She was then treated with PGE$_1$ in the dosage designed for the present study. Unfortunately, it was not possible to follow the ulcer development immediately after the PGE$_1$ treatment. However, 90 days later her ulcer, which before PGE$_1$ had continuously worsened, was unchanged. She was then treated with 0.5 μg/min PGE$_1$ by continuous iv infusion, which was five times the dosage used in the double-blind study. This was associated with ulcer improvement and finally healing. It is possible that the small dose PGE$_1$ arrested the ulceration, whereas the large dose was needed to induce healing.

4. Some ulcers may not respond to treatment with PGE$_1$. Different metabolic, hemodynamic and microvascular factors probably underlie an ischemic ulcer. It is important to distinguish between the type of ischemic ulcer for which PGE$_1$ is beneficial and the type for which it is of no value. Thus, larger controlled studies with higher dosage and longer treatment periods are needed to demonstrate the healing effect of PGE$_1$.

ACKNOWLEDGMENTS

This study was supported by grants from Tore Nilsons Fund and from the Swedish Medical Research Council (No. 19X-204).

REFERENCES

1. Carlson L.A., Eriksson I.: Femoral-artery infusion of prostaglandin E$_1$ in severe peripheral vascular disease. *Lancet* I:155, 1973.
2. Carlson L.A., Olsson A.G.: Intravenous prostaglandin E$_1$ in severe peripheral vascular disease. *Lancet* 2:810, 1976.
3. Carlson L.A., Olsson A.G.: PGE$_1$ in ischaemic peripheral vascular disease, in *The Practical Applications of Prostaglandins and Their Synthesis Inhibitors*. Lancaster, England, S.M.M. Karim MTP Press Limited, 1979, pp. 39–51.
4. Eriksson G., Eklund A.-E., Torlegård K., Dauphin E.: Evaluation of leg ulcer treatment with stereophotogrammetry. *Br. J. Dermatol.* 101:123–131, 1979.
5. Snedecor G.S.: *Statistical Methods*. Ames, Iowa, Iowa State University Press, 1961.

Long-Term Prostacyclin (PGI$_2$) Therapy in Peripheral Arterial Disease—Influence on Some Vascular and Platelet Regulation Mechanisms

K. SILBERBAUER, H. SINZINGER,
CH. PUNZENGRUBER

Second Department of Internal Medicine
University of Vienna, Austria

Introduction

Prostacyclin (PGI$_2$) is synthetized from arachidonic acid in the vessel wall and has been shown to have vasodilating and platelet-inhibiting activities.[1] The generation of PGI$_2$ by atherosclerotic arteries in animals[2] and man[3] is severely suppressed. Recent data indicate that PGI$_2$ infusion in patients with peripheral vascular disease might be of therapeutic benefit.[4] The administration of this endogenous compound in pharmacologic dosage could alter in vivo vascular and platelet regulation mechanisms.[5]

We assessed the effect of a continuous intra-arterial PGI$_2$-infusion on some properties of the cardiovascular system, on the renin-angiotensin-aldosterone system, and on platelet function in patients with peripheral arterial disease.

Patients and Methods

PATIENTS.—Ten patients with peripheral arterial disease of the lower extremities were treated with a continuous intra-arterial infusion of PGI$_2$ for four days. The diagnosis of atherosclerosis obliterans was confirmed by angiography (patient data are listed in Table 20–1). All but one patient stopped smoking at least one month before the treatment.

PROSTACYCLIN TREATMENT.—The sodium salt of PGI_2 in glycine buffer was obtained from Dr. O'Grady (Wellcome, Beckenham, Kent, UK). Biologic identification was always done in our laboratory by estimation of platelet antiaggregatory activity in vitro at least twice a day. The stability of the infused PGI_2 was verified by comparing the platelet antiaggregatory activity from an aliquot taken from the remaining part of each infusion syringe with the activity of a newly prepared standard. A solution of lyophilized sodium salt of PGI_2 in glycine buffer (pH 10.5; cooled at 4°C) was infused by a constant rate infusion pump at a mean dosage of 5 ng/kg body weight/min (range: 1.5 to 7 ng). During the infusion, the electrocardiogram (ECG) and the heart rate were monitored continuously, while blood pressure was measured by the Korotkoff method by the same observer. Blood flow in the lower extremities was measured daily in the morning with strain gauges placed around the calf, and was expressed as ml/ 100 ml tissue/minute. In addition, reactive hyperemia as peak flow was measured in both limbs after compression of the thigh with 250 mm Hg prior to the infusion period, immediately after, and one week thereafter. The systolic blood pressure at the ankle (posterior tibial and dorsalis pedis pulses) and the upper extremity (brachial pulse) were evaluated by an ultrasound Doppler blood flow detector device daily.

BLOOD SAMPLING.—Blood was drawn daily in the morning after a 12-hour overnight fast. Plasma renin activity (PRA; ng/ml/hr), angiotensin II (pg/ml), and aldosterone (pg/ml) were measured in the venous blood by standard radioimmunoassay. Plasma norepinephrine,

TABLE 20–1.—TREATMENT OF PERIPHERAL ARTERIAL DISEASE WITH PGI_2

PATIENT	AGE	SEX	DIABETES	HYPERTENSION	STAGE (FONTAINE) Before	After
1 B.A.	42	M	+	–	IV	Amputation
2 K.L.	71	F	+	+	IV	II
3 W.G.	59	M	–	–	II	II
4 P.O.	63	M	–	–	IV	II
5 K.L.	72	F	+	+	IV	Bypass surgery
6 S.K.	66	M	+	–	III	II
7 T.J.	68	M	+	+	III	III
8 K.E.	78	F	+	+	III	III
9 S.K.	66	M	+	–	III	Bypass surgery
10 K.K.	66	M	–	–	III	II

epinephrine, and dopamine were determined radioenzymatically. The platelet count and platelet aggregation response to ADP (1 μM; Born-type-aggregometer, platelet-rich plasma—PRP; 3.8% sodium citrate as anticoagulant) were examined within 30 minutes of sampling. In addition, platelet sensitivity to synthetic PGI_2 in vitro (expressed in ID_{50}, i.e., the amount of PGI_2 in ng/ml necessary to suppress the ADP-induced platelet aggregation 50%) was tested. Routine plasmatic coagulation parameters, such as prothrombin time, activated partial thromboplastin time, and clottable fibrinogen were measured. Routine biochemical screening (SMAC-Technicon) and urine excretion of potassium and sodium were examined daily.

Statistical evaluation was carried out by Student's t-test for paired data.

Results

Systolic and diastolic blood pressure showed a falling tendency, whereas heart rate (HR) increased to a moderate degree only (Fig 20–1). In general, during PGI_2-infusion no significant premature beats or any other form of arrhythmia were observed. However, in

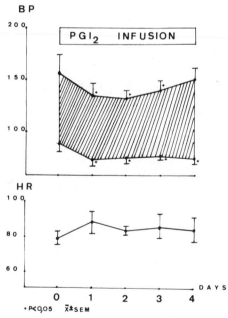

Fig 20–1.—Effect of PGI_2 infusion on blood pressure (*BP*) and heart rate (*HR*).

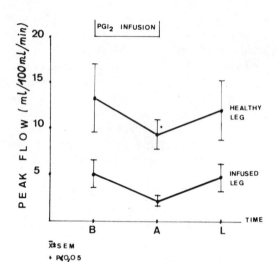

Fig 20–2.—Peak muscle blood flow before *(B)* and after *(A)* treatment, and complete restoration to peak flow within one week *(L)*.

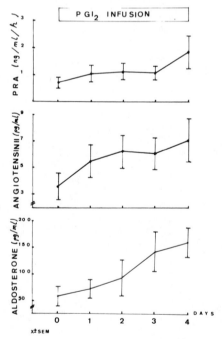

Fig 20–3.—Measurement of plasma renin activity (PRA), angiotensin II, and aldosterone during PGI_2 infusion.

one patient, a ventricular bigeminus was observed on the fourth day of infusion, but it disappeared after reduction of the PGI_2-dosage from 5 to 3 ng/kg/minute.

In spite of a moderate reduction of the systemic blood pressure, Doppler indices and the resting muscle blood flow measured by strain gauge technique did not change significantly. However, peak flow after ischemic stimulus was reduced in the infused and contralateral limbs immediately after PGI_2 infusion (Fig 20–2). Within one week a complete restoration of peak flow to initial values was noted. PRA, angiotensin II, and aldosterone rose slightly during PGI_2 infusion, but not to a significant degree (Fig 20–3). In patients who received a lower PGI_2 dose, the PRA was not altered (Fig 20–4). The serum concentrations of sodium and potassium, as well as their 24-hour excretion, did not alter significantly. Body weight remained unchanged. Plasma catecholamines showed only moderate fluctuation (Fig 20–5). However, in the patient with transient ventricular bigeminus, very high values (390% of the initial) of noradrenaline were observed. In all the patients, the peripheral platelet count increased constantly during PGI_2 infusion (Fig 20–6). Three out of 10 showed suppressed ADP-induced aggregation 24 hours after starting the PGI_2 infusion (Fig 20–7). Subsequently, however, platelet aggregation returned to baseline levels. Moreover, in four patients, an in-

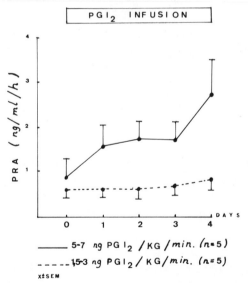

Fig 20–4.—Comparison of low- and high-dosage of PGI_2 on plasma renin activity (PRA).

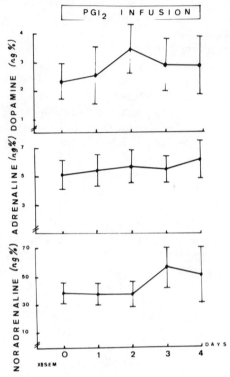

Fig 20–5.—Moderate fluctuation of plasma catecholamines during PGI$_2$ infusion.

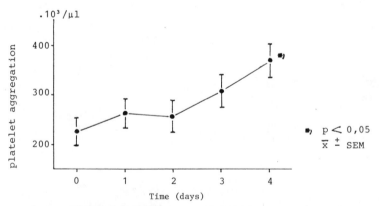

Fig 20–6.—Platelet count during PGI$_2$ infusion.

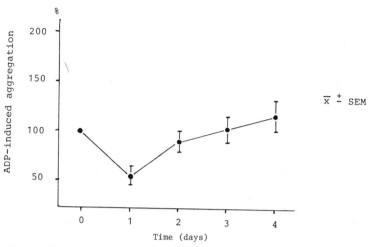

Fig 20–7.—Percent change of ADP-induced platelet aggregation after 1 μM ADP during PGI$_2$ infusion.

crease of platelet aggregability was seen between the second and the third day, whereas the sensitivity of platelets to the inhibitory potency of PGI$_2$ in vitro decreased significantly (Fig 20–8). The platelet sensitivity to PGI$_2$ in vitro decreased to about 40% (i.e., an increase of ID$_{50}$). All values returned to initial levels within 1 week after the end of the PGI$_2$ infusion. PGI$_2$ infusion caused no distinct change in prothrombin time or in activated partial thromboplastin time. However, clottable fibrinogen increased significantly (Fig 20–9). Two patients out of four with stage IV ischemia (according to Fontaine) im-

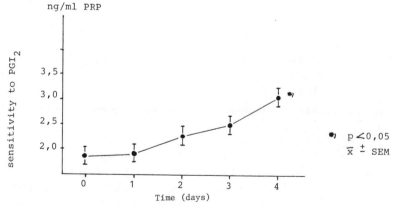

Fig 20–8.—Effect of PGI$_2$ infusion on platelet sensitivity to PGI$_2$ in vitro.

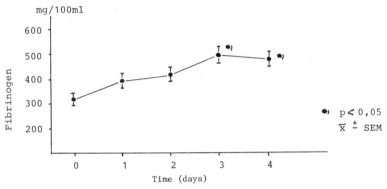

Fig 20–9.—Effect of PGI_2 infusion on plasma fibrinogen levels.

proved to stage II, whereas one patient with extensive gangrene of the lower leg required amputation.

In the fourth patient, femorocrural bypass surgery was performed. Of five patients with stage III ischemia, one improved to stage II, one required femorocrural bypass surgery, and two showed no clinical effect. One patient with stage II ischemia did not change (see Table 20–1).

Discussion

During continuous PGI_2 infusion in 10 patients with advanced obliterative arterial disease, we observed, besides vasodilatory and platelet effects, some counterregulatory responses. The moderate increase in heart rate, the reduction of blood pressure, and the appearance of erythema of the infused limb in some patients were consistent with the vasodilatory properties of PGI_2. An increase of blood flow, measured by strain gauge technique, could not be demonstrated in general. However, the reactive hyperemia, as measured by peak flow, was markedly diminished immediately after cessation of the PGI_2 infusion. It has been shown that reactive hyperemia is caused partly by the action of endogenously produced prostaglandins, especially PGI_2.[6]

Our observations suggest that long-term administration of synthetic PGI_2 in pharmacologic dosage may suppress the reactivity of smooth muscle cells in the vessel wall in response to the ischemic stimulus and may desensitize these cells to endogenously produced PGI_2. In spite of a positive clinical effect in about 50% of the patients, these data should be taken into account during long-term infusion of PGI_2 in patients with obliterative arterial disease, because PGI_2 infusion may suppress vascular compensation mechanisms. Recent studies have shown that short-term infusion of PGI_2 in high dosage in men causes a substantial rise in circulating plasma renin-activity and angiotensin II.[6] Our data indicate that PGI_2 infusion induces a dose-related increase in plasma renin-activity and angiotensin II,[7] which may antagonize to some extent the vasodilator effects of PGI_2.

In vitro incubation studies have demonstrated that PGI_2 can stimulate renin release directly from cortical slices[8] and from renal medulla tissue.[9] However, hemodynamic changes produced by the infusion of PGI_2 might account for the rise in plasma renin activity and angiotensin II. Furthermore, systemic PGI_2 can reduce renal vascular resistance and increased renal blood flow,[10] which tends to increase renin. The tendency of plasma aldosterone to increase is probably secondary to the increase in circulating angiotensin II.

The failure of plasma catecholamines to rise significantly suggests that the systemic baroreflex was not activated by the moderate fall in blood pressure. However, in one patient the occurrence of a ventricular bigeminus was associated with high plasma noradrenalin concentrations. This variation in individual sensitivity to infused PGI_2 necessitates a continuous monitoring of cardiovascular responses. In earlier studies, contradictory findings have been reported concerning the antiplatelet effects of PGI_2 infusion. During a short-term PGI_2 infusion of 15 ng/kg/min in healthy volunteers, inhibition of ADP-induced platelet aggregation was demonstrable.[7] In another study, platelet activity, assessed by ADP-induced aggregation and circulating platelet aggregates, was suppressed during the infusion of PGI_2, but returned to normal shortly after termination of the infusion.[11] In a recent communication, no inhibition of aggregation could be demonstrated in nine patients with peripheral vascular disease. However, when papaverine was included in the citrate anticoagulant, 50% showed inhibition of ADP-induced platelet aggregation during a 72-hour infusion.[12] In contrast to these data, we have reported a different behavior of platelets during long-term prostacyclin infusion.[13] Initially, platelet activity decreased, as assessed by ADP-induced platelet aggregation and by platelet sensitivity to exogenous synthetic PGI_2 in vitro. However, 24-48 hours after the beginning of the infusion of PGI_2, platelet aggregability was enhanced. Moreover, platelet sensitivity to PGI_2 decreased, indicating a desensitization of platelets to exogenous and probably also to the endogenously produced PGI$_2$. An important factor in disturbed platelet-vessel wall interactions might be a change in platelet sensitivity to PGI$_2$ produced by vascular tissue.[14] It is important to note that the alteration in sensitivity is much more pronounced for PGI$_2$ and PGE$_1$ than for PGD$_2$. These findings[15] support the view that the antiaggregatory prostaglandins PGI$_2$ and PGE$_1$ share the same receptor on the platelet surface. In diabetics there is not only decreased platelet sensitivity to PGI$_2$[16] but also decreased vascular prostacyclin formation.[17] This could be interpreted as a double error in thromboregulatory functions. The decreased sensitivity of platelets to PGI$_2$ during infusion might explain the lack of beneficial effect in some cases and may constitute a limiting factor for the continuation of the infusion itself. It is not yet clear whether this phenomenon is due to a stimulation of an endogenous inhibitor of PGI$_2$. On the other hand, recently it has been recognized that chronically elevated or decreased levels of hormones tend to be associated with changes in the hormone responsiveness of target tissues. These changes include hormone refractoriness or changes in the qualitative pattern of effects.[18] The decreased sensitivity of platelets, and probably smooth muscle cells in the vessel wall, to PGI$_2$ might be the result of an alteration of surface receptors. In addition, the mechanism of the increase in platelet count during the PGI$_2$ infusion requires explanation.

If we assume that a continuous consumption of platelets takes place in peripheral vascular disease, the rise of the platelet count might indicate reduced intravascular platelet consumption. However, the possibility that PGI$_2$ releases platelets directly or indirectly from splenic or nonsplenic pools can not be excluded. The influence of PGI$_2$ on platelet production is not known. We are also unable to explain the increase in fibrinogen concentration associated with PGI$_2$ infusion. The clinical importance of the reported vascular and platelet responses following PGI$_2$ infusion remains unclear. One should keep in mind that treatment with PGI$_2$ in pharmacologic doses can influence and disturb regulatory and balance mechanisms. To date, however, no thrombotic event or other effect associated with platelet response has been reported by investigators utilizing PGI$_2$ to treat advanced atherosclerosis.

Future studies with PGI$_2$ should employ shorter infusion periods or intermittent treatment, and platelet and vascular reactivity should be closely monitored in order to prevent possible side effects. Such studies will be necessary to assess fully the clinical importance of this compound in peripheral vascular disease.

REFERENCES

1. Moncada S., Gryglewski R.J., Bunting S., Vane J.R.: An enzyme isolated from arteries transforms prostaglandin endoperoxides to an unstable substance that inhibits platelet aggregation. *Nature* 263:663–665, 1976.
2. Gryglewski R.J., Dembinska-Kiec A., Zmuda A., Gryglewska T.: Prostacyclin and thromboxane A_2-biosynthesis capacities of heart, arteries and platelets at various stages of experimental atherosclerosis in rabbits. *Atherosclerosis* 31:385–394, 1978.
3. Sinzinger H., Feigl W., Silberbauer K.: Prostacyclin generation in human atherosclerotic arteries. *Lancet* II:469–470, 1979.
4. Szczeklik A., Nizankowski R., Skawinski S., Szczeklik J., Gluszko P., Gryglewski R.J.: Successful therapy of advanced arteriosclerosis obliterans with prostacyclin. *Lancet* I:1111–1114, 1979.
5. Neri Serneri G., Masotti G., Poggesi L., et al: Release of prostacyclin into the bloodstream and its exhaustion in human local blood flow changes (ischemia and venous stasis). *Thromb. Res.* 17:197–208, 1980.
6. Miyamori I., Fitzgerald G.A., Brown M.J., Lewis P.J.: Prostacyclin stimulates the renin angiotensin aldosterone system in men. *J. Clin. Endocrinol. Metabol.* 49:943–944, 1979.
7. Silberbauer K., Sinzinger H., Schernthaner G., Leithner Ch., Kaliman J., Elliott M., Burghuber O.: Prostacyclin infusion in men: effects on hormones and on cardiovascular system. *Prostaglandins and Thromboxanes*, 345–349, 1980.
8. Whorton A.R., Mison K., Hollifield J., Frölich J.C., Inagami T., Oates J.A.: Prostaglandins and renin release: II. Stimulation of renin release from rabbit renal cortical slices by PGI_2. *Prostaglandins* 14:1095–1101, 1978.
9. Silberbauer K., Sinzinger H., Winter M.: Prostacyclin (PGI_2) activity in rat kidney stimulated by angiotensin II. *Exp. Molec. Pathol.* 30:242–254, 1979.
10. Bolger P.M., Eisner G., Ramwell P.W., Slotkoft L.M.: Renal actions of prostacyclin. *Nature* 271:467–469, 1978.
11. Szczeklik A., Gryglewski R.J., Nizankowski R., Skawinski J., Gluszko P., Korbut R.: Prostacyclin therapy in peripheral arterial disease. *Thromb. Res.* 19:191–199, 1980.
12. Machin S.J., Chamone P.A.F., Detreyn G., Vermylen J.: The effect of clinical prostacyclin infusions in advanced arterial disease on platelet function and plasma 6-keto-PGF$_1$ alpha levels. *Br. J. Haematol.* 47:413–422, 1981.
13. Sinzinger H., Silberbauer K., Horsch A.K., Gall A.: Decreased sensitivity of human platelets to PGI_2 during long-term intra-arterial prostacyclin infusion in patients with peripheral vascular disease—a rebound phenomenon. *Prostaglandins* 18:56–57, 1981.
14. Klein K., Sinzinger H., Kaliman J., Silberbauer K.: Plättchensensitivität für PGI_2—ein Maß für die Prostacyclinrezeptoren der Plättchen. *VASA* 7:241–245, 1980.
15. Sinzinger H., Horsch A.K., Silberbauer K.: Platelet function during pros-

tacyclin treatment in patients with peripheral vascular disease. *Thromb. Haemost.* 1981 (in press).

16. Klein K., Sinzinger H., Kaliman J., Schernthaner G.: Decreased platelet sensitivity to PGI_2 in maturity onset diabetes. *Pharm. Res. Comm.* (In press).

17. Silberbauer K., Schernthaner G., Sinzinger H., Piza-Katzer H., Winter M.: Decreased vascular prostacyclin in juvenile-onset diabetes. *N. Engl. J. Med.* 300:366–367, 1979.

18. Tell G.P., Haour F., Saez J.M.: Hormonal regulation of membrane receptors and cell responsiveness: A review. *Metabolism* 27:1566–1592, 1978.

PART IV

PROSTAGLANDINS IN ASTHMA AND THE PULMONARY CIRCULATION

Role of Prostaglandins in Asthma

ROY PATTERSON AND KATHLEEN E. HARRIS

Department of Medicine
Northwestern University Medical School
Chicago, Illinois

Introduction

For a variety of reasons, prostaglandins have been considered as potential mediators in asthma. Histamine, a mediator released from IgE antibody-sensitized mast cells, may not be of major importance in asthma, as evidenced by the failure of antihistamines to inhibit IgE-mediated asthma. Prostaglandin synthetase inhibitors, including aspirin and indomethacin, can produce extremely severe acute asthma in a small number of asthmatics. One explanation suggested for this response is that these agents result in an imbalance in prostaglandins, with an excess of bronchoconstricting prostaglandins, such as $PGF_{2\alpha}$, and diminished bronchodilating prostaglandins, such as PGE_1. In rare cases of asthma, aspirin and related compounds may result in clinical improvement.[1, 2]

Various in vitro studies of IgE-mediated mast cell reactions have shown that $PGF_{2\alpha}$, PGD_2, PGE_1, and thromboxanes are released or generated by mast cells or other cells.[3, 4] $PGF_{2\alpha}$ produces bronchospasm in man,[5] and asthmatics are more sensitive than normals to the bronchoconstricting action of $PGF_{2\alpha}$.[6] Increased concentrations of PGD_2 have been found in patients with mast cell disease.[7] In contrast to $PGF_{2\alpha}$, PGE_1 results in relaxation of smooth muscle,[8] and a potential therapeutic role for PGE_1 as a bronchodilator in asthma has been considered.

In order to study the effects of prostaglandins and other products of arachidonic acid metabolism under controlled laboratory conditions, we have used the rhesus monkey model of primate asthma.

RHESUS MODEL OF IgE-MEDIATED ASTHMA.—Some characteristics of the rhesus monkey model of asthma due to IgE antibody to ascaris antigen are: (1) stable colony of animals observed for years;[22] (2) re-

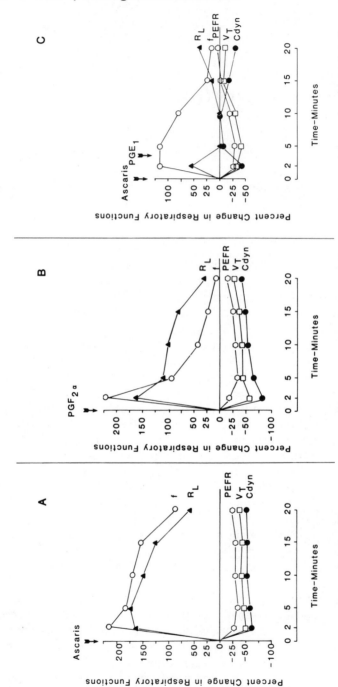

Fig 21–1.—Characteristic airway responses of a rhesus monkey. *A*, *Ascaris serum* antigen; *B*, prostaglandin F₂ₐ; *C*, effect of prostaglandin E₁ on an ascaris-induced respiratory response. Abbreviations: f = breathing frequency; R_L = pulmonary resistance; PEFR = peak expiratory flow rate; V_T = tidal volume; C_dyn = dynamic compliance.

actions that are consistently reproducible;[21] (3) airway responses that are acute, with onset of immediate type reactions occurring within 10 minutes; (4) physiologic functions that may be monitored, including pulmonary resistance, dynamic compliance, tidal volume, breathing frequency, peak expiratory flow rate, and arterial blood gases; (5) agents that inhibit asthma and may be studied by (a) inhibition of degree of abnormalities of pulmonary function following a standard antigen challenge,[19] and (b) shift in the threshold concentration of antigen required to produce an airway response;[19] and (6) agents that may act as mediators of asthma and may be studied by determining the degree to which they reproduce the antigen-induced airway response.[12, 13] The availability of this model permitted us to compare the response of the primate airway to prostaglandins with an antigen-induced response,[9] a histamine response, and a carbocholine response.[10] A typical antigen-induced airway response is shown in Figure 21–1*A*. Further, agents that might interfere with arachidonic acid metabolism could be studied to determine whether inhibition of an antigen-induced response occurred.

STUDIES OF PROSTAGLANDINS.—Selected prostaglandins were evaluated, depending on availability and possible potential for involvement in IgE-mediated reactions. $PGF_{2\alpha}$ resulted in airway responses that qualitatively simulated antigen responses more closely than the anticholinergic agent, carbocholine, or the anticholinesterase, physostigmine.[11] The airway response to $PGF_{2\alpha}$ is shown in Figure 21–1*B*. Neither PGD_2 nor PGI_2 simulated antigen-induced responses as closely as $PGF_{2\alpha}$.[12] PGD_2 resulted in an increase in frequency and pulmonary resistance and a decrease in peak expiratory flow rate, tidal volume, and dynamic compliance, but in contrast to $PGF_{2\alpha}$ and antigen, PGD_2 had a major effect on pulmonary resistance and a lesser effect on frequency. PGI_2 increased frequency and decreased peak expiratory flow rate, tidal volume, and dynamic compliance. In contrast to $PGF_{2\alpha}$ and PGD_2, PGI_2 resulted in no change in pulmonary resistance, suggesting a deficiency in receptor sites in large airways for PGI_2. When PGD_2 and PGI_2 were aerosolized to the airway simultaneously in equal concentrations, the airway response simulated an antigen or $PGF_{2\alpha}$ airway response, and an airway response could be obtained at one-tenth the concentration required for a response from either agent alone, suggesting synergistic action.[12] The results indicate that $PGF_{2\alpha}$, PGD_2, and PGI_2 are agents that could, singly or in combination, result in bronchospasm if bronchial concentrations of these agents were sufficient.

PGE_1 was evaluated to determine its potential for reversing acute bronchospastic airway responses to antigen or pharmacologic agents (histamine, $PGF_{2\alpha}$, carbocholine, and physostigmine) and compared with the beta agonist isoproterenol. In contrast to isoproterenol, which partially or completely reverses all pulmonary function abnormalities, PGE_1 selectively reversed abnormalities of pulmonary resistance and dynamic compliance. Further, this bronchodilator effect was highly transient, lasting 2 to 10 minutes in various experiments.[13] The effect of aerosolized PGE_1 on the rhesus antigen-induced airway response is shown in Figure 21–1C. If these results are applicable to human asthma, the transient nature of the bronchodilator effect would clearly limit clinical efficacy.

SLOW REACTING SUBSTANCE (SRS).—The lack of general availability of SRS permitted only limited experiments in our rhesus colony. Using aerosolized SRS generated from rat peritoneal mast cells, airway responses occurred, but the only abnormalities of pulmonary function seen were increased pulmonary resistance and decreased dynamic compliance, not the complete antigen-induced response in Figure 21–1A.[14] Whether leukotrienes, which have not yet been available for us to study, can reduplicate an antigen-induced response is unknown. An immediate-type cutaneous reaction to SRS in rhesus skin was obtained and could be blocked in a dose-response pattern by FPL55712, the SRS blocking agent.[14]

ARACHIDONIC ACID.—Arachidonic acid is the precursor of multiple potentially bioactive agents. Through the cyclo-oxygenase metabolic pathway, such products as the prostaglandins are produced, and through the lipoxygenase pathway, such products as leukotrienes (slow-reacting substances) are produced. We found that arachidonic acid was inert in the rhesus airway.[15] Further, the ionophore, A23187, which activates rhesus bronchial mast cells to release histamine,[16] resulted in no airway response, but the combination of arachidonic acid and ionophore produced an airway response qualitatively similar to an antigen-induced response.[15] In in vitro studies done by others,[4, 17] using mast cells from various sources, the combination of ionophore and arachidonic acid results in synthesis of a variety of bioactive materials including PGD_2, PGE_2, $PGF_{2\alpha}$, thromboxanes,[4] and SRS.[17] The ionophore-arachidonic acid airway response in rhesus monkeys is inhibited by 5, 8, 11, 14-eicosatetraynoic acid (ETYA), an inhibitor of the lipoxygenase and cyclo-oxygenase pathways of arachidonic acid, suggesting that the airway response is due to the prostaglandins, related compounds, and SRS, singly or in combination. Arachidonic acid, aerosolized prior to challenge with antigen in rhesus monkeys, resulted in a selective increase in pulmonary resistance.[18]

The effect of aerosolized indomethacin was similar: a selective increase in pulmonary resistance under the conditions of the antigen challenge system used.[18]

EFFECT OF ETYA ON ANTIGEN-INDUCED AIRWAY RESPONSES.—Using the IgE-mediated, ascaris-induced airway response in rhesus monkeys, the effect of ETYA as a lipoxygenase and cyclo-oxygenase inhibitor was evaluated. ETYA clearly inhibited the antigen-induced airway responses. Further, the ETYA inhibited the immediate-type skin reactivity induced by antigen in the sensitive monkeys.[19] Both of these inhibitory effects could have been due to inhibition of the generation of prostaglandins or SRS, both of which stimulate airway responses and immediate type skin reactions. Other than the beta agonist, isoproterenol, and the mast cell inhibitor, disodium cromoglycate, ETYA is the first pharmacologic agent we have found that inhibits the primate, antigen-induced, airway response.

BW755C.—Another compound, 3-amino-1-(3-trifluoromethyl-phenyl)-2-pyrazoline hydrochloride (BW755C), was studied because it had been reported to inhibit rat lung cyclo-oxygenase and lipoxygenase.[20] BW755C was found to be an agent that would release histamine from peripheral blood basophils, bronchial lumen, and skin mast cells.[21] We found that BW755C inhibited two pulmonary function abnormalities, pulmonary resistance and dynamic compliance of antigen-induced rhesus monkey asthma. Although BW755C had been shown to be a histamine-releasing agent, it did not induce an airway response. Further, the histamine$_1$ blocking agent, pyrilamine maleate, does not inhibit the antigen-induced airway reactions.[21] These results suggest additional evidence that histamine is not a major mediator of asthma. The reason the lipoxygenase and cyclo-oxygenase inhibitor, ETYA, inhibits all abnormalities of pulmonary function in the immediate-type airway response and BW755C inhibits only 2 abnormalities of pulmonary function is unknown.

Summary and Interpretation

Bioactive mediators resulting from IgE-mediated mast cell activation result in asthmatic airway responses. Products of the metabolism of arachidonic acid appear to play a major role in the airway response. The bioactive materials could be prostaglandins and other products of the cyclo-oxygenase metabolic pathway or of the lipoxygenase pathway of arachidonic acid metabolism. Because of general lack of clinical efficacy of cyclo-oxygenase inhibitors in asthma and the results with indomethacin reported here, a major role for bioactive products of the lipoxygenase pathway appears likely. End-organ antagonists for these products, lipoxygenase inhibitors, or phospholipase inhibitors may have potential therapeutic roles in asthma.

ACKNOWLEDGMENTS

This study was supported by USPHS Grant AI-11759 and the Ernest S. Bazley grant.

REFERENCES

1. Kordansky D., Adkinson N.F. Jr., Norman P.S., Rosenthal R.R.: Asthma improved by nonsteroidal anti-inflammatory drugs. Ann. Int. Med. 88:508–511, 1978.
2. Szczeklik A., Gryglewski R.J., Nizankowska E.: Asthma and nonsteroidal anti-inflammatory drugs. Ann. Int. Med. 90:126, 1979. (Letter)
3. Jakschik B.A., Parker C.W., Needleman P.: Production of prostaglandin (PG) D_2 by rat basophilic leukemia (RBL-1) cells and purified rat mast cells. Fed. Proc. 37:384, 1978. (Abstract Number 906)
4. Roberts L.J. II, Lewis R., Hansbrough R., Austen K.F., Oates J.A.: Biosynthesis of prostaglandins, thromboxanes, and 12-hydroxy -5, 8, 10, 14-eicosatetraenoic acid by rat mast cells. Fed. Proc. 37:384 1978. (Abstract Number 908)
5. Hedqvist P., Holmgren A., Mathé A.A.: Effect of prostaglandin $F_{2\alpha}$ on airway resistance in man. Acta Physiol. Scand. 82:29A, 1971.
6. Mathé A.A., Hedqvist P., Holmgren A., Svanborg N.: Bronchial hyperactivity to prostaglandin $F_{2\alpha}$ and histamine in patients with asthma. Br. Med. J. 1:193–196, 1973.
7. Roberts L.J., Sweetman B.J., Lewis R.A., Folarin V.F., Austen K.F., Oates J.A.: Markedly increased synthesis of prostaglandin D_2 in mastocytosis. Clin. Res. 28:552A, 1980.
8. Cuthbert M.F.: Effect on airways resistance of PGE_1 given by aerosol to healthy and asthmatic volunteers. Br. Med. J. 4:723–726, 1969.
9. Kelly J.F., Cugell D.W., Patterson R., Harris K.E.: Acute airway obstruction in rhesus monkeys induced by pharmacologic and immunologic stimuli. J. Lab. Clin. Med. 83:738–749, 1974.
10. Patterson R., Harris K.E.: The effect of cholinergic and anticholinergic agents on the primate model of allergic asthma. J. Lab. Clin. Med. 87:65–72, 1976.
11. Miller M., Patterson R., Harris K.E.: A comparison of immunologic asthma to two types of cholinergic respiratory responses in the rhesus monkey. J. Lab. Clin. Med. 88:995–1007, 1976.
12. Patterson R., Harris K.E., Greenberger P.A.: Effect of prostaglandin D_2 and I_2 on the airways of rhesus monkeys. J. Allerg. Clin. Immunol. 65:269–273, 1980.
13. Patterson R., Harris K.E.: Effect of PGE_1 on immediate-type immunologic and pharmacologic respiratory responses of the rhesus monkey. J. Lab. Clin. Med. 90:18–24, 1977.
14. Patterson R., Orange R., Harris K.E.: A study of the effect of slow react-

ing substance of anaphylaxis on the rhesus monkey airway. *J. Allerg. Clin. Immunol.* 62:371–377, 1978.

15. Patterson R., Harris K.E., Greenberger P.A.: Ionophore and arachidonic acid stimulation of airway responses in rhesus monkeys. *J. Clin. Invest.* 64:49–55, 1979.

16. Patterson R., Mc Kenna J.M., Suszko I.M., Solliday N.H., Pruzansky J.J., Roberts M., Kehoe T.J.: Living histamine-containing cells from the bronchial lumens of humans. Description and comparison of histamine content with cells of rhesus monkeys. *J. Clin. Invest.* 59:217–225, 1977.

17. Yecies L.D., Wedner H.J., Johnson S.M., Parker C.W.: Characterization of a slow reacting substance from rat peritoneal mast cells. *Fed. Proc.* 37:1667, 1978. (Abstract)

18. Patterson R., Harris K.E., Greenberger P.A.: The effect of arachidonic acid on airway responses of rhesus monkeys. *Life Sci.* 22:389–400, 1978.

19. Patterson R., Harris K.E.: Inhibition of IgE mediated, antigen-induced monkey asthma and skin reactions by 5, 8, 11, 14 - eicosatetranoic acid. *J. Allerg. Clin. Immunol.* 67:146–152, 1981.

20. Higgs G.A., Copp F.C., Denyer C.V., Flower R.J., Tateson J.E., Vane J.R., Walker J.M.G.: Reduction of leucocyte migration by a cyclo-oxygenase and lipoxygenase inhibitor. *Proceedings of Seventh International Congress in Pharmacology.* Oxford, Pergamon Press, p. 334, 1978. (Abstract 843)

21. Patterson R., Pruzansky J.J., Harris K.E.: An agent which releases basophil and mast cell histamine but blocks cyclo-oxygenase and lipoxygenase metabolism of arachidonic acid inhibits IgE mediated asthma in rhesus monkeys. *J. Allerg. Clin. Immunol.* 67:444–449, 1981.

22. Patterson R., Harris K.E., Suszko I.M., Roberts M.: Reagin-mediated asthma in rhesus monkeys and relation to bronchial cell histamine release and airway reactivity to carbocholine. *J. Clin. Invest.* 57:586–593, 1976.

Persistent Fetal Circulation

P. M. OLLEY AND F. COCEANI

Research Institute, Hospital for Sick Children
Toronto, Canada

Introduction

The term—persistent fetal circulation (PFC)—was originally applied to a syndrome of central cyanosis secondary to right-to-left shunts through the foramen ovale and the ductus arteriosus occurring in term infants without structural cardiac defects.[1] Subsequently, the concept was expanded to include premature infants, and infants with certain pulmonary or hematologic abnormalities who exhibit a similar clinical picture.[2] Furthermore, some overlap with the syndromes of transient tachypnea of the newborn and transient myocardial ischemia has been recognized.[3, 4] Common to all these conditions is an abnormally high pulmonary vascular resistance in the absence of structural heart disease. Because these patients lack placental oxygenation of the blood, some authors have proposed alternative names for the syndrome, such as "persistent transitional circulation"[5] or "persistent pulmonary hypertension of the newborn."[2] Perhaps the most appropriate designation should be "abnormal pulmonary vascular resistance of the newborn."

Perinatal Pulmonary Vascular Characteristics

Reid has studied normal growth and development of the lung in great detail.[6] The fetal pulmonary vasculature is characterized by abundant smooth muscle in preacinar arteries, whereas intra-acinar vessels are only partially muscular or are nonmuscular. Wall thickness exceeds that in the adult for vessels of all sizes. Furthermore, there are fewer blood vessels per unit lung volume, which significantly reduces total cross-sectional area. As term approaches pulmonary vascular resistance falls, largely because the number of vessels increases. The multiplication of intra-acinar vessels per unit lung vol-

253

ume continues after birth and through early childhood to keep pace with the increasing number of alveoli.

The fetal pulmonary vasculature is extremely responsive to changes in pulmonary arterial blood oxygen tension and to pharmacologic agents. Fetal hypoxia induces pulmonary vasoconstriction, presumably to maximize blood flow through the ductus arteriosus and thence to the placenta. This sensitivity to hypoxia increases with gestational age, at least in lambs.[7] Acetylcholine, tolazoline, isoproteronol, bradykinin, and E type prostaglandins dilate the fetal pulmonary vascular bed. In the newborn, this pulmonary hyper-reactivity persists while the vessels remain muscular. Acidosis enhances the vasoconstrictor response to hypoxia.[8]

The morphologic features of the fetal pulmonary circulation ensure that pulmonary blood flow is low, being less than 10% of the total cardiac output.[9] Pulmonary and systemic arterial pressures equalize because of the widely patent ductus arteriosus. At birth, pulmonary vascular resistance normally decreases markedly, resulting in a dramatic increase in pulmonary blood flow, and as the ductus arteriosus constricts, pulmonary artery pressure also falls to about 25% of systemic pressure.

This fall in resistance is partly achieved by expansion of the lungs and replacement of alveolar fluid by air, but mainly reflects pulmonary vasodilation induced by alveolar oxygen. These acute adaptive changes are followed by a more gradual regression in the vascular smooth muscle content, which decreases fairly rapidly during the first week of life and then more slowly over the next one to two months. This effect is enhanced by a concurrent increase in vessel number.[6] While the evidence favors a direct action for oxygen in inducing pulmonary vasodilation, certain vasoactive agents, especially bradykinin and E-type prostaglandins, have been proposed as having a role in these adaptive events.

Etiologic Factors in PFC

The cause of PFC is unclear, although there are some clues from both experimental and clinical observations. Abnormal pulmonary vascular resistance may occur in a normal pulmonary vascular bed or in one that is abnormal. A normal vasculature may fail to relax postnatally, may exhibit a normal constrictor response to an abnormal stimulus, or may undergo an abnormal constrictor reaction. The possible mechanisms of abnormal pulmonary vascular resistance in the newborn are (1) in the normal pulmonary vasculature, failure to relax postnatally, normal constrictor response to an abnormal stimulus, abnormal constrictor response, or increased blood viscosity; and (2) in the abnormal pulmonary vasculature, abnormal muscle content or reduced vessel number. Hypoxia, especially when associated with acidemia, produces intense pulmonary vasoconstriction, and consequently any acute perinatal insult, such as fetal asphyxia, meconium aspiration, airway obstruction, or alveolar hypoventilation, may predispose to PFC.

Evidence favoring the presence of abnormal circulating pulmonary vasoconstrictors in this condition is lacking, although it has been suggested that certain bacterial infections might induce the release of such agents from platelets or other cells. Surfactant deficiency in eight patients with PFC and normal chest radiographs has recently been reported.[10]

Blood viscosity may be an important factor in some patients. Red cell number, plasma proteins, and red cell deformability determine whole blood viscosity,[11] of which red cell number is the chief factor in the neonate. An increase in hematocrit above 60 to 65% results in an exponential rise in blood viscosity. Fouron and Herbert demonstrated a progressive increase in pulmonary vascular resistance with increasing hematocrit in newborn lambs, coinciding with reversed shunting through the ductus arteriosus and a rapid fall in systemic vascular resistance and pressure.[12] Gross et al. studied 18 polycythemic newborns and pointed out the importance of erythrocyte deformability to hyperviscosity.[3] Reduced deformability, caused by both hypoxia and acidosis, increases blood viscosity. Intrauterine hypoxia may cause polycythemia by increasing erythropoietin production,[14] and placental, or twin-to-twin, transfusion can also cause neonatal polycythemia. Hyperviscosity may exist with a hematocrit in the upper limits of normal;[13] hence whole blood viscosity should be measured in clinically suspect neonates.

The pulmonary vascular bed may also be abnormal, either because of increased muscle content or because of decreased cross-sectional area. Haworth and Reid studied three infants who died with unexplained pulmonary hypertension in the first three months of life.[15] Quantitative examination of the lungs revealed both increased thickness of the muscle coat in normally muscular vessels and an abnormal extension of muscle into smaller intra-acinar arteries. Although these patients were considered to be examples of PFC, the age at presentation in two was atypical, being 48 hours and one month respectively.

Chronic maternal hypoxia in rats causes increased medial thickness in the small pulmonary arteries of the progeny,[16] which may also be found in infants who are small for gestational age or who are polycythemic.[17] Fetal systemic hypertension, produced by unilateral renal artery constriction or partial occlusion of the ductus arteriosus, induces chronic pulmonary hypertension with a significant increase in pulmonary arterial smooth muscle.[18]

Prostaglandin synthetase blockade in pregnant ewes, with aspirin or indomethacin, constricts the ductus arteriosus,[19] and it has been suggested that intrauterine constriction of the ductus may be an etiologic factor in PFC. Levin et al. observed not only increased pulmonary vascular smooth muscle in the lambs of ewes treated with indomethacin, but also evidence of right ventricular degenerative changes.[20]

Newborn rats from dams given 2 mg/kg/day of indomethacin from the seventeenth day of pregnancy to delivery differed from controls by developing medial hypertrophy and newly muscularized arterioles in the pulmonary circulation.[21]

Indomethacin is being used to inhibit labor by blocking prostaglandin formation, and a PFC-like syndrome occurred in two infants of mothers so treated.[22] A further five such patients were observed by Csaba et al.[23] The lungs of two infants whose mother took, respectively, aspirin throughout pregnancy and indomethacin 25 mg/day for three days, two weeks before delivery, showed increased pulmonary vascular smooth muscle. In addition, the infant with chronic aspirin exposure had a decreased vessel count per unit lung volume. Both infants died with features of PFC.[24] Persistent pulmonary hypertension, with a closed patent ductus arteriosus and abnormally low plasma concentrations of prostaglandin E, occurred in twins and in a single infant born at 30 weeks gestation to mothers given naproxen (d-2(6' methoxy-2-naphthyl) proprionic acid) to retard labor.[25] Finally, Perkin et al. measured serum salicylate concentrations in newborn infants with PFC.[26] These concentrations were significantly elevated in patients with pulmonary hypertension but no right-to-left ductal shunt. No such elevation was found in infants with pulmonary hypertension associated with right-to-left ductal shunt. We may conclude that, while circumstantial, the evidence strongly favors maternal ingestion of prostaglandin synthetase inhibitors as a causative factor in some cases of persistent fetal circulation.

Total cross-sectional area of the pulmonary vasculature may be reduced by intrauterine factors that interfere with lung growth or by space-occupying lesions in the chest. The most commonly encountered problem of this nature is a congenital diaphragmatic hernia, in which the hemodynamic situation resembles PFC.

Pathophysiology

Increased pulmonary vascular resistance causes pulmonary hypertension and maintains the right-to-left fetal direction of blood flow through the ductus arteriosus. Systemic hypoxia lowers systemic resistance, thus further encouraging right-to-left ductal shunting. Pulmonary blood flow and, therefore, left atrial filling are reduced, and right atrial pressure remains greater than left atrial pressure, both because of reduced left atrial filling and because of continued right ventricular hypertension. Right-to-left flow through the foramen ovale becomes probable and causes systemic hypoxia in the upper half of the body. Tissue hypoxia often leads to metabolic acidosis, and the combination of hypoxia and acidosis may further constrict the pulmonary vasculature and compound the hemodynamic problem. Pulmonary artery hypertension, caused by distention of the proximal vessels, may induce reflex vasoconstriction of the more distal muscular arteries, causing the increased resistance to become self-perpetuating.[27]

Myocardial function, especially of the right ventricle, may be impaired because of increased work load and inadequate coronary perfusion with blood of low oxygen content. This impaired function may include tricuspid or mitral insufficiency due to papillary muscle dysfunction and poor contractility. Ischemic changes may develop in the electrocardiogram. The poor cardiac function further worsens the pul-

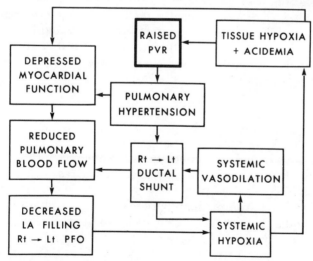

Fig 22-1.—Schema of events in persistent fetal circulation. Once established, several mechanisms perpetuate the hemodynamic changes.

monary and systemic flow and causes a progressive deterioration. Therapy is aimed at reversing this self-sustaining situation.

Clinical Picture and Diagnosis

A history of fetal distress, meconium staining of the amniotic fluid or skin, and low Apgar score are common. The onset is usually within a few hours of birth, and clinical features include central cyanosis with variable respiratory distress in a poorly perfused infant. Cardiac murmurs, due to either tricuspid or mitral insufficiency, may be heard, and the right ventricle may be hyperdynamic. The electrocardiogram is often normal or shows right ventricular hypertrophy. S-T segment or T wave changes suggestive of myocardial ischemia can develop. The chest roentgenogram may show a normal sized heart with underperfused lungs or cardiomegaly with pulmonary edema. Primary pulmonary disease may be present. The echocardiogram is extremely valuable in excluding cardiac malformations, in assessing myocardial function, in confirming the presence of pulmonary hypertension, and in following the efficacy of therapy.[28, 29] Hematocrit, blood glucose, and serum calcium should be estimated and corrected if abnormal.

Arterial Po_2 is usually low, although early in the course it may be sufficiently high to make cyanotic heart disease unlikely. There is usually a poor response to a hyperoxic test. Evidence for right-to-left ductal shunting may be adduced by measuring arterial or cutaneous Po_2 from sites above and below the ductus. A difference of more than 10 torr is significant, but in the presence of profound hypoxia, there may be little difference even when a major ductal shunt is present. When reliable echocardiography is available, cardiac catheterization is seldom required.

Treatment

Hypoglycemia, hypocalcemia, and metabolic acidosis should be corrected as quickly and as completely as possible.

Hypoxia often proves refractory to all measures, which should include a high F_{Io_2} and positive pressure ventilation. Continuous positive airway pressure may help patients with pulmonary edema or a respiratory distress syndrome component to their illness.

Hyperviscosity should be corrected by an exchange transfusion and volume expansion, the rate of which is controlled by monitoring central venous pressure.

PULMONARY VASODILATORS.—If the basic mechanism in most patients with PFC is pulmonary vasoconstriction, then the most rational therapy should be a pulmonary vasodilator. Unfortunately, no agent specific to the pulmonary circulation exists, and concomitant systemic vasodilation may be extremely dangerous. However, certain agents have been used in PFC with some reported success.

Tolazoline (Priscoline) has been used with benefit in hypoxic newborns with pulmonary vasoconstriction.[30] Goetzman reported that 15 of 46 patients treated showed no response, and 14 infants experienced complications possibly related to tolazoline. In unsedated newborn lambs, tolazoline has a direct pulmonary vasodilating action on the pulmonary circulation during hypoxia; however, it does not lower the pulmonary-to-systemic resistance ratio even when injected directly into the pulmonary artery. Despite this lack of selective action on the pulmonary circuit, tolazoline may still improve arterial oxygenation by increasing cardiac output,[31] and it merits a therapeutic trial in patients who fail to improve with high FI_{O_2} and ventilation. Tolazoline should be used with caution, because of its potential for causing profound systemic hypotension. The initial dose is 1 to 2 mq/kg given slowly over five minutes. Ideally, central venous pressure should be monitored and hypovolemia corrected before tolazoline is used.

Several lines of evidence suggest that prostaglandins (PG) may actively control or modulate pulmonary vascular tone in the neonate. In conscious lambs, aged 2 to 3 weeks, PGD_2 and $PGF_{2\alpha}$ are direct pulmonary vasoconstrictors, whereas PGE_1, PGE_2, and PGI_2 are direct dilators. Hypoxia augments the vasodilation of PGE_1 and PGI_2 and diminishes the constriction due to PGD_2 and $PGF_{2\alpha}$. The E-type PGs differ from PGI_2 in that their systemic dilatory action exceeds the pulmonary action, even during hypoxia. In contrast, the PGI_2-induced fall in pulmonary resistance exceeded the fall in systemic resistance during hypoxia, suggesting that PGI_2 is a relatively more specific pulmonary vasodilator than are the E-type prostaglandins.[32]

6-Keto-PGE_1, a possible derivative of either PGI_2 or its relatively inactive metabolite, 6-keto-$PGF_{1\alpha}$, was found to be a direct dilator of the pulmonary and systemic circulations under both normoxia and hypoxia in newborn conscious lambs. Although it is equally effective on both circulations during hypoxia, the systemic effect predominates under normoxic conditions.[33] Tod and Cassin studied the effects of 6-keto-PGE_1 in open-chest anesthetized newborn lambs.[34] They confirmed the pulmonary and systemic dilator effects, but in contrast to the studies of Lock et al.,[33] found no difference under normoxic conditions. This contrast may be explained by methodologic differences. Lock et al. employed bolus injections of 2 μg/kg, whereas Tod and Cassin used one-minute infusions (0.078 to 5.15 μg/kg/min) into the pulmonary artery. The infusion technique maximizes the pulmonary actions while tending to minimize systemic effects.

Murphy et al. reported the unsuccessful use of PGE_1 in five patients with PFC. Only one patient demonstrated a rise in the Po_2 in the descending aorta, and this rise was not sustained.[35] Four patients with PFC were treated with peripherally administered PGE_1 by Schober et al., Pao_2 rose significantly in one and fell in the remaining three.[36]

PGI_2 was used with excellent effect in one patient with PFC,[37] but subsequent experience has proved to be less encouraging, and several patients treated with PGI_2 have developed profound systemic hypotension and bradycardia.

Although PGD_2 is a pulmonary vasoconstrictor, it may be a relaxant in the first 24 hours of life, at least in primates.[38] If this finding is confirmed, then PGD_2 may merit clinical trial in PFC.

Myocardial Support

Most patients with PFC show some degree of impaired myocardial function and may have the full features of transient myocardial ischemia.[39] Patients with clinical, electrocardiographic, or echocardiographic evidence of impaired myocardial function should be digitalized, but diuretics should only be used after hypovolemia has been excluded or corrected. Dopamine in a medium dose (2 to 10 μg/kg/min) has been effective in four infants with myocardial dysfunction associated with PFC.[40]

Hyperventilation-induced alkalosis is currently under evaluation in the management of PFC.

Peckham and Fox treated 10 infants with severe pulmonary hypertension by hyperventilation to reduce $Paco_2$ from 46.9 ± 5.6 mm Hg to 28.6 ± 1.5 mm Hg; pH rose from 7.43 ± 0.05 to 7.6 ± 0.10. Pulmonary artery pressures fell significantly and oxygenation improved.[41]

In another report, hyperventilation alkalosis (pH > 7.6) reversed right-to-left ductal shunting and decreased the ratio of pulmonary artery mean pressure to systemic artery mean pressure to less than one. The effects of tolazoline and dopamine were unpredictable.[42]

Summary

Persistent fetal circulation or abnormal pulmonary vascular resistance of the newborn is probably of multiple etiology. The role of prostaglandins in its development is speculative. Prostaglandins may control or modulate the normal transition of the pulmonary circulation from its high-resistance fetal state to its low-resistance postnatal condition. Furthermore, prostaglandins may be important in controlling normal pulmonary vascular tone. Failure of either function could cause a PFC-like illness. Circulating vasoconstrictor PGs released from platelets or other tissues under the influence of infection might also be implicated. Strong circumstantial evidence connects maternal ingestion of prostaglandin synthetase inhibitors with some cases of PFC, and such drugs should be used with great caution during pregnancy until more information is available.

PGs and their analogues, which relax pulmonary vessels, are potential therapeutic agents, but require careful evaluation in animal experiments before being applied clinically. All presently available agents have both pulmonary and systemic effects.

Current therapy aims to correct metabolic abnormalities and to maximize oxygenation by increasing FI_{O_2} and using positive pressure ventilation. Tolazoline is effective in some patients, probably by increasing cardiac output. Myocardial support is frequently necessary. In spite of these measures, the mortality in severe PFC remains high.

ACKNOWLEDGMENTS

Work done at the Hospital for Sick Children was supported by the Ontario Heart Foundation and the Upjohn Company.

REFERENCES

1. Gersony W.M., Duc G.V., Sinclair J.C.: "PFC" syndrome (persistence of the fetal circulation). *Circulation* 40(Suppl. III):3–87, 1969.
2. Levin D.L., Heymann M.A., Kitterman J.A., Gregory G.A., Phibbs R.H., Rudolph A.M.: Persistent pulmonary hypertension of the newborn infant. *J. Pediatr.* 89:626–630, 1976.
3. Rowe R.D.: Abnormal pulmonary vasoconstriction in the newborn. *Pediatrics* 59:319–321, 1977.
4. Riemenschneider T.A., Nielsen H.C., Ruttenberg H.D., Jaffe R.B.: Disturbances of the transitional circulation: spectrum of pulmonary hypertension and myocardial dysfunction. *J. Pediatr.* 89:622–625, 1976.
5. Brown R., Pickering D.: Persistent transitional circulation. *Arch. Dis. Child.* 49:883–885, 1974.
6. Reid L.: The lung: Its growth and remodeling, in health and disease. *Am. J. Roentgenol. Rad. Ther. Nucl. Med.* 129:777–788, 1977.
7. Lewis A.B., Heymann M.A., Rudolph A.M.: Gestational changes in pulmonary vascular responses in fetal lambs in utero. *Circ. Res.* 39:536–541, 1976.
8. Rudolph A.M., Yuan S.: Response of the pulmonary vasculature to hy-

poxia and H⁺ ion concentration changes. *J. Clin. Invest.* 45:399–411, 1966.

9. Rudolph A.M., Heymann M.A.: Fetal and neonatal circulation and respiration. *Ann. Rev. Physiol.* 36:187–207, 1974.
10. Hallman M., Kankaanpää K.: Evidence of surfactant deficiency in persistence of the fetal circulation. *Eur. J. Pediatr.* 134:129–134, 1980.
11. Merrill E.W.: Rheology of blood. *Physiol. Rev.* 49:863–888, 1969.
12. Fouron J.C., Hébert F.: The circulatory effects of hematocrit variations in normovolemic newborn lambs. *J. Pediatr.* 82:995–1003, 1973.
13. Gross G.P., Hathaway W.E., McGaughey H.R.: Hyperviscosity in the neonate. *J. Pediatr.* 82:1004–1012, 1973.
14. Walker J., Turnbull E.P.N.: Haemoglobin and red cells in the human foetus and their relation to the oxygen content of the blood in the vessels of the umbilical cord. *Lancet* II:312–318, 1953.
15. Haworth S.G., Reid L.: Persistent fetal circulation: Newly recognized structural features. *J. Pediatr.* 88:614–620, 1976.
16. Goldberg S.J., Levy R.A., Siassi B., Betten J.: The effects of maternal hypoxia and hyperoxia upon the neonatal pulmonary vasculature. *Pediatrics* 48:528–533, 1971.
17. Behrman R.E.: *The High-Risk Infant in Neonatology Diseases of the Fetus and Infant.* St. Louis, The C.V. Mosby Company, 1973.
18. Levin D.L., Hyman A.I. Heymann M.A., Rudolph A.M.: Fetal hypertension and the development of increased pulmonary vascular smooth muscle: A possible mechanism for persistent pulmonary hypertension of the newborn infant. *J. Pediatr.* 92:265–269, 1978.
19. Olley P.M., Bodach E., Heaton J., Coceani F.: Further evidence implicating E-type prostaglandins in the patency of the lamb ductus arteriosus. *Eur. J. Pharmacol.* 34:247–250, 1975.
20. Levin D.L., Mills L.J., Weinberg A.G.: Hemodynamic, pulmonary vascular, and myocardial abnormalities secondary to pharmacologic constriction of the fetal ductus arteriosus. A possible mechanism for persistent pulmonary hypertension and transient tricuspid insufficiency in the newborn infant. *Circulation* 60:360–364, 1979.
21. Harker L.C., Kirkpatrick S.E., Friedman W.F., Bloor C.M.: Effects of indomethacin on fetal rat lungs: A possible cause of persistent fetal circulation (PFC). *Pediatr. Res.* 15:147–151, 1981.
22. Manchester D., Margolis H.S., Sheldon R.E.: Possible association between maternal indomethacin therapy and primary pulmonary hypertension of the newborn. *Am. J. Obstet. Gynecol.* 126:467–469, 1976.
23. Csaba I.F., Sulyok E., Ertl T.: Relationship of maternal treatment with indomethacin to persistence of fetal circulation syndrome. *J. Pediatr.* 92:484, 1978.
24. Levin D.L., Fixler D.E., Morriss F.C., Tyson J.: Morphologic analysis of the pulmonary vascular bed in infants exposed in utero to prostaglandin synthetase inhibitors. *J. Pediatr.* 92:478–483, 1978.
25. Wilkinson A.R., Aynsley-Green A., Mitchell M.D.: Persistent pulmonary hypertension and abnormal prostaglandin E levels in preterm infants after maternal treatment with naproxen. *Arch. Dis. Child.* 54:942–945, 1979.
26. Perkin R.M., Levin D.L., Clark R.: Serum salicylate levels and right-to-

left ductus shunts in newborn infants with persistent pulmonary hypertension. *J. Pediatr.* 96:720–726, 1980.

27. Hyman A.L.: Pulmonary vasoconstriction due to non-occlusive distention of large pulmonary arteries in the dog. *Circ. Res.* 23:401–413, 1968.

28. Riggs T., Hirschfeld S., Fanaroff A., Liebman J., Fletcher B., Meyer R.: Persistence of fetal circulation syndrome: An echocardiographic study. *J. Pediatr.* 91:626–631, 1977.

29. Johnson G.L., Cunningham M.D., Desai N.S., Cottrill C.M., Noonan J.A.: Echocardiography in hypoxemic neonatal pulmonary disease. *J. Pediatr.* 96:716–720, 1980.

30. Goetzman B.W., Sunshine P., Johnson J.D., Wennberg R.P., Hackel A., Merten D.F., Bartoletti A.L., Silverman N.H.: Neonatal hypoxia and pulmonary vasospasm: Response to tolazoline. *J. Pediatr.* 89:617–621, 1976.

31. Lock J.E., Coceani F., Olley P.M.: Direct and indirect pulmonary vascular effects of tolazoline in the newborn lamb. *J. Pediatr.* 95:600–605, 1979.

32. Lock J.E., Olley P.M., Coceani F.: Direct pulmonary vascular responses to prostaglandins in the conscious newborn lamb. *Am. J. Physiol.* 238:631–638, 1980.

33. Lock J.E., Olley P.M., Coceani F., Hamilton F., Doubilet G.: Pulmonary and systemic vascular responses to 6-Keto-PGE$_1$ in the conscious lamb. *Prostaglandins* 18:303–309, 1979.

34. Tod M.L., Cassin S.: Effects of 6-Keto-prostaglandin E$_1$ on perinatal pulmonary vascular resistance (41037). *Proc. Soc. Exp. Biol. Med.* 166:148–152, 1981.

35. Murphy J.D., Freed M.D., Lang P., Epstein M., Frantz I.: Prostaglandin-E$_1$ infusion in neonatal persistent pulmonary hypertension. *Pediatr. Res.* 14:606, 1980.

36. Schöber J.G., Kellner M., Mocellin R., Schumacher G., Buhlmeyer K.: Indications and pharmacological effects of therapy with prostaglandin E$_1$ in the newborn, in Samuelsson B., Ramwell P.W., Paoletti R. (eds.): Advances in Prostaglandin and Thromboxane Research 7. New York, Raven Press, 1980, pp. 905–911.

37. Lock J.E., Olley P.M., Coceani F., Swyer P.R., Rowe R.D.: Use of prostacyclin in persistent fetal circulation. *Lancet* I:1343, 1979.

38. Heymann M.A.: Personal communication.

39. Rowe R.D., Hoffman T.: Transient myocardial ischemia of the newborn infant: A form of severe cardiorespiratory distress in full-time infants. *J. Pediatr.* 81:243–250, 1972.

40. Fiddler G.I., Chatrath R., Williams G.J., Walker D.R., Scott O.: Dopamine infusion for the treatment of myocardial dysfunction associated with a persistent transitional circulation. *Arch. Dis. Child.* 55:194–198, 1980.

41. Peckham G.J., Fox W.W.: Physiologic factors affecting pulmonary artery pressure in infants with persistent pulmonary hypertension. *J. Pediat.* 93:1005–1010, 1978.

42. Drummond W.H., Gregory G.A., Heymann M.A., Phibbs R.A.: The independent effects of hyperventilation, tolazoline, and dopamine on infants with persistent pulmonary hypertension. *J. Pediatr.* 98:603–611, 1981.

The Role of the Ductus Arteriosus in the Control of Pulmonary Blood Flow in Newborn Infants

MICHAEL A. HEYMANN

Cardiovascular Research Institute and the Department of Pediatrics and Department of Obstetrics, Gynecology, and Reproductive Sciences, University of California, San Francisco

Introduction

Our knowledge of the factors that control patency of the ductus arteriosus during fetal life and allow for its closure after birth has advanced dramatically in the past few years. We also have come to realize the important role played by the ductus arteriosus either in providing adequate pulmonary blood flow in infants with certain congenital heart malformations or in producing or aggravating pulmonary disease in prematurely born infants. Studies of the basic physiology of the ductus arteriosus have provided information that has allowed for new therapeutic approaches to the management of these infants. Some of these studies and their clinical application will be reviewed.

Physiologic Principles

After birth closure of the ductus arteriosus occurs in two stages. Initial functional closure is brought about by contraction of the smooth muscle in the wall of the ductus. Permanent closure is produced by destruction of the endothelium, by proliferation of the subintimal layers, and by connective tissue formation.

RESPONSES TO OXYGEN

Many studies have shown the importance of oxygen as a stimulus for constriction of the ductus arteriosus probably by direct action on the smooth muscle cells.[1-4] Several in vitro studies have suggested that delayed closure of the ductus arteriosus in premature infants is related to an ineffective contractile response to an increase in oxygen tension (Po_2).[3, 5-8] Isometrically contracting rings of ductus arteriosus from immature fetal lambs (100 days gestation) have a significantly lower response to oxygen than do those from near term animals. This diminished response may be secondary to developmental alterations in smooth muscle receptors for oxygen or to a developmental alteration in the sensitivity of the vessel to, or metabolism of, locally produced relaxing substances.

ROLE OF PROSTAGLANDINS

Since stimulation of smooth muscle contraction by prostaglandins had been shown to require the presence of oxygen,[9] Coceani and Olley investigated the possible role of prostaglandins in postnatal constriction of the ductus arteriosus.[10] They showed that in the presence of a low Po_2, exogenous prostaglandins E_1, (PGE_1), and E_2 (PGE_2) dilate, rather than constrict, the fetal lamb ductus arteriosus. Recently, prostacyclin (PGI_2) also has been invoked as a possible dilator of the ductus arteriosus.[8, 11-13] Since administration of inhibitors of prostaglandin synthesis to pregnant animals near term produces constriction of the ductus arteriosus in the fetuses,[13-16] it is likely that prostaglandins play an active role in maintaining the ductus arteriosus in a dilated state during normal fetal life.

The exact sites of production of the prostaglandins responsible for maintaining the ductus arteriosus in a dilated state in vivo are unknown. According to one current view, prostaglandins are formed intramurally and exert their action locally on the muscle cells.[17] Several studies have shown that tissue homogenates or intact rings of ductus arteriosus produce PGE_2, PGI_2, and $PGF_{2\alpha}$.[11, 12, 17] PGI_2 appears to be the major prostaglandin released by the ductus arteriosus, and endogenous PGE_2 production is about one-tenth to one-twentieth the PGI_2 production.[8] Although PGI_2 is a potent vasodilator of several vascular tissues,[18] it is two to three orders of magnitude less potent than PGE_2 in relaxing the lamb ductus arteriosus.[19] Therefore, even though PGE_2 is a lesser product of arachidonic acid metabolism and prostaglandin production in the lamb ductus arteriosus, the greater sensitivity of the tissue to PGE_2 probably makes it the most important endogenous prostaglandin in the regulation of patency of the ductus. However, another possibility exists.

Prostaglandins are detectable only in very low concentrations in the plasma of adults and therefore are not thought to act as circulating hormones because of their rapid catabolism in the lungs. The fetus, however, has high circulating concentrations of prostaglandins and particularly of PGE_2.[20] This probably reflects the low pulmonary blood flow and therefore decreased prostaglandin catabolism in the lungs of the fetus, as well as the fact that the placenta produces prostaglandins. It is likely, therefore, that PGE_2 plays a hormonal role in the fetus and that it is involved in maintaining the ductus arteriosus in a dilated state during normal fetal life.

At birth, the placental source of production is removed and the large increase in pulmonary blood flow would allow effective removal of any circulating PGE_2, thus enabling the ductus arteriosus to constrict. It thus appears that physiologic patency or closure of the ductus arteriosus represents a balance between the constricting effects of oxygen and perhaps certain vasoconstrictive substances and the relaxing effects of several prostaglandins.

Role of Ductus in Providing Adequate Pulmonary Flow

CONGENITAL RIGHT VENTRICULAR OUTFLOW OBSTRUCTION

Newborn infants with congenital heart malformations that produce severe (or complete) obstruction to right ventricular outflow (Fig 23–1) depend mainly on a patent ductus arteriosus to provide an adequate pulmonary blood flow and thereby adequate oxygen supply.[21] Shortly after birth, the ductus arteriosus constricts despite the low systemic arterial blood oxygen tension (Pao_2). This produces a fall in pulmonary blood flow with increasing hypoxemia and perhaps acidemia. The exact mechanisms responsible for this constriction of the ductus arteriosus, despite reduced pulmonary blood flow and often severe hypoxemia, are not clear. In infants with these malformations, it is usual to find the ductus arteriosus diameter reduced because of the very low flow through it during fetal life. This may permit minor degrees of constriction to produce a significantly larger reduction in cross sectional area than in a larger, more normal ductus arteriosus.

Several palliative surgical procedures have been used to improve pulmonary blood flow in these extremely ill infants. In many in-

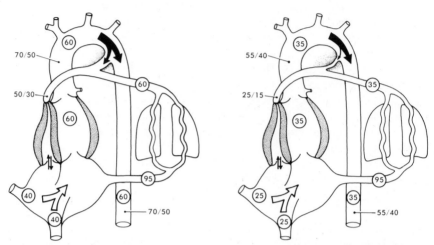

Fig 23–1.—Diagrammatic representation of the heart and great arteries in an infant with pulmonary atresia. Pressures, blood oxygen saturations (in circles), and flow patterns are shown while the ductus arteriosus is patent (on the left) and after it has constricted (on the right). (From Engle M.A. (ed.): *Pediatric Cardiovascular Disease.* Cardiovascular Clinics, Philadelphia, F.A. Davis Publishing Co., 1981, pp. 301–310.)

stances, however, the results have not been good. Since PGE$_1$ and PGE$_2$ had been shown to dilate the ductus arteriosus in experimental animals,[10] the possibility that one of these agents would dilate the ductus arteriosus and thereby improve pulmonary blood flow in infants with cyanotic congenital heart disease was investigated by Elliot and associates.[22] They showed an increase in arterial blood oxygen saturation following PGE$_1$ infusion. Subsequently, several reports have shown an increase in Pao$_2$ during infusion of either PGE$_1$ or PGE$_2$ in groups of infants with congenital right ventricular outflow obstruction.[23–25]

Once a diagnosis is confirmed and the infusion is started, surgery may be delayed for several hours; this allows for stabilization of the infant, excretion of angiographic contrast medium, correction of metabolic acidemia, and return to normal electrolyte balance. The infusion may be continued after surgery to improve pulmonary blood flow as much as possible in the postoperative period. In specific instances, such as small preterm infants or infants with very small branch pulmonary arteries where surgery is not feasible, long-term infusions for several weeks or even months have been performed allowing the infant to grow prior to eventual surgery.

MONITORING.—Since PGE$_1$ may produce systemic hypotension, it is important to monitor systemic arterial blood pressure throughout the infusion. Heart rate, rectal temperature, electrocardiogram, and respiratory rate should be monitored continuously, and the infant should be observed closely for clinical signs of respiratory depression or central nervous system irritation. Arterial blood pH, P_{O_2}, and P_{CO_2} should be monitored intermittently throughout the infusion.

In general in these infants, PGE_1 infusion has become an extremely valuable adjunct to management and improved oxygenation is almost invariable.

Role of the Ductus in Overcirculation of the Lungs

PERSISTENT PATENCY OF THE DUCTUS ARTERIOSUS IN PRETERM INFANTS

A significant proportion of prematurely born infants, and particularly those with a birth weight less than 1250 grams, have a persistently patent ductus arteriosus (PDA). Many of these infants have appreciable left-to-right shunting of blood through the PDA with overcirculation of the lungs and a high pulmonary arterial pressure. Left ventricular decompensation and pulmonary edema occur fairly commonly and, when added to the underlying primary pulmonary disease of prematurity, may severely compromise pulmonary function. More recently, even a moderate shunt within the first several days after birth has been considered to be a factor in the development and persistence of pulmonary disease in preterm infants.[26]

Many of these infants, particularly the most immature, are unresponsive to fluid restriction and the administration of digitalis and diuretics and, in the past, required surgical ligation. Since the foregoing experimental evidence indicated that inhibition of prostaglandin synthesis in fetal animals produced constriction of the ductus, we considered that this may be a useful approach to the management of PDA in these infants.

INDICATIONS FOR TREATMENT

Originally, indomethacin was introduced for the treatment of infants with a large left-to-right shunt in whom standard medical management was ineffective and in whom surgical ligation was contemplated.[27, 28] As experience expanded, it appeared that indomethacin, properly utilized, had few side-effects, and these only transient. Now many infants are treated before serious hemodynamic deterioration is apparent. The realization that digitalis, particularly in the smaller infants (1250 grams and less), had little effect and frequently led to problems of toxicity has provided a further stimulus to the use of indomethacin.

RESPONSES

Variable success has been reported because of the diverse manner in which indomethacin has been used. The poorest responses have been in the most mature infants and in those infants treated very late in the course of their disease (usually between 2 and 3 weeks after birth). In addition, the definition of "success" has been variable, and several studies have considered only the early responses in the analysis. In general, as reported by McCarthy et al.,[29] the best overall response can be expected in infants treated before about 10 days of age and whose gestational age at birth was between 28 and 34 weeks. There is no apparent difference in response between oral and intravenous administration.[30]

Between 50% and 75% of infants show a significant constriction or complete closure of the ductus arteriosus following the first course of one to three doses. Some infants have shown complete closure initially, and then again develop evidence of a left-to-right shunt several days later. Many of these infants respond to a second course; however, some do not and may require surgical ligation. Other infants may show only a partial initial response; some of these require no further specific treatment because of a reduction in the adverse hemodynamic effects; others may require a second course or even surgical ligation.

In most infants there is a significant reduction in the left-to-right shunt and, consequently, in pulmonary blood flow. This generally leads to improvement in pulmonary function.

The potential risks of indomethacin administration must be weighed against those of conservative medical management or of surgical ligation. Currectly, it appears that the administration of indomethacin, although not always effective, is a safe approach. Current investigations are aimed at determining whether early treatment of a PDA, i.e., prior to the presence of major symptomatology, will lead to a reduction in incidence or severity of secondary pulmonary disease. This important question remains to be answered by further careful clinical studies.

ACKNOWLEDGMENTS

This work was supported in part by Program Project Grants HL06285 and HL24056 from the National Institutes of Health.

REFERENCES

1. Kovalcik V.: The response of the isolated ductus arteriosus to oxygen and anoxia. *J. Physiol. Lond.* 169:185–197, 1963.
2. Fay F.S.: Guinea pig ductus arteriosus. I. Cellular and metabolic basis for oxygen sensitivity. *Am. J. Physiol.* 221:470–479, 1971.
3. McMurphy D.M., Heymann M.A., Rudolph A.M., Melmon K.L.: Developmental changes in constriction of the ductus arteriosus: Responses to oxygen and vasoactive substances in the isolated ductus arteriosus of the fetal lamb. *Pediatr. Res.* 6:231–238, 1972.
4. Heymann M.A., Rudolph A.M.: Control of the ductus arteriosus. *Physiol. Rev.* 55:62–78, 1975.
5. Oberhansli-Weiss I., Heymann M.A., Rudolph A.M., Melmon K.L.: The pattern and mechanisms of response to oxygen by the ductus arteriosus and umbilical artery. *Pediatr. Res.* 6:693–700, 1972.
6. Noel S., Cassin S.: Maturation of contractile response of ductus arteriosus to oxygen and drugs. *Am. J. Physiol.* 231:240–243, 1976.
7. Clyman R.I., Mauray F., Wong L., Heymann M.A., Rudolph A.M.: The developmental response of the ductus arteriosus to oxygen. *Biol. Neonate* 34:177–181, 1978.
8. Clyman R.I.: Ontogeny of the ductus arteriosus response to prostaglandins and inhibitors of their synthesis. *Semin. Perinatol.* 4:115–124, 1980.
9. Eckenfels A., Vane J.R.: Prostaglandins, oxygen tension and smooth muscle tone. *Br. J. Pharmacol.* 45:451–462, 1972.
10. Coceani F., Olley P.M.: The response of the ductus arteriosus to prostaglandins. *Can. J. Physiol. Pharmacol.* 51:220–225, 1973.
11. Pace-Asciak C.R., Rangaraj G.: The 6-ketoprostaglandin $F_{1\alpha}$ pathway in the lamb ductus arteriosus. *Biochim. Biophys. Acta* 486:583–585, 1977.
12. Clyman R.I., Mauray F., Koerper M.A., Wiemer F., Heymann M.A., Rudolph A.M.: Formation of prostacyclin (PGI_2) by the ductus arteriosus of fetal lambs at different stages of gestation. *Prostaglandins* 16:633–642, 1978.
13. Coceani F., Olley P.M.: Role of prostaglandins, prostacyclin, and thromboxanes in the control of prenatal patency and postnatal closure of the ductus arteriosus. *Sem. Perinatol.* 4:109–113, 1980.
14. Sharpe G.L., Larsson K.S., Thalme B.: Studies on closure of the ductus arteriosus. XII. In utero effect of indomethacin and sodium salicylate in rats and rabbits. *Prostaglandins* 9:585–596, 1975.
15. Coceani F., Olley P.M., Bodach E.: Lamb ductus arteriosus: Effect of prostaglandin synthesis inhibitors on the muscle tone and the response to prostaglandin E_2. *Prostaglandins* 9:299–308, 1975.
16. Heymann M.A., Rudolph A.M.: Effects of acetylsalicylic acid on the ductus arteriosus and circulation in fetal lambs in utero. *Circ. Res.* 38:418–422, 1976.
17. Terragno N.A., Terragno A.: Prostaglandin metabolism in the fetal and maternal vasculature. *Fed. Proc.* 38:75–77, 1979.
18. Omini C., Moncada S., Vane J.R.: The effects of prostacyclin (PGI_2) on tissues which detect prostaglandins. *Prostaglandins* 14:625–632, 1977.
19. Clyman R.I., Mauray F., Roman C., Rudolph A.M.: PGE_2 is a more potent vasodilator of the lamb ductus arteriosus than is either PGI_2 or 6 keto $PGF_{1\alpha}$. *Prostaglandins* 16:259–264, 1978.

20. Challis J.R.G., Dilley S.R., Robinson J.S., Thorburn G.D.: Prostaglandins in the circulation of the fetal lamb. *Prostaglandins* 11:1041–1052, 1976.
21. Heymann M.A., Rudolph A.M.: Effects of congenital heart disease on fetal and neonatal circulation. *Prog. Cardiovasc. Dis.* 15:115–143, 1972.
22. Elliott R.B., Starling M.B., Neutze J.M.: Medical manipulation of the ductus arteriosus. *Lancet* I:140–142, 1975.
23. Olley P.M., Coceani F., Bodach E.: E-type prostaglandins: A new emergency therapy for certain cyanotic congenital heart malformations. *Circulation* 53:728–731, 1976.
24. Heymann M.A., Rudolph A.M.: Ductus arteriosus dilatation by prostaglandin E$_1$ in infants with pulmonary atresia. *Pediatrics* 59:325–329, 1977.
25. Neutze J.M., Starling M.B., Elliott R.B., Barratt-Boyes B.G.: Palliation of cyanotic congenital heart disease in infancy with E-type prostaglandins. *Circulation* 55:238–241, 1977.
26. Jacob J., Gluck L., DiSessa T., Edwards D., Kulovich M., Kurlinski J., Merritt T.A., Friedman W.F.: The contribution of PDA in the neonate with severe RDS. *J. Pediatr.* 96:79–87, 1980.
27. Heymann M.A., Rudolph A.M., Silverman N.H.: Closure of the ductus arteriosus in premature infants by inhibition of prostaglandin synthesis. *N. Engl. J. Med.* 295:530–533, 1976.
28. Friedman W.F., Hirschklau M.J., Printz M.P., Pitlick P.T., Kirkpatrick S.E.: Pharmacological closure of the patent ductus arteriosus in premature infants. *N. Engl. J. Med.* 295:526–529, 1976.
29. McCarthy J.S., Zies L.G., Gelband H.: Age-dependent closure of the patent ductus arteriosus by indomethacin. *Pediatrics* 62:706–711, 1978.
30. Bhat R., Vidyasagar D., Fisher E., Hstreiter A., Ramirez J.L., Burns L., Evans M.: Pharmacokinetics of oral and intravenous indomethacin in preterm infants. *Dev. Pharmacol. Ther.* 1:101–110, 1980.

PART V

PROSTAGLANDINS IN CORONARY ARTERY DISEASE

Coronary Prostacyclin and Thromboxane Levels in Patients with Coronary Artery Disease

PAUL D. HIRSH, L. DAVID HILLIS,
WILLIAM B. CAMPBELL, BRIAN G. FIRTH,
JAMES T. WILLERSON

*Departments of Internal Medicine (Cardiovascular
Division) and Pharmacology, University of Texas Health
Science Center at Dallas*

Introduction

There has been recent speculation concerning the role of prostacyclin and thromboxane in ischemic heart disease.[1,2] These naturally occurring compounds are potent modulators of vascular smooth muscle tone and platelet aggregability.[3] Prostaglandin I_2 (PGI_2), a powerful vasodilator and inhibitor of platelet aggregation, is the predominant prostaglandin synthesized by the heart.[4,5] In contrast, thromboxane A_2 (TXA_2) is a potent vasoconstrictor released by platelets which, in turn, causes further aggregation of circulating platelets.[6] Both PGI_2 and TXA_2 are unstable and spontaneously convert to the inactive metabolites, 6-keto-prostaglandin $F_{1\alpha}$ (6-keto-$PGF_{1\alpha}$) and thromboxane B_2 (TXB_2), respectively.[6,7]

Several investigators have suggested that prostaglandins and thromboxane may counterbalance one another in the normal regulation of coronary blood flow.[8,9] Derangements of platelet function as well as alterations in prostaglandin and thromboxane production and release have been reported in association with many of the risk factors related to coronary artery disease.[10-14] Therefore, the present study was performed to assess prostaglandin and thromboxane release into the coronary circulation in patients with unstable angina pectoris, stable angina pectoris, nonischemic chest pain syndromes,

273

and various nonischemic cardiac diseases. In particular, we tested the hypothesis that patients with unstable angina pectoris have increased transcardiac thromboxane levels in close proximity to the last episode of chest pain.

Methods

From September, 1979, to September, 1980, blood samples from the coronary sinus (CS) and ascending aorta (AO) were obtained in 60 individuals (31 women and 29 men, aged 20 to 76) during cardiac catheterization at Parkland Memorial Hospital, Dallas, Texas. There was no attempt to control or to alter the patients' medications prior to catheterization, but careful records were kept of all medications administered within one week prior to study. None of the patients received premedication prior to catheterization. Following informed consent, a No. 7 or 8 French woven dacron (Goodale-Lubin) catheter was advanced to the coronary sinus via a brachial vein under fluoroscopic control, and its location was confirmed by both fluoroscopy and blood sampling for oxygen saturation. A No. 7 or 8 French polyurethane pigtail catheter was introduced percutaneously into the femoral artery and advanced to the ascending aorta adjacent to the coronary ostia. In all patients, blood samples were obtained prior to systemic heparinization or injection of radiographic contrast material.

PATIENT GROUPS

On the basis of the history, noninvasive evaluation, and results of cardiac catheterization, and without knowledge of the prostacyclin, thromboxane, or lactate results, each patient was assigned by agreement of two of the authors to one of five groups. For the purposes of this study, patients with ischemic heart disease were defined as those with (1) fixed atherosclerotic coronary artery disease in which at least one coronary artery had $\geq 50\%$ luminal diameter narrowing, (2) angiographically documented coronary arterial spasm, and/or (3) electrocardiographic evidence of previous myocardial infarction with a corresponding segmental wall-motion abnormality by left ventriculography.

Group A (n = 6) had nonischemic heart disease, including a variety of congenital and acquired noncoronary cardiac lesions. Specifically, these patients had patent ductus arteriosus, atrial septal defect, mitral stenosis, mitral regurgitation, idiopathic (nonischemic) cardiomyopathy, and cor pulmonale secondary to primary pulmonary hypertension. Group B (n = 14) was composed of patients with a syndrome of chest pain without objective evidence of cardiac disease by resting electrocardiogram, ambulatory two-channel electrocardiographic monitoring, exercise tolerance testing with simultaneous radionuclide equilibrium gated blood pool scintigraphy, and cardiac catheterization, including selective coronary arteriography with ergonovine provocation. In Group C (n = 18), each patient had ischemic heart disease with the most recent episode of chest pain more than 96 hours prior to study. In Group D (n = 15), each patient had ischemic heart disease, and the most recent chest pain occurred 24 to 96 hours prior to study. Finally, group E (n = 7) was composed of patients with unstable angina pectoris and chest pain within 24 hours prior to study. One patient who sustained an acute subendocardial myocardial infarction 12 hours following the study (confirmed by serum enzymes including CK-B[15] and serial technetium-99m stannous pyrophosphate myocardial scintigraphy[16]) was included in group E. There were two patients with evidence of coronary arterial spasm (one in group D, one in group E).

CHEMICAL ANALYSES

The blood specimens for prostacyclin and thromboxane analysis were drawn simultaneously into heparinized plastic syringes and transferred quickly into iced 10-ml tubes containing indomethacin (10 μg) and heparin (1000 U). They were immediately centrifuged at 2000 × g for 15 min at 4°C. The supernatants were separated and stored at −20°C for subsequent analysis. 6-keto-prostaglandin $F_{1\alpha}$ and TXB_2 concentrations in aortic and coronary sinus blood were analyzed in all 60 patients, and lactate concentrations were measured in the first 45 patients.

Prostaglandins were measured by radioimmunoassay using the method of Dray et al.[17] as modified by Campbell et al.[18] Briefly, this method consists of adding ^3H-6-keto-$PGF_{1\alpha}$ or ^3H-TXB_2 to 4 ml of plasma and extracting the plasma with 20 ml of petroleum ether. The aqueous phase is then extracted with 20 ml of ethyl acetate:cyclohexane (50:50) after acidification to pH 3 with glacial acetic acid. The organic phase is removed and evaporated to dryness under a stream of nitrogen at 30°C. Then the extract is separated into its prostaglandin components by silicic acid chromatography with solvents of increasing polarity. Free fatty acids, PGA_2, and PGB_2 are first eluted from the silicic acid with toluene:ethyl acetate

(60:40). Then, 6-keto-PGF$_{1\alpha}$ and TXB$_2$ are eluted in the second fraction with toluene:ethyl acetate:methanol:water (60:40:5:1). The second fraction is evaporated to dryness under nitrogen, reconstituted in phosphate-buffered saline containing gelatin, and assayed for prostaglandins by radioimmunoassay.

The antibodies for the radioimmunoassay were produced in our laboratory in rabbits. The rabbits were immunized against a prostaglandin-thyroglobulin conjugate produced by the mixed anhydride method of Jaffe and Behrman.[19] The levels of sensitivity of the assays are less than 5 pg for 6-keto-PGF$_{1\alpha}$ and less than 1 pg for TXB$_2$. The anti-6-keto-PGF$_{1\alpha}$ serum cross-reacted 2% with PGE$_1$, 14% with PGF$_{1\alpha}$, and less than 0.6% with the other known prostaglandins and 6-keto-PGF$_{1\alpha}$ metabolites. The anti-TXB$_2$ serum cross-reacted less than 0.003% with all known prostaglandins. The results obtained by radioimmunoassay were corrected for recoveries (65.4 ± 12.0%, mean ± SD) and expressed as picograms per milliliter of plasma.

The blood samples for lactate determination were immediately deproteinated in iced perchloric acid, centrifuged, decanted, and stored frozen. Lactate concentration was assayed enzymatically using the Sigma Chemical Co. kit (St. Louis, Missouri); spectrophotometric measurements were made at 340 nm.

STATISTICAL ANALYSIS

Because of unequal variances among groups, the CS and AO concentrations as well as CS/AO concentration ratios for the prostaglandins and thromboxane were analyzed for inter-group differences using a nonparametric analysis (the Kruskal-Wallis procedure).[20] An analysis of variance was performed to test for inter-group differences in mean % myocardial lactate extraction.

All values are expressed as mean ± standard deviation, with the median and range reported for additional comparison because of the skewed distribution of some groups.

Results

THROMBOXANE B$_2$

When the CS and AO concentrations of TXB$_2$ were expressed as the ratio CS/AO, significant inter-group differences were observed (Fig 24–1). Group A (valvular and congenital nonischemic heart disease)

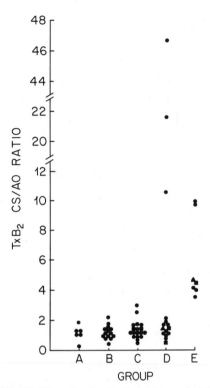

Fig 24–1.—The TXB$_2$ CS/AO ratios for the five groups of patients. Each point represents the data from one patient. Squares identify patients who received a cyclo-oxygenase inhibitor within 5 days of study, and triangles identify patients with coronary arterial spasm. In groups A (valvular and congenital nonischemic heart disease), B (chest pain syndrome without ischemic heart disease), and C (ischemic heart disease without chest pain for at least 96 hours), all patients had TXB$_2$ CS/AO ratios ≤ 3.1. Group D (ischemic heart disease with chest pain 24 to 96 hours prior to study) had a bimodal distribution: 12 patients had low TXB$_2$ CS/AO ratios, while 3 had very high ratios. Group E (ischemic heart disease and chest pain within 24 hours prior to study) had TXB$_2$ CS/AO ratios (range 3.5 to 9.9) which were higher than groups A, B, and C (p<0.05). (From Hirsh P.D., et al.: *N. Engl. J. Med.* 304:685–691, 1981. Used by permission.)

had a TXB$_2$ CS/AO ratio of 1.2±0.6 (median 1.2, range 0.2–1.9); group B (chest pain syndrome without ischemic heart disease) had a TXB$_2$ CS/AO ratio of 1.2±0.4 (median 1.2, range 0.4–2.2); and group C (ischemic heart disease without chest pain for at least 96 hours) had a TXB$_2$ CS/AO ratio of 1.3±0.6 (median 1.2, range 0.5–3.0). Although the overall mean TXB$_2$ CS/AO ratio for group D (ischemic heart disease with chest pain 24 to 96 hours prior to study) was 6.3±12.5 (median 1.5, range 0.5 to 46.6), this group demonstrated a distinct bimodal distribution: 12 patients had low TSB_2 CS/AO ratios (mean 1.3 ± 0.4, range 0.5 to 2.1), whereas 3 patients had markedly elevated values (mean 26.2 ± 18.5, range 10.5 to 46.6). The patients in group D with low and high TXB_2 CS/AO ratios could not be distinguished from each other on the basis of any clinical criteria. Group E (ischemic heart disease and chest pain within 24 hours prior to study) had a TXB_2 CS/AO ratio of 5.8 ± 2.8 (median 4.5, range 3.5–9.9), significantly higher ($p < 0.05$) than groups A, B, and C.

The aortic concentrations of TXB_2 allowed no distinction among groups A to E. As shown in Table 24–1, there was no association between the aortic TXB_2 concentration and the presence or degree of clinical activity of ischemic heart disease. Similarly, neither the coronary sinus TXB_2 concentrations alone nor the absolute changes in TXB_2 concentration across the coronary bed corresponded to the clinical grouping of the patients (Table 24–1).

6-KETO-PGF$_{1\alpha}$

The CS/AO ratios of prostaglandin 6-keto-PGF$_{1\alpha}$ (a chemical degradation product of PGI_2) showed no significant inter-group differences (Fig 24–2 and Table 24–1). As observed with the absolute TXB_2 values, the absolute 6-keto-PGF$_{1\alpha}$ concentrations from the coronary sinus and aortic blood (Table 24–1) as well as the absolute difference across the coronary bed failed to demonstrate any significant differences among groups A to E.

TXB$_2$/6-KETO-PGF$_{1\alpha}$ RATIO

The CS/AO ratio of TXB_2 divided by the CS/AO ratio of 6-keto-PGF$_{1\alpha}$ did not allow better discrimination among the five groups of patients than the TXB_2 CS/AO ratio alone (Table 24–1).

LACTATES

The % myocardial lactate extraction was calculated by the formula $100 \times (AO-CS)/AO$, where AO = aortic lactate concentration and CS = coronary sinus lactate concentration. All 45 patients had positive values indicating net myocardial lactate extraction.[21] There were no significant intergroup differences in terms of lactate concentrations. Specifically, the % myocardial lactate extraction for the various groups expressed as the mean $\pm$ SD were: group A, 18.2 ± 8.5; group B, 21.4 ± 11.9; group C, 20.8 ± 13.7; group D, 18.3 ± 10.6; and group E, 13.0 ± 7.2.

TABLE 24–1.—THROMBOXANE AND PROSTACYCLIN PROFILE OF THE FIVE PATIENT GROUPS

GROUPS*		CS (pg/ml)	THROMBOXANE B$_2$ AO (pg/ml)	CS/AO†	CS (pg/ml)	6-KETO-PGF$_{1\alpha}$ AO (pg/ml)	CS/AO†	TXB$_2$ CS/AO / 6-keto-PGF$_{1\alpha}$ CS/AO
A	Mean ± SD	133 ± 104	117 ± 69	1.2±0.6‡	167 ± 74	240±177	0.8±0.2	1.5±0.8
	Median	99	102	1.2‡	157	166	0.9	1.8
	Range	30–314	47–246	0.2–1.9	64–257	60–515	0.5–1.1	0.2–2.2
B	Mean ± SD	98±57	97±72	1.2±0.4‡	115±53	140±71	0.9±0.3	1.5±0.9
	Median	79	72	1.2‡	118	117	1.0	1.3
	Range	41–245	27–274	0.4–2.2	19–205	51–277	0.2–1.5	0.3–4.0
C	Mean ± SD	104±105	74±65	1.3±0.6‡	143±99	135±58	1.1±0.6	1.5±0.8
	Median	73	52	1.2‡	127	131	0.9	1.2
	Range	13–375	10–267	0.5–3.0	47–492	57–253	0.6–3.1	0.5–3.6
D	Mean ± SD	228±290	108±224	6.3±12.5	144±78	139±122	1.2±0.5	4.4±7.0
	Median	123	42	1.5	125	119	1.1	1.4
	Range	8–980	13–908	0.5–46.6	57–333	49–565	0.4–2.1	0.6–22.2
E	Mean ± SD	405±381	67±60	5.8±2.8‡	168±86	129±55	1.4±0.5	4.7±2.6
	Median	329	54	4.5‡	174	145	1.2	4.4
	Range	54–1044	11–180	3.5–9.9	78–324	53–205	0.9–2.1	2.2–8.3

*Patient groups A–E as described in detail within the text. Total n=60 (Group A, n=6; Group B, n=14; Group C, n=18; Group D, n=15; Group E, n=7).
†These calculations represent the mean, median, and range of the individual patient CS/AO ratios for each group.
‡Group E is different (p<0.05) from Groups A, B, and C.
(From Hirsh P.D., et al.: N. Engl. J. Med. 304:685–691, 1981. Used by permission.)

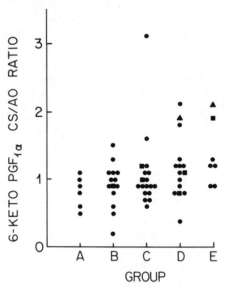

Fig 24-2.—The 6-keto-PGF$_{1\alpha}$ CS/AO ratios for the five groups of patients. Each point represents the data from one patient. Squares identify patients who received a cyclo-oxygenase inhibitor within 5 days of study, and triangles identify patients with coronary arterial spasm. The five groups are not different statistically from one another. (From Hirsh P.D., et al.: *N. Engl. J. Med.* 304:685–691, 1981. Used by permission.)

EFFECTS OF MEDICATIONS

Of the 60 patients, 47 (78%) were receiving long-acting nitrates, 21 (35%) were receiving propranolol (dose range 30 to 240 mg/24 hours, mean 120 mg/24 hours), and 2 (3%) were receiving lopressor (100 mg/ 24 hours) at the time of catheterization. In addition, six patients had received cyclooxygenase inhibitors within five days of study (aspirin in two, aspirin plus ibuprofen in one, sulfinpyrazone in one, indomethacin in one, and sulindac in one). These patients were approximately equally distributed among groups A to E (Fig 24–1). Exclusion of these six patients did not alter the conclusions based on statistical analysis at the $p<0.05$ confidence level.

Discussion

Recently, there has been great interest in the role of prostacyclin and thromboxane as mediators of unstable angina pectoris and acute myocardial infarction.[1,2] Hemodynamic, scintigraphic, and arteriographic studies in patients with angina at rest or acute myocardial infarction have shown that some episodes of ischemia or infarction are caused by a primary reduction of coronary arterial flow, due either to increased coronary arterial tone[22-24] or to phasic platelet aggregation at the site of a coronary stenosis.[25-27] Thus, in the patient with angina at rest or acute myocardial infarction, a reduction of coronary blood flow due to coronary arterial spasm and/or intermittent platelet aggregation is an attractive pathophysiologic hypothesis. Since prostacyclin and thromboxane are powerful modulators of vascular smooth muscle tone and platelet aggregability, their potential role as mediators of unstable angina pectoris and acute myocardial infarction is conceptually appealing. Figure 24–3 provides a schematic representation of this hypothesis.

The half-life of PGI_2 in blood at 37 C is two to three minutes and that of TXA_2 is approximately 30 seconds.[3] Because of their short

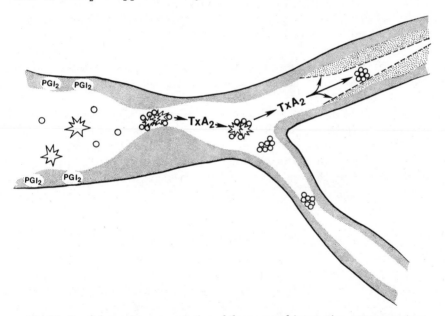

Fig 24–3.—Schematic representation of the proposed interaction among prostacyclin, thromboxane, platelets and vascular smooth muscle in the pathophysiology of unstable angina pectoris and acute myocardial infarction. Circulating platelets *(circles)* become activated *(stars)*, and adhere to exposed collagen at the site of an atherosclerotic lesion. Adhering platelets undergo a release reaction: thromboxane A_2 (TXA_2) is produced and released, and platelet aggregation is initiated. Platelet aggregates may "plug" a distal coronary artery at the site of a stenosis, or TXA_2 may cause vasoconstriction, allowing platelet "plugs" to obstruct even a normal coronary artery. Prostacyclin may prevent platelet adherence to normal vascular endothelium, and its absence in diseased vessels may be important in the initiation of this pathologic process.

half-lives, these compounds exert their effects on the tissues where they are synthesized, acting as local hormones. For this reason, the examination of the transcardiac changes in the concentrations of these compounds may be necessary to assess their role in various clinical syndromes of ischemic heart disease. This assumption is supported by the findings of the present study. Specifically, when examined individually, the absolute coronary sinus or ascending aortic concentrations of TXB_2 and 6-keto-$PGF_{1\alpha}$ did not reveal significant intergroup differences (Table 24–1). However, when the transcardiac changes in the concentrations of these compounds were evaluated, the CS/AO ratios of TXB_2 were significantly elevated in patients studied within 24 hours of ischemic chest pain (group E) in comparison to patients with anginal chest pain more than 96 hours prior to study (group C) and the two nonischemic control groups (groups A and B). Patients who experienced ischemic chest pain 24 to 96 hours prior to study (group D) demonstrated a bimodal distribution of the TXB_2 CS/AO ratio: the majority had normal CS/AO ratios, but a minority had markedly elevated TXB_2 CS/AO ratios. Although these findings suggest that TXB_2 is released acutely in the coronary vascular bed in association with angina, it is presently unknown whether it is cause or consequence.

Although other studies have suggested that alterations in platelet function develop as platelets traverse an atherosclerotic vascular bed,[28-30] the transcardiac changes in TXB_2 observed in the present study bear no relationship to the presence or degree of atherosclerotic coronary artery disease (Fig 24–4). Consequently, the stimulus to platelet thromboxane production does not appear to be related to the extent of coronary atherosclerosis. However, it is possible that an episode of myocardial ischemia induces alterations in the coronary circulation, with resultant intracoronary platelet sensitization. Thus, the increase in TXB_2 levels from ascending aorta to coronary sinus may have occurred in the coronary circulation or in the coronary sinus catheter, and the present study cannot distinguish between these two possibilities. Nevertheless, since recent studies have shown intracoronary platelet aggregates in a variety of clinical ischemic heart syndromes,[31, 32] it seems possible that sensitized platelets release TXA_2 into the coronary circulation, with resultant intracoronary aggregation. Thromboxane A_2 could cause this not only by a direct effect on platelets, but also by increasing coronary vascular resistance, thereby reducing coronary blood flow locally, with subsequent platelet aggregation.

Prostaglandin I_2, synthesized in coronary vascular tissue, serves as

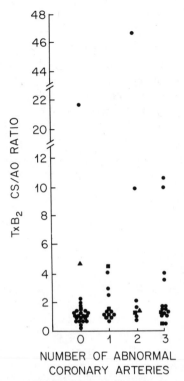

Fig 24–4.—The TXB_2 CS/AO ratios plotted for the presence and degree of coronary artery disease. Each point represents the data from one patient. Squares identify patients who received a cyclo-oxygenase inhibitor within 5 days of study, and triangles identify patients with coronary arterial spasm. The TXB_2 CS/AO ratios are similar among those with and without underlying coronary artery disease. (From Hirsh P.D., et al.: *N. Engl. J. Med.* 304:685–691, 1981. Used by permission.)

a physiologic TXA_2 antagonist.[33] Although an endogenous TXA_2-PGI_2 balance has been postulated,[34, 35] there has been no previous systematic investigation of this in individuals with cardiac disease. The present study fails to demonstrate a clinical basis for this concept. Specifically, there are no differences in the CS/AO ratio of the PGI_2 metabolite, 6-keto-$PGF_{1\alpha}$, among the five groups of patients studies. Furthermore, inspection of individual patient values suggests that a deficiency of coronary PGI_2 synthesis in the presence of an elevated transcardiac TXA_2 concentration is not the mechanism responsible for the syndrome of unstable angina. For example, the patient in group D with the highest TXB_2 CS/AO ratio (46.6) had only a mildly elevated 6-keto-$PGF_{1\alpha}$ CS/AO ratio, but he had no chest pain within 24 hours of study. Therefore, it appears PGI_2 may not be important pathophysiologically in this regard. However, there are several possible alternative explanations. First, metabolic products of PGI_2 other than 6-keto-$PGF_{1\alpha}$ have been described and, under certain conditions, 6-keto-$PGF_{1\alpha}$ may not reflect the total changes in PGI_2.[36] Second, localized alterations in PGI_2 may exert important effects without altering the PGI_2 concentration in coronary sinus blood, at least as measured with current techniques. Nevertheless, it still seems likely that despite its in vitro pharmacologic effects, PGI_2 may not play an important role in normal coronary vascular homeostasis. Indeed, Curwen et al. have suggested that PGI_2 generation by the vascular endothelium may not be important in preventing platelet adherence to the normal vessel wall.[37] The theoretical role assigned to PGI_2 based on in vitro studies may not prove correct in vivo. However, we cannot exclude a transient imbalance between TXA_2 and PGI_2 as being associated temporally with the development of unstable angina.

The principal question of whether TXA_2 plays a causal role in the patient with unstable angina remains unanswered even by the present study, since the data obtained demonstrate a temporal but not necessarily causal relationship. One approach to this problem would be assessment of selective pharmacologic inhibition of TXA_2 production in such patients. However, there is no selective thromboxane synthetase inhibitor available for human investigation at this time. Cyclo-oxygenase inhibitors, such as indomethacin and ibuprofen, are nonspecific inhibitors of all prostaglandin and thromboxane production. Aspirin, even in low doses, has the same effect,[38–40] although PGI_2 synthesis recovers somewhat faster than TXA_2 synthesis following aspirin administration. Thus, selective inhibition of thromboxane synthetase is not yet clinically feasible.

In conclusion, the transcardiac TXB_2 concentration is increased in patients with unstable angina pectoris who have experienced chest pain within 24 hours of study, whereas it is not elevated in individuals with (1) arteriosclerotic coronary artery disease without chest pain for at least 96 hours, (2) nonischemic chest pain syndromes, and (3) valvular or congenital nonischemic cardiac disease. In patients with ischemic heart disease and chest pain 24 to 96 hours before study, the transcardiac thromboxane B_2 concentrations are heterogeneous; some are greatly elevated, whereas others are normal. In contrast, the transcardiac concentrations of 6-keto-$PGF_{1\alpha}$ demonstrate no relationship to the presence or degree of clinical activity of ischemic heart disease. That transcardiac thromboxane B_2 is increased in close temporal proximity to an anginal episode, but is independent of transcardiac lactate production, suggests that the ongoing release of thromboxane B_2 may not be a result of persistent myocardial ischemia. Whether transcardiac increases in thromboxane B_2 are of etiologic importance in the development of unstable angina pectoris and acute myocardial infarction remains to be determined.

ACKNOWLEDGMENTS

Supported in part by a research grant (HL-17669) from the National Institutes of Health (NIH) Ischemic Heart Disease Specialized Center, a grant (HL-25471) from the National Heart, Lung, and Blood Institute (NHLBI), and a grant from the Texas affiliate of the American Heart Association. Dr. Hirsh's work was supported by NHLBI training grant HL-07360. Dr. Campbell is the recipient of a Research Career Development Award from the NIH (K04-HL-00801). Prostaglandins for this study were furnished by Dr. John E. Pike of the Upjohn Company.

REFERENCES

1. Braunwald E.: Coronary spasm and acute myocardial infarction—new possibility for treatment and prevention. *N. Engl. J. Med.* 299:1301–1303, 1978.
2. Borer J.S.: Unstable angina: a lethal gun with an invisible trigger. *N. Engl. J. Med.* 302:1200–1202, 1980.
3. Moncada S., Vane J.R.: Pharmacology and endogenous roles of prostaglandin endoperoxides, thromboxane A_2, and prostacyclin. *Pharmacol. Rev.* 30:293–331, 1979.
4. Isakson P.C., Ray A., Denny S.E., Pure E., Needleman P.: A novel prostaglandin is the major product of arachidonic acid metabolism in rabbit heart. *Proc. Natl. Acad. Sci. USA* 74:101–105, 1977.
5. deDeckere E.A.M., Nugteren D.H., TenHoor F.: Prostacyclin is the major prostaglandin released from the isolated perfused rabbit and rat heart. *Nature* 268:160–163, 1977.
6. Hamberg M., Svensson J., Samuelsson B.: Thromboxanes: a new group of biologically active compounds derived from prostaglandin endoperoxides. *Proc. Natl. Acad. Sci. USA* 72:2994–2998, 1975.
7. Wong P.Y.-K., Sun F.F., McGiff J.C.: Metabolism of prostacyclin in blood vessels. *J. Biol. Chem.* 253:5555–5557, 1978.
8. Needleman P., Kaley G.: Cardiac and coronary prostaglandin synthesis and function. *N. Engl. J. Med.* 298:1122–1128, 1978.
9. Moncada S., Vane J.R.: Arachidonic acid metabolites and the interactions between platelets and blood-vessel walls. *N. Engl. J. Med.* 300:1142–1147, 1979.
10. Carvalho A.C.A., Colman R.W., Lees R.S.: Platelet function in hyperlipoproteinemia. *N. Engl. J. Med.* 290:434–438, 1974.
11. Bizios R., Wong L.K., Vaillancourt R., Lees R.S., Carvalho A.C.: Platelet

prostaglandin endoperoxide formation in hyperlipidemias. *Thromb. Haemostas.* 38:228, 1977.

12. Tremoli E., Folco G., Agradi E., Galli C.: Platelet thromboxanes and serum-cholesterol. *Lancet* I:107–108, 1979.

13. Stuart M.J., Gerrard J.M., White J.G.: Effect of cholesterol on production of thromboxane B_2 by platelets in vitro. *N. Engl. J. Med.* 302:6–10, 1980.

14. Butkus A., Skrinska V.A., Schumacher O.P.: Thromboxane production and platelet aggregation in diabetic subjects with clinical complications. *Thromb. Res.* 19:211–223, 1980.

15. Willerson J.T., Stone M.J., Ting R., et al.: Radioimmunoassay of creatine kinase-B isoenzyme in human sera: results in patients with acute myocardial infarction. *Proc. Natl. Acad. Sci. USA* 74:1711–1715, 1977.

16. Parkey R.W., Bonte F.J., Meyer S.L., Atkins J.M., Curry G.C., Willerson J.T.: A new method for radionuclide imaging of acute myocardial infarction in humans. *Circulation* 50:540–546, 1974.

17. Dray F., Charbonnel B., Maclouf J.: Radioimmunoassay of prostaglandins F_α, E_1, and E_2 in human plasma. *Eur. J. Clin. Invest.* 5:311–318, 1975.

18. Campbell W.B., Gomez-Sanchez C.E., Adams B.V.: Role of prostaglandin E_2 in angiotensin-induced aldosterone release. *Hypertension* 2:471–476, 1980.

19. Jaffe B.M., Behrman H.R.: Prostaglandins E, A, and F, in Jaffe B.M., Behrman H.R. (eds.): Methods of Hormone Radioimmunoassay. New York, Academic Press, 1974, pp. 19–34.

20. Zar J.H.: Biostatistical Analysis. Englewood Cliffs, N.J., Prentice-Hall, 1974, pp. 139–142.

21. Parker J.O., Chiong M.A., West R.O., Case R.B.: Sequential alterations in myocardial lactate metabolism, S-T segments, and left ventricular function during angina induced by atrial pacing. *Circulation* 40:113–131, 1969.

22. Oliva P.B., Brenkinridge J.C.: Arteriographic evidence of coronary arterial spasm in acute myocardial infarction. *Circulation* 56:366–374, 1977.

23. Maseri A., L'Abbate A., Baroldi G., et al.: Coronary vasospasm as a possible cause of myocardial infarction: a conclusion derived from the study of preinfarction angina. *N. Engl. J. Med.* 299:1271–1277, 1978.

24. Chierchia S., Brunelli C., Simonetti I., Lazzari M., Maseri A.: Sequence of events in angina at rest: primary reduction in coronary flow. *Circulation* 61:759–768, 1980.

25. Folts J.D., Crowell E.B. Jr., Rowe G.G.: Platelet aggregation in partially obstructed vessels and its elimination with aspirin. *Circulation* 54:365–370, 1976.

26. Aiken J.W., Gorman R.R., Shebuski R.J.: Prevention of blockage of partially obstructed coronary arteries with prostacyclin correlates with inhibition of platelet aggregation. *Prostaglandins* 17:483–494, 1979.

27. Neill W.A., Wharton T.P. Jr., Fluri-Lundeen J., Cohen I.S.: Acute coronary insufficiency—coronary occlusion after intermittent ischemic attacks. *N. Engl. J. Med.* 302:1157–1162, 1980.

28. Mehta J., Mehta P., Pepine C.J.: Platelet aggregation in aortic and coronary venous blood in patients with and without coronary disease. III.

Role of tachycardia stress and propranolol. *Circulation* 58:881–886, 1978.
29. Mehta P., Mehta J., Pepine C.J., Miale T.D., Burger C.: Platelet aggregation across the myocardial vascular bed in man. I. Normal versus diseased coronary arteries. *Thromb. Res.* 14:423–432, 1979.
30. Mehta J., Mehta P., Pepine C.J., Conti C.R.: Platelet function studies in coronary artery disease. VII. Effect of aspirin and tachycardia stress on aortic and coronary venous blood. *Am. J. Cardiol.* 45:945–951, 1980.
31. Haerem J.W.: Platelet aggregates in intramyocardial vessels of patients dying suddenly and unexpectedly of coronary artery disease. *Atherosclerosis* 15:199–213, 1972.
32. El-Maraghi N., Genton E.: The relevance of platelet and fibrin thromboembolism of the coronary microcirculation with special reference to sudden cardiac death. *Circulation* 62:936–944, 1980.
33. Moncada S., Gryglewski R., Bunting S., Vane J.R.: An enzyme isolated from arteries transforms prostaglandin endoperoxides to an unstable substance that inhibits platelet aggregation. *Nature* 263:663–665, 1976.
34. Moncada S., Gryglewski R.J., Bunting S., Vane J.R.: A lipid peroxide inhibits the enzyme in blood vessel microsomes that generates from prostaglandin endoperoxides the substance (prostaglandin X) which prevents platelet aggregation. *Prostaglandins* 12:715–737, 1976.
35. Moncada S., Higgs E.A., Vane J.R.: Human arterial and venous tissues generate prostacyclin (prostaglandin X) a potent inhibitor of platelet aggregation. *Lancet* I:18–20, 1977.
36. Oates J.A., Roberts L.J. II, Sweetnam B.J., Maas R.L., Gerkens J.F., Taber D.F.: Metabolism of the prostaglandins and thromboxanes, in Samuelsson B., Ramwell P.W., Paoletti R. (eds.): Advances in Prostaglandin and Thromboxane Research. New York, Raven Press, 1980, pp. 35–41.
37. Curwen K.D., Gimbrone M.A. Jr., Handin R.I.: In vitro studies of thromboresistance: the role of prostacyclin (PGI$_2$) in platelet adhesion to cultured normal and virally transformed human vascular endothelial cells. *Lab. Invest.* 42:366–374, 1980.
38. Jaffe E.A., Weksler B.B.: Recovery of endothelial cell prostacyclin production after inhibition by low doses of aspirin. *J. Clin. Invest.* 63:532–535, 1979.
39. Capurro N.L., Lipson L. C., Bonow R.O., Goldstein R.E., Shulman R., Epstein S.E.: Relative effects of aspirin on platelet aggregation and prostaglandin-mediated coronary vasodilatation in the dog. *Circulation* 62:1221–1227, 1980.
40. Preston F.E., Whipps S., Jackson C.A., French A.J., Wyld P.J., Stoddard C.J.: Inhibition of prostacyclin and platelet thromboxane A$_2$ after low-dose aspirin. *N. Engl. J. Med.* 304:76–79, 1981.

Prostaglandin E_1 in Ischemic Heart Failure: Demonstration of Salutary Actions on Myocardial Energetics and Ventricular Pump Performance

NAJAM A. AWAN, JAMES M. BEATTIE,
KATHLEEN E. NEEDHAM, MARK K. EVENSON,
DEAN T. MASON

*Section of Cardiovascular Medicine, Departments of
Medicine and Physiology, University of California at
Davis, School of Medicine and Sacramento Medical
Center, Davis and Sacramento, California*

Although sodium nitroprusside is regarded as the standard intravenous vasodilator for the vasodilator therapy of acute and chronic congestive heart failure,[1-6] the usefulness of this drug during active myocardial ischemia following acute myocardial infarction remains controversial.[7-9] Furthermore, increasing thiocyanate levels represent a persistent concern limiting the use of prolonged nitroprusside infusions.[10] Therefore, we evaluated cardiocirculatory actions of the vasodilator and platelet deaggregatory agent,[11, 12] prostaglandin E_1, by cardiac catheterization and forearm plethysmography in patients with extensive coronary artery disease and severe congestive heart failure.

Methods

All nine patients underwent right heart catheterization with placement of the balloon-tipped thermodilution Swan-Ganz catheter in the pulmonary artery for assessment of cardiac performance. Forearm plethysmography was performed in seven of these patients, using a mercury-filled rubber strain gauge placed around the mid-forearm as previously described.[6, 13] The study group comprised nine patients, seven males and two females, with a mean age of 54.6 years. All patients had previously demonstrated coronary artery disease with remote myocardial infarction (≥3 months) documented clinically, electrocardiographically, and angiographically. Patients with significant valvular heart disease were excluded from the study. All patients had severe congestive heart failure and were taking maximum doses of digoxin and diuretics.

After control hemodynamics and cardiac output were recorded and control forearm plethysmography was performed, prostaglandin E_1 (PGE_1) was gradually infused through a peripheral vein, starting at the low dose of 0.01 µg/kg and slowly titrating the dose upward in increments of 0.005/µg/kg under constant hemodynamic and electrocardiographic monitoring. Upward titration of PGE_1 was terminated and constant infusion rate was maintained when optimum hemodynamics ≥ 20% increase in cardiac output (CO) and/or ≥ 20% decline in left ventricular filling pressure (LVFP) were obtained. Following 15 minutes of this constant optimum dose PGE_1 infusion (mean dose 0.03 µg/kg), hemodynamics and cardiac output were again recorded and forearm plethysmography was repeated.

Results

CARDIAC EFFECTS

The control heart rate of 69 ± 2 bpm was unchanged by PGE_1, being 71 ± 1 bpm (p>0.05) during infusion of this drug. Mean systemic blood pressure was modestly reduced by PGE_1. The average MBP declined from the control of 85 ± 6 mmHg to 76 ± 5 mmHg (p< 0.025). A mild decline in this variable was noted in the majority of our heart failure patients. Additionally, the LV filling pressure of 19 ± 3 mmHg was reduced by PGE_1 to 15 ± 2 mmHg (p<0.01). This moderate reduction in LVFP was noted in seven of our nine patients.

The control index of 1.9 ± 0.2 L/min/M² was augmented by PGE_1 to 2.5 ± 0.2 (p<0.005). A marked increase in CI was seen in the majority of our patients, the average percent increase being 37%. Similarly, the stroke volume index of 28 ± 2.4 ml/beat/M² was elevated by PGE_1 to 35 ± 2.9 (p<0.01). Substantial increase in this index was also observed in most of the patients studied.

PGE_1 raised the stroke work index from 25 ± 4.3 to 30 ± 4.4

$gm/m/M^2$ (p<0.02), while total systemic vascular resistance declined from 1862 ± 192 to 1282 ± 100 $dynes/sec/cm^{-5}$ (p<0.02). The indirect index of myocardial oxygen consumption HR/SBP product, was reduced by PGE_1 from 9492 ± 666 to 8278 ± 493 mmHg/min (p<0.02), whereas the effective endocardial perfusion pressure (diastolic BP-LVFP), an index of myocardial perfusion, remained unchanged (control 47 ± 5, PGE_1 44 ± 5 mmHg; p>0.05). Thus, improvement in myocardial oxygenation likely occurred with PGE_1 infusion.

PERIPHERAL CIRCULATORY ACTIONS

Forearm blood flow (FBF) was raised by PGE_1 from 2.5 ± 0.5 to 3.4 ± 0.5 ml/100 gm/min (p<0.05), and forearm vascular resistance was reduced by PGE_1 from 36.1 ± 5.3 to 23.7 ± 3.7 mmHg/ml/100 gm/min (p<0.02), but forearm venous tone remained unchanged (control 18.8 ± 2.9, PGE_1 20.1 ±3.1 mmHg/ml; p>0.05).

Discussion

This investigation of the hemodynamic actions of prostaglandin E_1 clearly demonstrated that this agent markedly augments cardiac performance in patients with severe chronic congestive heart failure. Moreover, this enhancement in cardiac performance was accomplished with improved myocardial oxygenation, since the double product diminished while myocardial perfusion was maintained. Additionally PGE_1 raised myocardial pump efficiency as increased ventricular work was performed with less oxygen requirement. Further, this impressive modulation of cardiac function coincided with simultaneous concordant beneficial modification of peripheral circulatory function of reduced vascular resistance and enhanced peripheral blood flow.

These salutary improvements in cardiac function were probably produced by the vascular relaxing actions of the prostaglandin E_1 on the arteriolar resistance bed.[11] Thus, decreased left ventricular output impedance facilitated cardiac emptying, augmenting the ejection fraction and raising the cardiac output. Further enhancement in cardiac contractility, while possible,[14] probably represents a less important mechanism for the marked augmentation of ventricular pump output observed in our patients with severe congestive heart failure. It is likely that the modest decline in left ventricular filling pressure noted in our patients during PGE_1 infusion reflects an indirect effect of the enhanced left ventricular ejection fraction. Additionally, relief of myocardial ischemia in our coronary heart failure patients may have improved ventricular compliance contributing to the observed fall in the elevated left ventricular filling pressure. Importantly, our observation of no significant relaxing effects of prostaglandin E_1 on the systemic capacitance bed is consistent with the moderate decrease in ventricular preload observed in this study. Further, prostaglandin E_1 may have possibly caused marked venodilation in certain peripheral vascular beds, thereby modestly lowering the abnormally elevated ventricular preload in our severe heart failure patients.

Accordingly, the careful use of modest doses of prostaglandin E_1 in patients with marked left ventricular dysfunction caused by severe coronary heart disease may produce a marked augmentation of cardiac performance. Thus, our results indicate that prostaglandin E_1 may be beneficial for the vasodilator therapy of acute and chronic severe left ventricular dysfunction in coronary patients following myocardial infarction.

ACKNOWLEDGMENTS

This work was supported in part by Program Project Grant HL-14780 from the National Heart, Lung and Blood Institute, National Institutes of Health, and by research grants from the California chapters of the American Heart Association.

REFERENCES

1. Majid P.A., Sharma B., Taylor S.H.: Phentolamine for vasodilator treatment of severe heart failure. *Lancet* 2:719–724, 1971.
2. Franciosa J.A., Guiha, N.H., Limas C.J., Rodriguera E., Cohn J.N.: Improved ventricular function during nitroprusside infusion in acute myocardial infarction. *Lancet* 1:650–654, 1972.
3. Chatterjee K., Parmley W.W., Ganz W., Forrester J., Walinsky P., Crexells C., Swan H.J.C.: Hemodynamic and metabolic responses to vasodilator therapy in acute myocardial infarction. *Circulation* 48:1183–1193, 1973.
4. Chatterjee K., Parmley W.W., Swan H.J.C., Berman G., Forrester J., Marcus H.S.: Beneficial effects of vasodilator agents in severe mitral regurgitation due to dysfunction of the subvalvular apparatus. *Circulation* 48:684–690, 1973.
5. Miller R.R., Vismara L.A., Zelis R., Amsterdam E.A., Mason D.T.: Clinical use of sodium nitroprusside in chronic heart disease. *Circulation* 51:328–336, 1975.
6. Miller R.R., Vismara L.A., Williams D.O., Amsterdam E.A., Mason D.T.: Pharmacological mechanisms for left ventricular unloading in clinical congestive heart failure: Differential effects of nitroprusside, phentolamine and nitroglycerin on cardiac function and peripheral circulation. *Circ. Res.* 39:127–133, 1976.

7. DaLuz P.L., Forrester J.S., Wyatt H.L., Tyberg J.V., Chagrasulis R., Parmley W.W., Swan H.J.C.: Hemodynamic and metabolic effects of sodium nitroprusside on the performance and metabolism of regional ischemic myocardium. *Circulation* 52:400–407, 1975.

8. Awan N.A., Miller R.R., Vera Z., DeMaria A.N., Amsterdam E.A., Mason D.T.: Reduction of ST elevation with infusion of nitroprusside, in patients with acute myocardial infarction. *Am. J. Cardiol.* 38:435–439, 1976.

9. Chiarello M., Gold H.K., Leinbach R.C., Davis M.A., Maroko P.R.: Comparison between the effects of nitroprusside and nitroglycerin on ischemic injury during acute myocardial infarction. *Circulation* 54:766–773, 1976.

10. Boguez M., Maroz J., Karski J., Gierz J., Regiel A., Witrowska R., Golabek A.: Blood cyanide and thiocyanate level after therapeutic application of sodium nitroprusside. *Vet. Hum. Toxicol.* 21:66–67, 1979.

11. Gorman R.R.: Prostaglandins, Thromboxones and Prostacyclin, in Rickenberg H.V. (ed.): *Biochemistry and Mode of Action of Hormones II, Volume 20.* Baltimore, University Park Press, 1978, pp. 81–107.

12. Needleman P., Kaley G.: Medical progress: Cardiac and coronary prostaglandin synthesis and function. *N. Engl. J. Med.* 298:1122–1128, 1978.

13. Mason D.T., Braunwald E.: A simplified plethysmographic system for the measurement of systemic arterial pressure and peripheral blood flow. *Am. Heart J.* 64:796–804, 1962.

14. Solotkoff L.M., Angerio A.D., Kot P.A., Rose J.D.: Effect of PGA_1, nitroprusside, and diazoxide on myocardial contractility. *J. Cardiovasc. Pharmacol.* 1:245–252, 1979.

Prostaglandin E_1 Therapy in Unstable Angina Pectoris

MARK NEMEROVSKI AND WILLIAM E. SHELL

Division of Cardiology, Department of Medicine,
Cedars-Sinai Medical Center, UCLA School of
Medicine, Los Angeles, California

Introduction

The incidence of complete occlusion of a coronary artery by thrombus in the first several hours following acute transmural myocardial infarction approaches 80% to 90%.[1] However, autopsy studies have demonstrated complete coronary occlusion in less than 50% of patients dying with recent unstable angina pectoris or nontransmural myocardial infarction.[1-3] Coronary arteriography in patients with unstable angina demonstrates a high incidence of subtotal occlusion, which tends to progress to complete occlusion over time.[4] Several authors have proposed that the acute myocardial ischemic syndromes in man, other than transmural myocardial infarction, may be initiated by reversible intermittent coronary obstruction rather than thrombus formation.[5]

The syndrome of rest angina appears to occur without any antecedent change in the determinants of myocardial oxygen demand, implying that the pathophysiology of this syndrome involves a primary reduction in myocardial oxygen supply.[6] Maseri and colleagues studied 76 patients with rest angina, and consistently observed coronary vasospasm and reduction in myocardial blood flow during anginal episodes.[7] These findings were independent of the severity of coronary atherosclerosis and independent of whether the episodes of rest pain were associated with ST segment depression or elevation. None of the episodes was preceded by an increase in hemodynamic indices of myocardial oxygen demand.

The initiation of acute ischemic syndromes can be conveniently depicted as a "teeter-totter" representing the relationship between myocardial oxygen supply and demand (Fig 26–1). Nonischemic intervals are characterized by a balance between the two. Either decreased supply (second panel in figure) or increased demand (third panel) can shift the balance towards ischemia. Most cases of unstable angina pectoris, particularly rest angina, reflect acute reduction in oxygen supply (second panel) rather than abrupt increase in demand.

Several pathophysiologic mechanisms have been proposed to explain the genesis of angina. Experimental studies suggest that phasic platelet aggregation at the site of a subtotal occlusion may be responsible for acute ischemic syndromes.[8–10] This work has been supported by various studies which have demonstrated enhanced platelet aggregability[11–15] and release of platelet-specific proteins[16–18] in patients with ischemic heart disease. Intramyocardial platelet aggregation has been associated with sudden death in patients with coronary disease, but without thrombotic occlusion.[19–21]

Other observations favor a "spasm" theory for reduced coronary blood flow. In angiographic and hemodynamic studies, Oliva,[22] Maseri,[7] and others[23] have demonstrated a primary increase in coronary arterial tone (spasm) in patients with Prinzmetal's and other forms of rest angina. Although certain authors have expressed reservations regarding the contribution of altered vascular tone to the angiographic findings,[24] the predominant opinion is that coronary arterial spasm is a real and not uncommon phenomenon. In addition, in our laboratory, we have measured coronary blood flow by the continuous thermodilution technique in several patients with unstable angina associated with ST depression.[25] We have observed a primary in-

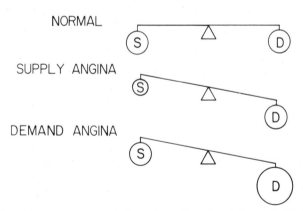

Fig 26–1.—Schematic representation of supply *(S)* and demand *(D)* forms of angina pectoris.

crease in coronary vascular resistance preceding spontaneous episodes of rest angina in these patients (unpublished observations).

Role of Prostaglandins

Since prostaglandins and thromboxanes are ubiquitous natural compounds which have both potent vasoactive and platelet-active properties,[26] several investigators have argued that coronary vascular tone may be modulated by the local balance between prostacyclin and thromboxane A_2.[27] Further, it has been proposed that an imbalance in this regulatory system may induce or modify coronary vasospasm and/or intracoronary platelet aggregation, leading to an acute ischemic crisis.[28]

Several lines of evidence implicate the prostaglandin-thromboxane system in the pathophysiology of ischemic heart disease in man. Prostacyclin (PGI_2) has potent effects on relaxation of vascular smooth muscle, including that of coronary arteries,[29] and is the most potent inhibitor of platelet aggregation yet discovered.[30] Further, prostacyclin is the predominant metabolite of arachidonic acid released from the isolated, perfused heart.[31] Thromboxane A_2 (TXA_2), which is synthesized by aggregated platelets, can be considered a physiologic antagonist to prostacyclin. Although the effects of TXA_2 in the intact coronary circulation have not yet been reported, it has potent vasoconstrictive effects on coronary arteries in vitro,[32] and can initiate and promote platelet aggregation.[24]

In patients with variant angina, thromboxane B_2 (the major stable metabolite of TXA_2) is released into the coronary sinus after two to three minutes of spontaneous ischemia, reaching its highest concentration some several minutes after resolution of the ST segment elevation.[35, 36] Markedly elevated plasma concentrations of thromboxane B_2[37–39] and urinary levels of dinorthromboxane A_2[35] have been reported in these patients.

Enhanced thromboxane A_2 production has also been associated with typical spontaneous rest angina associated with ST segment depression. Increased coronary sinus concentrations of TXB_2 have been found in these patients within 24 hours of the last episode of chest pain, but inconsistently when measured later.[39] Plasma levels of malondialdehyde (another stable metabolite of TXA_2) are also elevated.[40] Platelets isolated from these patients are hyperaggregable, and the amount of prostacyclin necessary to inhibit aggregation is highest during an acute anginal episode.[40]

Rapid atrial pacing to angina threshold in patients with angiographically proven coronary arterial stenoses results in significant increases in arterial and coronary sinus levels of thromboxane B_2, which return to control levels after ten minutes.[41] In this study, release of TXB_2 followed a similar time course to myocardial lactate production, and was not found when ischemia was not evoked. These results have recently been confirmed.[37]

Thus, the foregoing data support the hypothesis that local thromboxane A_2 production, presumably through potent arterial vasoconstriction and/or platelet aggregation, may play a pathophysiologic role in myocardial ischemia associated with both supply and demand angina.

Although prostacyclin and thromboxane A_2 are the most potent products of arachidonic acid metabolism, several other vasoactive metabolites have been reported. Based on the currently available evidence, a theoretical schema for the regulation of coronary vascular tone can be developed. Such a formulation is depicted in Figure 26–2.

According to this model, arachidonic acid is enzymatically cleaved from membrane lipoproteins in response to some stimulus, perhaps mechanical membrane deformation. Arachidonic acid then provides

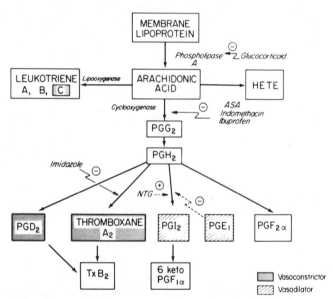

Fig 26–2.—The arachidonic acid cascade. Vasoconstricting compounds are denoted by solid shading and vasodilating compounds by cross-hatching. Enzyme inhibition is represented by ⊖ and potentiation by ⊕. The dashed lines are theoretical.

the substrate for synthesis of a variety of vasoactive derivatives. Among these compounds, thromboxane A_2, prostaglandin D_2, and leukotriene C have vasoconstrictive and proaggregatory properties, whereas prostacyclin and prostaglandin E_1 (Aprostadil) cause vasodilation and disaggregation. The concept of coronary vasoregulation as a teeter-totter balance between prostacyclin and thromboxane A_2 is obviously simplistic. Coronary vascular homeostasis is a complex biologic phenomenon that depends not only on an interplay among these several vasoactive humoral factors, but on poorly understood neural influences and calcium-dependent metabolic factors as well.

Pharmacologic Approaches

According to Figure 26–2, there are several sites at which pharmacologic therapy in ischemic heart disease can be directed. Inhibition of the pathway prior to biosynthesis of the cyclic endoperoxides PGG_2 and PGH_2 is illogical because synthesis of *both* vasodilating and vasoconstricting compounds will be inhibited in a nonselective way. Inhibition of cyclo-oxygenase by aspirin (noncompetitive) and sulfinpyrazone (competitive) have been generally disappointing in the secondary prevention of myocardial infarction.[42–49] Aspirin even in low doses inhibits both prostacyclin and TXA_2 production,[50, 51] although recovery of PGI_2 synthesis after withdrawal of the drug may precede recovery of TXA_2 synthesis.[52, 53] Ibuprofen and indomethacin have been demonstrated to actually antagonize the effects of nitroglycerin in vitro and in vivo.[54, 55]

Pharmacologic antianginal therapy can be more logically directed in the arachidonic acid cascade "distal to" the synthesis of the cyclic endoperoxides. Selective inhibition of the thromboxane synthetase is the most attractive possibility. Such an approach seems feasible since analogues of imidazole and thromboxane A_2[56, 57] appear to selectively inhibit production of thromboxane A_2. In animal models, 1-benzylimidazole prevents platelet accumulation on a de-endothelialized aortic wall, but only at doses much higher than those required to inhibit thromboxane synthetase.[58] Infusion of imidazole begun 30 minutes after experimental coronary artery occlusion in cats inhibited the rise in plasma thromboxane B_2 levels, decreased infarct size as estimated by ST segment elevation and CK curves, and significantly reduced the loss in myocardial CK and amino-nitrogen.[59] Pinane-thromboxane A_2 inhibits thromboxane synthesis, platelet aggregation, and coronary artery constriction induced by prostaglandin endoperoxide analogues.[57] Unfortunately, there are no currently available selective inhibitors of thromboxane synthetase for human use.

A second useful pharmacologic approach to the ischemic syndrome might be to administer certain prostaglandins or their analogues in an attempt to alter the local balance in favor of vasodilatation and platelet disaggregation. Logical choices for such therapy would be prostaglandin I_2 (prostacyclin) and prostaglandin E_1 (alprostadil), which are stable products and currently available for experimental use.

These agents have been shown in man to inhibit platelet aggregation at low doses,[30, 60] and hemodynamic studies confirm potent peripheral[26] and coronary[29, 61] vasodilator activity. Prostacyclin is about ten times more potent than alprostadil in both effects, but unfortunately can cause significant hypotension and reflex tachycardia.[62] Alprostadil appears to produce a significant reduction in peripheral vascular resistance without demonstrable changes in heart rate.[63] Although reported side-effects below 100 ng/kg/min include facial and generalized flushing, abdominal cramps, nausea, and headache, these symptoms are rare below 50 ng/kg/min.[64] Doses as high as 700 ng/kg/min have been administered without untoward effect,[65] and infusion has been continued as long as 4.5 months without apparent adverse effect.[66]

Several studies have suggested a role for prostacyclin in the preservation of ischemic myocardium following experimental coronary artery occlusion.[67-69] However, few studies have addressed its potential in unstable angina pectoris or nontransmural infarction. Infusion of prostacyclin can prevent thrombosis at the site of electrically induced coronary endothelial damage[70] and can prevent the phasic flow changes and subsequent occlusion induced by experimental subtotal coronary obstruction.[71] Inhibition of occlusion appears to correlate with inhibition of platelet aggregation, and can be achieved by local application of PGI_2 in doses small enough not to cause systemic effects.[71]

Unfortunately, prostacyclin induces profound systemic hemodynamic effects even at extremely low doses. Adverse effects on the myocardial oxygen supply/demand ratio associated with hypotension and tachycardia may preclude the general application of this agent to patients with ischemic heart disease.

In the few studies in which it has been used, the clinical data are conflicting. In one study of 12 patients with demand angina, PGI_2 decreased coronary vascular resistance but decreased blood pressure and increased heart rate significantly.[72] Platelet aggregation was inhibited, anginal threshold to atrial pacing was increased, and myocardial lactate metabolism at peak heart rate improved. Yet, in another group of 7 patients, infusion of PGI_2 at the same dose had no effect on angina induced by atrial pacing.[73]

The data are inconsistent for supply angina as well. One study found a salutory response on frequency of anginal attacks and nitroglycerin consumption,[73] whereas another study found no significant difference in number, duration, or severity of ischemic events.[74] These conflicting results may reflect variable effects on heart rate and coronary perfusion pressure induced by even small doses of prostacyclin.

Effects of Prostaglandin E₁ on Unstable Angina

Prostaglandin E_1 appears to induce somewhat less tachycardia than prostacyclin, even with comparable reduction in systemic vascular resistance. Intracoronary infusion of PGE_1 at doses too small to have important systemic effects results in significant coronary vasodilatation.[75]

Figure 26–3 demonstrates the angiographic effects of a 10 μg bolus injection of PGE_1 into the left anterior descending coronary artery of a normal dog. There was a 15% increase in luminal diameter as well as clearly improved visualization of several side branches. These angiographic findings were not the result of increased coronary perfusion pressure, since a 10% reduction in mean arterial blood pressure was observed. Dilatation of the larger caliber vessels seen with PGE_1 is similar to that seen with nitroglycerin. This finding is important, since agents that dilate only small caliber resistance arterioles may theoretically lead to so-called "coronary steal."[76]

Figure 26–4 presents the hemodynamic effects of intravenous prostaglandin E_1 in six patients with unstable angina pectoris. Following control hemodynamic measurements in the supine position, PGE_1 was administered by central vein at an initial dose of 10 ng/kg/min. After 15 minutes of infusion, hemodynamic measurements were recorded. The infusion rate was then doubled to 20 ng/kg/min, and once again hemodynamic variables were measured after 15 minutes. As shown in Figure 26–4, there was a dose-dependent decrease in systolic arterial pressure and an increase in cardiac index associated with a decrease in systemic vascular resistance. Of particular note, there was no demonstrable change in the heart rate at these doses. Thus, the increase in cardiac output was due to an increase in stroke volume without an associated change in heart rate.

Coronary blood flow was measured by the continuous thermodilu-

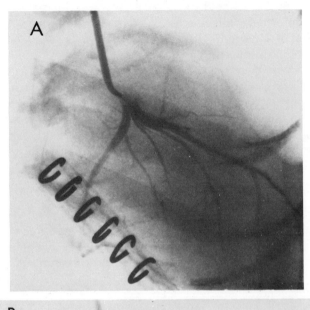

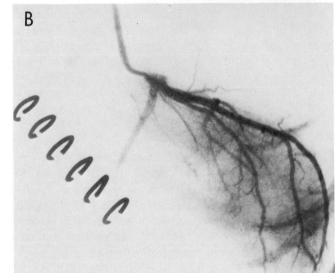

Fig 26–3.—Angiographic demonstration of coronary vasodilation following intracoronary prostaglandin E_1 administration. **A,** coronary angiogram taken under control conditions in a normal dog. **B,** angiogram performed immediately following a 10-μg intracoronary bolus injection of PGE_1.

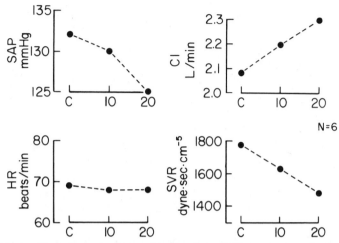

Fig 26–4.—Hemodynamic effects of intravenous PGE_1 in six patients with unstable angina pectoris. Values on the abscissa represent control, 10, and 20 ng/kg/min PGE_1. SAP = systolic arterial pressure (mmHg); CI = cardiac index (L/min/m²); HR = heart rate (beats/min); SVR = systemic vascular resistance (dyne-sec-cm⁻⁵).

tion technique in several of these patients.[25] At the same dosage levels as shown in Figure 26–4, there were significant increases in coronary blood flow associated with a decrease as much as 25% in coronary vascular resistance. These salutory hemodynamic effects (decreased systemic vascular and coronary vascular resistance, increase in cardiac output and coronary blood flow, no change in heart rate) should theoretically be useful in the amelioration of the ischemic process in patients with unstable angina.

Similar to prostacyclin, infusion of PGE_1 has been demonstrated to limit infarct size in experimental coronary artery occlusion in cats[77] and dogs,[78] and may lower the fibrillation threshold to acute ischemia.[78] It is particularly interesting that reduction of infarct size by PGE_1 appears to correlate with increased collateral flow to ischemic myocardium rather than with reduction in the rate-pressure product.[80] In preliminary studies in our animal laboratory, we have also found a limitation in anatomic infarct size following occlusion of the left anterior descending coronary artery in dogs when an infusion of PGE_1 was begun 10 minutes after the occlusion. Two-dimensional echocardiography in these animals has shown improvement in segmental contraction in the ischemic peri-infarction zones.

No careful studies regarding the potential use of PGE_1 in unstable angina pectoris in man have been reported. In an experimental model, however, an orally effective derivative of PGE_1 caused significant inhibition of platelet adhesiveness and suppressed ST segment depression induced by vasopressin in rats.[81]

We have infused PGE_1 by central vein in nine patients with unstable angina pectoris refractory to intravenous nitroglycerin and oral propranolol therapy. Although it appears that coronary effects may occur without important systemic effects, in this study we increased the infusion rate of prostaglandin E_1 in an incremental fashion until there was a 10% decrease in systolic blood pressure or 10% increase in heart rate. In all patients, the decrement in blood pressure was achieved without a significant effect on heart rate. In this group of patients, clinical efficacy in terms of reduction of anginal episodes was variable. However, in four patients with frequent recurrent rest pain refractory to intravenous nitroglycerin there was a dramatic reduction in the frequency of anginal attacks and in the frequency of associated elevations in pulmonary capillary wedge pressure.

The clinical response in one of these patients is shown in Figure 26–5. As is shown in the figure, this patient had frequent episodes of rest pain for the 60 hours prior to PGE_1 infusion. On day three, PGE_1 infusion was begun and titrated to a hemodynamic end point as described above. Intravenous nitroglycerin was discontinued. Over the subsequent 48 hours, the patient experienced complete abolition of recurrent chest pain. The infusion was discontinued on day five, and a single discrete episode of chest pain occurred approximately eight hours after discontinuation of the drug. This episode responded to single sublingual nitroglycerin tablet. On day six, chest pain recurred, but was less intense and less frequent compared to the pretreatment levels.

Following this experience, we have begun to administer oral antiplatelet agents during the last 24 hours of prostaglandin infusion and

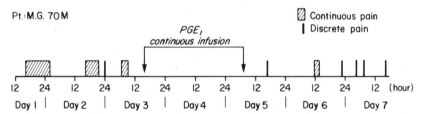

Fig 26–5.—Clinical efficacy of intravenous PGE_1 infusion in a patient with unstable angina pectoris refractory to maximal beta-blockade and intravenous nitroglycerin administration. Note the complete abolition of chest pain during PGE_1 infusion and the reduction in frequency and severity of anginal attacks after discontinuation of the PGE_1.

continue them when the infusion is discontinued. With this regimen, we have had encouraging clinical responses in several patients. The reasons for the unpredictable clinical effectiveness of PGE_1 infusion is not clear at this time. However, variability of response may reflect actual differences in the pathophysiologic mechanisms responsible for chest pain in these patients.

Summary

Abundant theoretical, experimental, and clinical data suggest that pharmacologic manipulation of the prostaglandin-thromboxane system might provide a powerful and clinically useful method for improving the natural history of acute myocardial ischemic syndromes. Prostaglandin E_1 infusion appears to be an attractive treatment option in patients with unstable angina pectoris. The drug has been shown to have salutory hemodynamic and clinical effects in this group of patients, and warrants further serious investigation in this regard.

REFERENCES

1. DeWood M.A., Spores J., Notske R., Mouser L.T., Burroughs R., Golden M.S., Lang H.T.: Prevalence of total coronary occlusion during the early hours of transmural myocardial infarction. *N. Engl. J. Med.* 303:897, 1980.
2. Chapman I.: The cause-effect relationship between recent coronary artery occlusion and acute myocardial infarction. *Am. Heart J.* 87:267, 1974.
3. Blumgart H.L., Schlesinger M.T., Davis D.: Studies on the relation of the clinical manifestations of angina pectoris, coronary thrombosis, and myocardial infarction to the pathologic findings. *Am. Heart J.* 19:1, 1940.
4. Neill W.A., Sharton T.P. Jr., Fluri-Lundeen J.F., Cohen I.S.: Acute coronary insufficiency—coronary occlusion after intermittent ischemic attacks. *N. Engl. J. Med.* 302:1157, 1980.
5. Neil W.A., Ritzmann L.W., Selden R.: The pathophysiologic basis of acute coronary insufficiency: observations favoring the hypothesis of intermittent reversible coronary obstruction. *Am. Heart J.* 94:439, 1977.
6. Chierchia S., Brunelli C., Simonetti I., Lazzari M., Maseri A.: Sequence of events in angina at rest: primary reduction in coronary flow. *Circulation* 61:759, 1980.
7. Maseri A. et al.: Coronary vasospasm as a possible cause of myocardial infarction: a conclusion derived from the study of "preinfarction" angina. *N. Engl. J. Med.* 299:1271, 1978.
8. Folts J.D., Crowell E.B., Rowe G.G.: Platelet aggregation in partially obstructed vessels and its elimination with aspirin. *Circulation* 54:365, 1976.
9. Folts J.D., Rowe G.G.: Platelet aggregation in stenosed coronaries: mechanism of sudden death? *Am. J. Cardiol.* 41:425, 1978. (Abstract)

10. Uchida Y., Yoshimoto N., Murao S.: Cyclic fluctuation in coronary blood pressure and flow induced by coronary artery constriction. *Jap. Heart J.* 16:454, 1975.
11. Schwartz M.B., Hawiger J., Timmons S., Friesinger G.C.: Platelet aggregates in ischaemic heart disease. *Thromb. Haemost.* 43:185, 1980.
12. Mehta J. et al.: Platelet aggregation in aortic and coronary venous blood in patients with and without coronary disease. 3. Role of tachycardia stress and propranolol. *Circulation* 58:881, 1978.
13. Mehta J., Mehta P.: Increased platelet prostaglandin generation and abnormal platelet sensitivity to prostacyclin and thromboxane A_2 in angina pectoris. *Am. J. Cardiol.* 45:454, 1980. (Abstract)
14. Salky N., Dugdale M.: Platelet abnormalities in ischemic heart disease. *Am. J. Cardiol.* 32:612, 1973.
15. Wu K.K., Hoak J.C.: A new method for the quantitative detection of platelet aggregates in patients with arterial insufficiency. *Lancet* II:924, 1974.
16. Sobel M., Salzman E.W., Davies G.C. et al.: Circulatory platelet products in unstable angina pectoris. *Circulation* 63:300, 1981.
17. Handin R.I., McDonough M., Lesch M.: Elevation of platelet factor four in acute myocardial infarction. *J. Lab. Clin. Med.* 91:340, 1978.
18. Denham M.J., Fischer M., James G. et al.: β-thromboglobulin and heparin-neutralising activity test in clinical conditions. *Lancet* I:1153, 1977.
19. El-Maraghi N., Genton E.: The relevance of platelet and fibrin thromboembolism of the coronary microcirculation, with special reference to sudden cardiac death. *Circulation* 62:936, 1980.
20. Haerem J.W.: Mural platelet microthrombi and major acute lesions of main epicardial arteries in sudden death. *Atherosclerosis* 19:529, 1974.
21. Haerem J.W.: Platelet aggregates in intramyocardial vessels of patients dying suddenly and unexpectedly of coronary artery disease. *Atherosclerosis* 15:199, 1972.
22. Oliva P.V., Potts D.E., Pluss R.G.: Coronary arterial spasm in Prinzmetal angina: documentation by coronary arteriography. *N. Engl. J. Med.* 288:745, 1973.
23. Guazzi M., Polese A., Fiorentini C., Magrini F., Bartorelli C.: Left ventricular performance and related hemodynamic changes in Prinzmetal's variant angina pectoris. *Br. Heart J.* 33:84, 1971.
24. Ganz W.: Coronary spasm in myocardial infarction: fact or fiction? *Circulation* 63:487, 1981. (Editorial)
25. Ganz W., Tamura K., Marcus H.S. et al.: Measurement of coronary sinus blood flow by continuous thermodilution. *Circulation* 44:181, 1971.
26. Dusting G.J., Moncada S., Vane J.R.: Prostaglandins, their intermediates and precursors: cardiovascular actions and regulatory roles in normal and abnormal circulatory systems. *Progr. Cardiovasc. Dis.* 21:405, 1979.
27. Needleman P., Kulkarni P.S., Raz A.: Coronary tone modulation: formation and action of prostaglandins, endoperoxides and thromboxanes. *Science* 195:409, 1977.
28. Borer J.S.: Unstable angina: a lethal gun with an invisible trigger. *N. Engl. J. Med.* 302:1200, 1980.
29. Dusting G.J., Moncada S., Vane J.R.: Prostacyclin (PGX) is the endogenous metabolite responsible for relaxation of coronary arteries induced by arachidonic acid. *Prostaglandins* 13:3, 1977.

30. Moncada S., Vane J.R.: Pharmacology and endogenous roles of prostaglandin endoperoxides, thromboxane A_2, and prostacyclin. *Pharmacol. Rev.* 30:293, 1979.

31. de Deckere E.A.M., Nugteren D.H., Ten Hoor F.: Prostacyclin is the major prostaglandin released from the isolated perfused rabbit and rat heart. *Nature* 268:160, 1977.

32. Ellis E.F., Oelz O., Roberts L.J. et al.: Coronary arterial smooth muscle contraction by a substance released from platelets: evidence that it is thromboxane A_2. *Science* 193:1135, 1976.

33. Needleman P., Minkes M., Ray A.: Thromboxanes: selective biosynthesis and distinct biological properties. *Science* 193:163, 1976.

34. Hamberg M., Svensson J., Samuelsson B.: Thromboxanes: a new group of biologically active compounds derived from prostaglandin endoperoxides. *Proc. Natl. Acad. Sci. USA* 72:2994–2998, 1975.

35. Robertson R.M., Robertson D., Roberts L.J., Maas R.L., Fitzgerald G.A., Friesinger G.C., Oates J.A.: Thromboxane A_2 in vasotonic angina pectoris: evidence from direct measurements and inhibitor trials. *N. Engl. J. Med.* 304:998, 1981.

36. Lewy R.I., Wiener L., Smith J.B., Walinsky P., Silver M.J., Saia J.: Comparison of plasma concentrations of thromboxane B_2 in Prinzmetal's variant angina and classical angina pectoris. *Clin. Cardiol.* 2:404, 1979.

37. Kuzuya T., Tada M., Inoue M. et al.: Increased levels of thromboxane A_2 in peripheral and coronary circulation in patients with angina pectoris. *Am. J. Cardiol.* 45:454, 1980.

38. Lewy R.I., Smith J.B., Silver M.J., Walinsky P., Wiener L.: Detection of thromboxane B_2 (TB_2) in peripheral blood of patients with Prinzmetal's angina. *Clin. Res.* 27:426A, 1979.

39. Lewy R.I. et al.: Prostacyclin: a potentially valuable agent for preserving patients with Prinzmetal's angina. *Prostaglandins Med.* 2:243, 1979.

40. Mehta J., Mehta P.: Increased platelet prostaglandin generation and abnormal platelet sensitivity to prostacyclin and thromboxane A_2 in angina pectoris. *Am. J. Cardiol.* 45:454, 1980.

41. Lewy R.I., Wiener L., Walinsky P., Lefer A.M., Silver M.J., Smith J.B.: Thromboxane release during pacing-induced angina pectoris: possible vasoconstrictor influence on the coronary vasculature. *Circulation* 61:1165, 1980.

42. McNicol G.P.: Antiplatelet drugs in the secondary prevention of myocardial infarction. *Lancet* II:736, 1980.

43. Elwood P.C., Cochrane A.C., Burr M.I. et al.: A randomized controlled trial of acetyl salicyclic acid in the secondary prevention of mortality after myocardial infarction. *Lancet* I:436, 1974.

44. Elwood P.C., Sweetnam P.M.: Aspirin and secondary mortality after myocardial infarction. *Lancet* II:1313, 1979.

45. Aspirin Myocardial Infarction Research Group: A randomized controlled trial of aspirin in persons recovered from myocardial infarction. *J.A.M.A.* 243:661, 1980.

46. Persantine-aspirin Reinfarction Study Research Group: Persantine and aspirin in coronary heart disease. *Circulation* 62:449, 1980.

47. Anturane Reinfarction Trial Research Group: Sulfinpyrazone in the prevention of sudden death after myocardial infarction. *N. Engl. J. Med.* 302:250, 1980.

48. Breddin K., Loew D., Lechner K., Uberla K., Walter E.: Secondary prevention of myocardial infarction: a comparison of acetylsalicylic acid, phenprocoumon and placebo. *Haemostatis* (in press).
49. Mitchell J.R.A.: Secondary prevention of myocardial infarction. *Br. Med. J.* 280:1128, 1980.
50. Preston F.E., Whipps S., Jackson C.A., French A.J., Wyld P.J., Stoddard C.K.: Inhibition of prostacyclin and platelet thromboxane A_2 after low-dose aspirin. *N. Engl. J. Med.* 304:76, 1981.
51. Capurro N.L., Lipson L.C., Bonow R.O., Goldstein R.E., Shulman N.R., Epstein S.E.: Relative effects of aspirin on platelet aggregation and prostaglandin-mediated coronary vasodilatation in the dog. *Circulation* 62:1221, 1980.
52. Masotti G., Galanti G., Poggesi L., Abbate R., Neri Sierneri G.G.: Differential inhibition of prostacyclin production and platelet aggregation by aspirin. *Lancet* II:1213, 1979.
53. Jaffe E.A., Weksler B.B.: Recovery of endothelial cell prostacyclin production after inhibition by low doses of aspirin. *J. Clin. Invest.* 63:532, 1979.
54. Anderson G.H. Jr., Hueber P., Sterling C., Tivnan E., Shroeder E.T.: Effect of nitroglycerin on prostacyclin production in rat aorta. *Circulation* 62(suppl III):326, 1980.
55. Van Dusen J., Fischl S.J.: Inhibition of nitroglycerin effect in humans by suppression of prostaglandin E. *Am. J. Cardiol.* 47:390, 1981.
56. Moncada S., Bunting S., Mullane K.M. et al.: Imidazole: a selective potent antagonist of thromboxane synthetase. *Prostaglandins* 13:611, 1977.
57. Nicolaou K.C., Magolda R.L., Smith J.B., Aharony D., Smith E.F., Lefer A.M.: Synthesis and biological properties of pinane-thromboxane A_2, a selective inhibitor of coronary artery constriction, platelet aggregation, and thromboxane formation. *Biochemistry* 76:2566, 1979.
58. Wu K.K., Chen Y.C., Fordham E., Raydidu G., Tsao C.H.: Effect of I-benzylimidazole on platelet-vessel wall (P-V) interaction in vivo. *Circulation* 62(suppl III):336, 1980. (Abstract)
59. Smith E.F. III, Lefer A.M., Smith B.J.: Influence of thromboxane inhibition on the severity of myocardial ischemia in cats. *Can. J. Pharmacol.* 58:294, 1980.
60. Elkeles R.S., Hampton J.R., Harrison M.J.G., Mitchell J.R.A.: Prostaglandin E₁ and human platelets. *Lancet* I:111, 1969.
61. Bloor C.M., White F.C., Sobel B.E.: Coronary and systemic haemodynamic effects of prostaglandins in the unanaesthetized dog. *Cardiovasc. Res.* 7:156, 1973.
62. Chierchia S., Crea F., Bernini W., et al.: Effects of prostacyclin (PGI₂) continuous infusion in angina at rest. *Circulation* 62(suppl III):310, 1980. (Abstract)
63. Popat K.D., Pitt B.: Prostaglandin E₁ infusion in acute myocardial infarction with left ventricular dysfunction. (abstr submitted) American Society for Clinical Investigation
64. Carlson L.A., Ekelund L., Oro L.: Clinical and metabolic effects of different doses of prostaglandin E₁ in man. *Acta Med. Scand.* 183:423, 1968.
65. Bergstrom S., Duner H., Euler U.S. von, et al.: Observations on the effects of infusion of prostaglandin E in man. *Acta Physiol. Scand.* 45:145, 1959.

66. Pitlick P., French J.W., Maze A., et al.: Long-term low-dose prostaglandin E₁ administration. (In press)
67. Ogletree M.L., Lefer A.M., Smith J.B., Nicolaou K.C.: Studies on the protective effect of prostacyclin in acute myocardial ischemia. *Eur. J. Pharmacol.* 56:95, 1979.
68. Lefer A.M., Ogletree M.L., Smith J.B., Silver M.J., Nicolaou K.C., Barnette W.E., Gasic G.P.: Prostacyclin: a potentially valuable agent for preserving myocardial tissue in acute myocardial ischemia. *Science* 200:52, 1978.
69. Araki H., Lefer A.M.: Role of prostacyclin in the preservation of ischemic myocardial tissue in the perfused cat heart. *Circ. Res.* 47:757, 1980.
70. Romson J.L., Haack D.W., Lucchesi B.R.: The antithrombotic and hemodynamic effects of prostacyclin infusion in the dog. *Circulation* 62(suppl III):165, 1980. (Abstract)
71. Aiken J.W., Gorman R.R., Shebuski R.J.: Prevention of blockage of partially obstructed coronary arteries with prostacyclin correlates with inhibition of platelet aggregation. *Prostaglandins* 17:483, 1979.
72. Bergman G., Rothman M.T., Daly K., Atkinson L., Richardson P., Jackson G., Jewitt D.: Haemodynamic, metabolic and platelet effects of intravenous prostacyclin in patients with coronary artery disease. *Circulation* 62(suppl III):327, 1980. (Abstract)
73. Szczeklik A., Szczeklik J., Nizankowski R., Gluszko P.: Prostacyclin for acute coronary insufficiency. *Artery* 8:7–11, 1980.
74. Chierchia S., Drea F., Bernini W., De Caterina R., Maseri A.: Effects of prostacyclin (PGI₂) continuous infusion in angina at rest. *Circulation* 62 (suppl III):310, 1980. (Abstract)
75. Rowe G.C., Afonso S.: Systemic and coronary hemodynamic effects of intracoronary administration of prostaglandins E₁ and E₂. *Am. Heart J.* 88:51, 1974.
76. Forman R., Kirk E.S., Downey J.M., Sonnenblick E.H.: Nitroglycerin and heterogeneity of myocardial blood flow. *J. Clin. Invest.* 52:905, 1973.
77. Ogletree M.L., Lefer A.M.: Prostaglandin-induced preservation of the ischemic myocardium. *Circ. Res.* 42:218, 1978.
78. Riemersma R.A., Talbot R.C., Ungar A., Mjost O.D., Oliver M.F.: Effects of prostaglandin-E₁ on ST segment elevation and regional myocardial blood flow during experimental myocardial ischaemia in dogs. *Eur. J. Clin. Invest.* 7:515, 1977.
79. Kelliher G.J., Lawrence T., Jurkiewicz N., Dix R.K.: Comparison of the effects of prostaglandins E₁ and A₁ on coronary occlusion induced arrhythmia. *Prostaglandins* 17:163, 1979.
80. Jugdutt B.I., Hutchins G.M., Bulkley B.H., Becker L.C.: Dissimilar effects of PGE₁ and PGE₂ on myocardial infarct size after coronary occlusion in conscious dogs, in Samuelsson B., Ramwell P.W., Paoletti R. (eds): *Advances in Prostaglandin and Thromboxane Research.* New York, Raven Press, 1980, p. 675.
81. Tsuboi T., Hatano N., Nakatsuji K., Fujitani B., Yoshida K., Shimizu M., Kawasaki A., Sakata M., Tsuboshima M.: Pharmacological evaluation of ONO 1206, a Prostaglandin E₁ derivative, as antianginal agent, in Samuelsson B., Ramwell P.W., Paoletti R. (eds.): *Advances in Prostaglandin and Thromboxane Research.* New York, Raven Press, 1980, p. 347.

PART VI

PROSTAGLANDINS IN THROMBOSIS

Prostaglandins and Thrombosis

JOHN C. HOAK

Cardiovascular Center and Specialized Center for
Research in Atherosclerosis, University of Iowa College
of Medicine, Iowa City

Introduction

A number of possible factors and mechanisms have been proposed to explain the nonthrombogenic properties of the vascular endothelium. Both the intact platelet and endothelial cell at physiologic pH have negatively charged membranes and are mutually repelled by each other. It is also believed that the surface of the endothelium is influenced by the presence of heparins and glycosoaminoglycans, which might facilitate the inactivation of thrombin and factor Xa by antithrombin III. An enzyme with ADPase activity has been found to be associated with the endothelial surface and would have an obvious role in preventing platelet aggregates from forming near intact endothelium.[1] The endothelium is known to produce an activator of plasminogen and carries the potential for activation of the fibrinolytic system to promote lysis of fibrin in thrombi.

An interesting new role for the endothelium has been suggested by the recent work of Lollar and Owen.[2] These workers have demonstrated that the binding of thrombin to the endothelium is an important primary mechanism for rapid removal of thrombin from the circulation and facilitates its subsequent association with antithrombin III to form a thrombin–AT III complex.

A most important nonthrombogenic property of the endothelium relates to its ability to produce and release prostacyclin. Moncada et al. have shown that arachidonate metabolic mechanisms exist in endothelial cells to convert arachidonic acid and cyclic endoperoxides to prostacyclin, a most potent inhibitor of platelet aggregation and adhesion.[3]

In relationship to the importance of prostacyclin in thrombosis, several key questions warrant attention: (1) Is prostacyclin responsible for the nonthrombogenic properties of the vascular endothelium? (2) What other antithrombotic mechanisms operate at the level of the blood vessel wall?

From the results of our own investigations and from recent reports in the literature, we will attempt to provide satisfactory answers to these questions.

Materials and Methods

The source and preparation of reagents and materials used in culture procedures, platelet adherence, and 6-keto-$PGF_{1\alpha}$ determinations have been described elsewhere.[4, 5]

Cultures of venous endothelium, arterial fibroblasts, and empty dish controls were prepared as previously described.[5]

Hemangioendothelioma cultures were prepared from a transplantable tumor originally obtained from Jackson Laboratory (Bar Harbor, ME). This hemangioendothelioma was shown to cause consumption of platelets and fibrinogen in the vascular channels of the tumor. The tumors, carried in the Jackson 129J strain mice, were removed aseptically, and connective tissue was dissected away. The remaining material was finely minced before incubating with 0.25% trypsin for 20 minutes at 37°C with stirring. The resulting cell suspension was filtered through sterile gauze. Clones of hemangioendothelioma were obtained by seeding a dilute cell suspension in multiwell plates. Only those wells that contained colonies without fibroblastic contaminants were used for subculturing. The resulting cell line when reinjected into the 129J strain mice produced hemangioendotheliomas in every animal. Morphology, as determined by light microscopy, was identical to that of the hemangioendothelioma produced by transplantation between mice. Hemangioendothelioma cultures derived from one clone were used in the passages 8–40 and contained 0.3 to 0.4 × 10^6 cells per dish.

The mouse fibroblasts used were from NCTC clone 929 of the parent L strain derived from normal subcutaneous areolar and adipose tissue of a 100-day-old C3H/An mouse. Subcultures were prepared as previously described for umbilical fibroblasts. Each 35-mm dish contained 2.5 to 3.5 × 10^6 cells.

Platelet adherence to the cell monolayers or the empty dish controls was determined by incubating ^{51}Cr-labeled human platelets with confluent monolayers in the presence or absence of 0.5 U bovine thrombin.[5] In experiments to determine the effect of exogenous PGI_2, monolayers and empty dishes were preincubated with 1 mM ASA for

30 minutes and washed twice, before adding PGI_2, thrombin, and platelets.[6]

Endogenous formation of PGI_2 was determined by measuring the 6-keto-$PGF_{1\alpha}$ concentration in the incubation medium after rocking the dishes for 30 minutes.[6] The 6-keto-$PGF_{1\alpha}$ levels in the supernatant were determined with a radioimmunoassay.[4]

Results

To delineate the role of prostacyclin, we have performed studies using a platelet adherence system with cultured vascular cell monolayers. Prostacyclin was measured in these studies using a radioimmunoassay for 6-keto-$PGF_{1\alpha}$, the stable end product of prostacyclin.[4, 5]

As reported earlier,[7] in the absence of thrombin, platelets did not adhere to any of the cell monolayers or to the empty dish control to any significant extent. However, in the presence of 0.5 U bovine thrombin, platelet adherence was greater than 75% to fibroblast monolayers or to the empty dish control. In contrast, it was only 4% to endothelium.

In order to test the effect of prostacyclin in the platelet adherence system, we eliminated it from the endothelium by using aspirin. Aspirin is known to acetylate the cyclo-oxygenase of the platelet and to inhibit thromboxane A_2 formation. Therefore, we chose to treat the endothelial monolayer with aspirin so that in a similar way the endothelial cyclo-oxygenase would be inhibited and prostacyclin production would cease. We tested this possibility using our assay for 6-keto-$PGF_{1\alpha}$ and the thrombin-induced platelet adherence system.

The results are shown in Figure 27–1. In the absence of thrombin, there was no increased platelet adherence despite inhibition of prostacyclin formation. In the presence of thrombin and in the absence of aspirin, 6-keto-$PGF_{1\alpha}$ increased and there was little platelet adherence. When the endothelium was treated with 0.01 mM aspirin, thrombin still caused significant release of 6-keto-$PGF_{1\alpha}$, and no increase in platelet adherence occurred. However, treatment of the endothelium with 1 mM aspirin prevented the formation of 6-keto-$PGF_{1\alpha}$ even in the presence of thrombin, and platelet adherence increased to 44%.

In each of the sets of experiments used to remove prostacyclin from the endothelium, baseline platelet adherence, in the absence of thrombin, did not increase. However, when thrombin was added to the incubation system, platelet adherence increased significantly, and this increase could be prevented by adding exogenous prostacyclin to

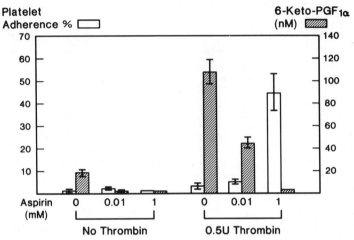

Fig 27–1.—Platelet adherence to untreated and aspirin (ASA)-treated endothelium compared with 6-keto-PGF$_{1\alpha}$ release. ASA or buffer control was incubated with the monolayer for 30 minutes at 37 C with rocking. The preincubation solution was removed and the dish was washed twice. Thrombin or buffer control was added, followed immediately by ^{51}Cr-platelets (for adherence) or unlabeled platelets (for PGI$_2$ determinations). The monolayer was rocked 30 minutes at 37 C. Percent adherence was calculated by dividing counts per minute of cells attached to the monolayer, multiplied by 100, by total counts per minute added to the dish. 6-keto-PGF$_{1\alpha}$ released into the supernate was determined by radioimmunoassay. (From Hoak J.C., et al.: *Philosophical Transactions of Royal Society*, 294:331–338, 1981. Used by permission.)

the incubation media. Thus, prostacyclin appeared to be an important component to maintain platelet adherence at a low value when thrombin was present in the incubation system with the endothelium.

Studies with Hemangioendothelioma Cells

We have reported earlier on the use of a murine model of the Kasabach-Merritt syndrome in which 129/J strain mice developed thrombocytopenia, microangiopathic hemolytic anemia, and a localized consumption coagulopathy in transplanted hemangioendotheliomas.[8, 9] It has been possible to grow these hemangioendothelioma cells in culture and to study their surface properties and their ability to produce prostacyclin.[7] The hemangioendothelioma monolayers did not produce prostacyclin in response to thrombin, and in comparison with venous endothelium, produced little prostacyclin upon addition of arachidonic acid or the endoperoxide, PGH$_2$.[7]

In order to study the effect of exogenous prostacyclin on platelet adherence to different types of vascular cells, the monolayers were

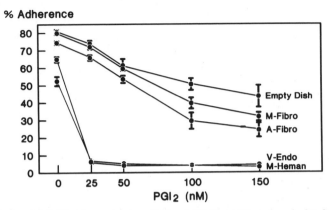

Fig 27–2.—Inhibition by exogenous PGI_2 of 0.5 thrombin-induced platelet adherence to 1 mM aspirin-treated cell layers. All monolayers were incubated 30 minutes with 1 mM aspirin in incubation medium. After rinsing twice, platelet adherence was determined, as described in Figure 27–1. PGI_2 was added just before thrombin and platelets to achieve the concentrations shown. Abbreviations are A-Fibro, arterial fibroblasts; V-Endo, venous endothelium; M-Heman, mouse hemangioendothelioma; M-Fibro, mouse L929 fibroblasts. (From Fry G.L., et al.: *Blood* 55:271–275, 1980. Published with permission.)

pretreated with 1 mM aspirin to block endogenous production of prostacyclin by thrombin. In order to determine whether some cell types were more sensitive to prostacyclin, concentrations from 25 to 150 mM were used. Fibroblasts were chosen as a representative cell type from the subendothelium, since values for smooth muscle and fibroblasts were not significantly different. Mouse fibroblasts were used as a control for the hemangioendothelioma. As can be seen in Figure 27–2, thrombin-induced platelet adherence to the venous endothelium and hemangioendothelioma cells decreased dramatically with as little as 25 μM prostacyclin. In contrast, platelet adherence to fibroblasts in the presence of thrombin was extremely resistant to the effect of prostacyclin.

Discussion and Conclusion

The endothelium has a number of important functions.[10] In this report, its normal role in platelet-vessel wall interactions has been emphasized. Prostacyclin appears to play a key role in the prevention of platelet aggregate formation and their adherence to vascular wall cells when a thrombogenic stimulus such as thrombin is present. It appears to be an important component of the nonthrombogenic effect exhibited by the endothelium. Removal of prostacyclin from the endothelium did not increase baseline platelet adherence, but did increase thrombin-induced platelet adherence from 4% to 60%. Addition of exogenous prostacyclin, at low concentrations, reversed the enhanced thrombin-induced platelet adherence under these conditions.

The failure of high concentrations of prostacyclin to completely block thrombin-induced platelet adherence to smooth muscle cells and fibroblasts suggests that these cells either lack a component normally found in endothelium or produce a substance that promotes adherence. Possible differences include collagen production (type and amount) by smooth muscle and fibroblasts or, in the case of endothelium, interactions at the surface that enhance the effect of prostacyclin. Monolayers derived from normal endothelium or from neoplastic endothelium (hemangioendothelioma) exhibit some property in addition to prostacyclin that prevents thrombin-induced platelet adherence. Therefore, despite its ability to decrease platelet adherence to all of the cell types tested, it is unlikely that prostacyclin is the sole factor regulating platelet adherence.

In Figure 27–3, mechanisms that may operate at the level of the vessel wall to inhibit thrombosis are shown. As demonstrated by the observations of Lollar and Owen,[3] thrombin binds with high affinity to the vascular endothelium. Thus, the endothelium can serve as a mechanism to remove thrombin from the circulation. In addition, binding of thrombin to the endothelial surface appears to accelerate the binding of thrombin to antithrombin III. This effect may be mediated by heparin on the endothelium.

As indicated earlier, thrombin causes the formation and release of prostacyclin from human umbilical vein endothelium.[4]

Of particular interest have been the observations released to the

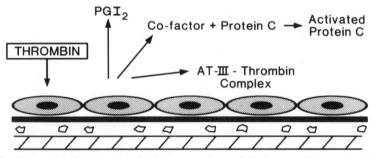

Fig 27–3.—Mechanisms in which the vascular endothelium participates in the development of antithrombotic activity.

potential antithrombotic effects of protein C. Protein C is a vitamin K-dependent factor which has an anticoagulant effect as a result of its ability to inactivate factors Va and VIIIa.[11] It has also been reported to produce enhanced fibrinolytic activity.[11] In vitro, thrombin can activate protein C but only at a very slow rate. When thrombin is incubated with inactive protein C in the presence of vascular endothelium, either in culture or in vivo, the protein C is activated rapidly.[12] Recent studies indicate that the endothelium supplies an essential co-factor for this activation process.[12]

In conclusion, it is appropriate to confirm that prostacyclin can play an important role in platelet-vessel wall interactions. It is unlikely that it plays a major role in maintaining the nonthrombogenic character of the endothelium under normal conditions. More likely, it comes into play when the endothelium is subjected to injury or thrombogenic stimuli. Other mechanisms, several of only recent discovery, appear to have an equally interesting and important role in maintaining the patency of blood vessels and circulation of blood elements in them.

ACKNOWLEDGMENTS

Research for this chapter was supported in part by grants HL-14230 and HL-22408 from the National Heart, Lung, and Blood Institute.

REFERENCES

1. Heyns A.DuP., Potgieter G.M., Retief F.P.: The inhibition of platelet aggregation by an aorta intima extract. *Thromb. Diath. Haemorrh.* 32:417–431, 1974.
2. Lollar P., Owen W.G.: Clearance of thrombin from circulation in rabbits by high affinity binding sites on endothelium. *J. Clin. Invest.* 66:1222–1230, 1980.
3. Moncada S., Gryglewski R., Bunting S., Vane J.R.: An enzyme isolated from arteries transforms prostaglandin endoperoxides to an unstable substance that inhibits platelet aggregation. *Nature* 263:663–665, 1976.
4. Czervionke R.L., Smith J.B., Hoak J.C., Fry G.L., Haycraft D.L.: Use of a radioimmunoassay to study thrombin-induced release of PGI_2 from cultured endothelium. *Thromb. Res.* 14:781–786, 1979.
5. Czervionke R.L., Hoak J.C., Fry G.L.: Effect of aspirin on thrombin-induced adherence of platelets to cultured cells from the blood vessel wall. *J. Clin. Invest.* 62:847–856, 1978.
6. Czervionke R.L., Smith J.B., Fry G.L., Hoak J.C., Haycraft D.L.: Inhibition of prostacyclin by treatment of endothelium with aspirin. *J. Clin. Invest.* 63:1089–1092, 1979.
7. Fry G.L., Czervionke R.L., Hoak J.C., Smith J.B., Haycraft D.L.: Platelet

adherence to cultured vascular cells: Influence of prostacyclin. *Blood* 55:271–275, 1980.

8. Hoak J.C., Warner E.D., Cheng H.F., Fry G.L., Hankenson R.R.: Hemangioma with thrombocytopenia and microangiopathic anemia (Kasabach-Merritt syndrome): An animal model. *J. Lab. Clin. Med.* 77:941–950, 1971.

9. Warner E.D., Hoak J.C., Fry G.L.: Hemangioma, thrombocytopenia and anemia. The Kasabach-Merritt syndrome in an animal model. *Arch. Path.* 91:523–528, 1971.

10. Hoak J.C., Czervionke R.L., Fry G.L., Haycraft D.L., Brotherton A.A.: Role of the vascular endothelium. *Phil. Trans. R. Soc. Lond.* B 294:331–338, 1981.

11. Kisiel W., Ericsson L.H., Davies E.W.: Proteolytic activation of protein C from bovine plasma. *Biochemistry* 15:4893–4900, 1976.

12. Esmon C.T., Owen W.G.: Identification of an endothelial cell cofactor for thrombin-catalyzed activation of protein C. *Proc. Natl. Acad. Sci. USA* 78:2249–2252, 1981.

Prostacyclin in Thrombotic Thrombocytopenic Purpura and Hemolytic Uremic Syndrome

GIUSEPPE REMUZZI AND NORBERTO PERICO

Division of Nephrology and Dialysis
Ospedali Riuniti di Bergamo, Bergamo, Italy

Introduction

Thrombotic thrombocytopenic purpura and hemolytic uremic syndrome are both characterized by thrombocytopenia, microangiopathic hemolytic anemia, renal disease, and microthrombi occluding arterioles and capillaries of different organs. Because of the simultaneous occurrence of thrombosis and microangiopathic anemia, the term "thrombotic microangiopathy" (TMA) has been used to describe both syndromes.[1] TMA can also occur as a complication of pre-eclampsia and systemic lupus erythematosus.

Thrombotic Thrombocytopenic Purpura and Hemolytic Uremic Syndrome

In 1977, Byrnes and Khurana described a case of TTP in which the infusion of normal plasma was followed by clinical remission.[2] This observation suggested that normal plasma might contain a factor, possibly a physiologic inhibitor of platelet aggregation, which in some way prevents the uncontrolled intravascular platelet activation characteristic of TTP. Subsequently, we employed plasma infusion in the treatment of 11 patients with HUS.[3] Our results confirm the therapeutic effectiveness of plasma infusions and underscore the potential role of plasma factor(s) in the regulation of platelet vessel-wall interactions.

In three of the patients with HUS, we measured the amount of prostacyclin activity released from vascular specimens during the acute phase of the disease.[4] None was detected, suggesting that PGI_2 might be the physiologic inhibitor of platelet aggregation, presumed to be lacking in TTP.[2] We also examined the plasma of seven patients with TTP and HUS and measured their ability to stimulate prostacyclin production in normal rat vascular tissue.[5-8] Plasma from five of these patients on admission did not adequately stimulate vascular PGI_2 synthesis. However, in two patients, including one "nonresponder" to plasma infusion, the PGI_2-stimulating capacity of plasma appeared normal throughout the course of the disease.

The hypothesis that TMA is due to a "missing factor" has gained further support from recent observations that plasma levels of 6 keto $PGF_{1\alpha}$ (the stable breakdown derivative of PGI_2) are very low in patients with TTP or HUS.[9-11] In some patients, the deficiency of plasma factor persists long after clinical remission.[8, 12] A low level of plasma PGI_2-stimulating factor was also observed in family members who had no past history of microangiopathic episodes.[8, 12, 13] This suggests that decreased PGI_2-stimulating factor in plasma does not result "per se" in clinical disease, but reflects a genetic predisposition to TMA that may become clinically evident following exposure to a specific etiologic agent such as endotoxin.[14] In HUS and TTP, the reduced PGI_2 synthetic capacity could also be the consequence of an altered balance between oxidant and antioxidant factors in plasma.[14] This possibility is suggested by studies that indicate that free radicals derived from PGG_2 inactivate PGI_2 synthetase[15] and by other studies that demonstrate that microangiopathy in animals is associated with enhanced lipid peroxidation.[16] Further support for the possibility that uncontrolled lipid peroxidation may induce hemolysis and endothelial damage was obtained in two patients with HUS who demonstrated increased levels of fluorescent lipid-peroxidation products in their plasma.[17]

Pre-eclampsia

Pre-eclampsia is characterized by hypertension, edema, and proteinuria. In severe cases consumptive coagulopathy complicated by TMA may be present. In normal pregnancy, increased PGI_2 production by fetal and maternal vessels may account for the low peripheral resistance that is seen despite high plasma renin activity. If true, then the hypertension and microvascular thrombosis seen in pre-eclampsia could be due to reduced PGI_2 synthetic capacity of vascular tissues. Recently we reported that PGI_2 production in umbilical and placental vascular tissues from patients with severe pre-eclampsia is significantly depressed.[18] These findings were subsequently confirmed by other investigators in studies of umbilical artery,[19] amniotic fluid,[20] and maternal vessels.[21] Very recently Lewis et al. observed a decline in maternal PGI_2 prior to the onset of proteinuria, reduction in fetal growth, and worsening of hypertension.[22]

The plasmatic regulation of vascular PGI_2 in pregnancy has also been studied.[23, 24] The plasma factor stimulating PGI_2 is normal during early pregnancy, but reduced during late pregnancy. However, this plasmatic activity is significantly higher in pre-eclampsia than in normal pregnancy. This unexpected result is difficult to reconcile with the positive correlation obtained in other clinical conditions between the amount of vascular PGI_2 generated in in vitro systems and the stimulatory activity of plasma.[4, 25] Possibly the control of vascular PGI_2 in pregnancy is more complex. In this context, an excessive activity of the circulating prostaglandin synthesis inhibitor (EIPS), described by Saeed et al.,[26] could contribute to the decreased PGI_2 production observed in pre-eclampsia.[24] However, EIPS activity in normal pregnancy and pre-eclampsia did not differ significantly. More studies are needed to fully define the role of factors modulating prostaglandin synthesis in normal pregnancy and in pre-eclampsia.

Systemic Lupus Erythematosus

Systemic lupus is frequently complicated by microvascular thrombosis with glomerular thrombi signaling a poor prognosis in lupus nephritis.[27] Paradoxically, thrombosis in SLE is frequently associated with the presence of a "lupus anticoagulant,"[28] an immunoglobulin that inhibits the prothrombin activation complex and interferes with the prospholipid fraction.[29] Very recently, Carreras et al., demonstrated in a patient with "lupus anticoagulant" and recurrent thrombosis that a plasmatic activity linked to the IgG fraction inhibited the formation of PGI_2 in an in vitro system.[30] The patient's plasma level of 6-keto-$PGF_{1\alpha}$ was also reduced. The authors therefore suggested that the antibody interfering with the phospholipid fraction in blood coagulation could also inhibit the release of arachidonic acid from phospholipids in the endothelial cell membrane. This inhibitory activity was confirmed in additional patients by the same authors[31] and by Marchesi et al.[32] Although other mechanisms may account for thrombotic complications in systemic lupus,[32] in selected patients a direct role of the "lupus anticoagulant" in the pathogenesis of thrombosis seems likely.

Conclusions

Recent prostaglandin research has led to the concept that an imbalance between the opposing actions of thromboxane and prostacyclin may play a role in thrombotic microvascular diseases. The abnormal PGI_2 synthetic capacity found in HUS, TTP, pre-eclampsia, and systemic lupus may, at least partially, explain the occurrence of widespread microvascular platelet aggregation, a crucial event in the pathogenetic sequence of thrombotic microangiopathy. Several factors modulate platelet and vascular prostaglandin synthesis. Whether such factor(s) are identical to the factors in normal human plasma that stimulate[5, 6] or inhibit[26] prostaglandin formation is still to be defined. Studies should be performed to determine whether the impaired arachidonic acid metabolism observed in these disorders is the consequence of an imbalance between the formation and removal of free radicals in plasma.[14, 33] It will also be important to evaluate the usefulness of PGI_2 administration in patients in whom endogenous production of PGI_2 seems to be acutely deficient.[34] Thus far, the intravenous infusion of PGI_2 in TTP, HUS, or pre-eclampsia produced beneficial effects in some patients,[11, 35, 36] but not in others.[37, 38] These conflicting results suggest that thrombotic microangiopathy is a heterogeneous category of disease that contains many distinct subgroups yet to be identified.

ACKNOWLEDGMENTS

This study was supported by the Associazione Bergamasca per lo Studio delle Malattie Renali and by the Italian National Research Council (programs: Tecniche Sostitutive di Funzioni d'Organo and Farmacologia Clinica e Malattie Rare).

REFERENCES

1. Remuzzi G., Rossi E.C., Misiani R., Marchesi D., Mecca G., de Gaetano G., Donati M.B.: Prostacyclin and thrombotic microangiopathy. *Semin. Thromb. Hemostas.* 6:391–394, 1980.
2. Byrnes J.J., Khurana M.: Treatment of thrombotic thrombocytopenic purpura with plasma. *N. Engl. J. Med.* 297:1386–89, 1977.
3. Misiani R., Appiani A.C., Edefonti A., Gotti E., Bettinelli A., Giani M., Rossi E., Remuzzi G., Mecca G.: Hemolytic uremic syndrome: therapeutic effect of plasma infusion. (Submitted for publication)
4. Remuzzi G., Misiani R., Marchesi D., Livio M., Mecca G., de Gaetano G., Donati M.B.: Hemolytic-uremic syndrome: Deficiency of plasma factor(s) regulating prostacyclin activity? *Lancet* II:871–872, 1978.
5. MacIntyre D.E., Pearson J.D., Gordon J.L.: Localisation and stimulation

of prostacyclin production in vascular cells. *Nature* 271:549–551, 1978.

6. Remuzzi G., Livio M., Cavenaghi A.E., Marchesi D., Mecca G., Donati M.B., de Gaetano G.: Unbalanced prostaglandin synthesis and plasma factors in uremic bleeding. A hypothesis. *Thromb. Res.* 13:531–536, 1978.

7. Defreyn G., Vergara Dauden M., Machin S.J., Vermylen J.: A plasma factor in uraemia which stimulates prostacyclin release from cultured endothelial cells. *Thromb. Res.* 19:695–699, 1980.

8. Jørgensen K.A., Pedersen R.S.: Familial deficiency of prostacyclin production stimulating factor in the hemolytic uremic syndrome of childhood. *Thromb. Res.* 21:311–315, 1981.

9. Hensby C.N., Fitzgerald G.A., Friedman L.A., Lewis P.J., Dollery C.T.: Measurement of 6-oxo-PGF$_{1\alpha}$ in human plasma using gas chromatography-mass spectrometry. *Prostaglandins* 18:731–736, 1979.

10. Machin S.J., Defreyn G., Chamone D.A.F., Vermylen J.: Plasma 6-keto-PGF$_{1\alpha}$ levels after plasma exchange in thrombotic thrombocytopenic purpura. *Lancet* I:661, 1980.

11. Webster J., Rees A.J., Lewis P.J., Hensby C.N.: Prostacyclin deficiency in haemolytic-uremic syndrome. *Br. Med. J.* 281:271, 1980.

12. Remuzzi G., Marchesi D., Misiani R., Mecca G., de Gaetano G., Donati M.B.: Familial deficiency of a plasma factor stimulating vascular prostacyclin activity. *Thromb. Res.* 16:517–525, 1979.

13. Proesmans W.: Personal communication.

14. Donati M.B., Misiani R., Marchesi D., Livio M., Mecca G., Remuzzi G., de Gaetano G.: Hemolytic-uremic syndrome, prostaglandins and plasma factors, in Remuzzi G., Mecca G., de Gaetano G. (eds.): *Hemostasis, Prostaglandins and Renal Disease.* New York, Raven Press, 1980, pp. 283–290.

15. Ham E.A., Egan R.W., Soderman D.D., Gale P.H., Kuehl F.A. Jr.: Peroxidase-dependent deactivation of prostacyclin synthetase. *J. Biol. Chem.* 254:2191–2194, 1979.

16. Stamler F.W.: Fetal eclamptic disease of pregnant rats fed antivitamin E stress diet. *Am. J. Pathol.* 35:1207–1231, 1959.

17. Lunec J., Dormandy T.L.: Fluorescent lipid-peroxidation products in synovial fluid. *Clin. Sci.* 56:53–59, 1979.

18. Remuzzi G., Marchesi D., Zoja C., Muratore D., Mecca G., Misiani R., Rossi E., Barbato M., Capetta P., Donati M.B., de Gaetano G.: Reduced umbilical and placental vascular prostacyclin in severe pre-eclampsia. *Prostaglandins* 20:105–110, 1980.

19. Downing I., Shepherd G.L., Lewis P.J.: Reduced prostacyclin production in pre-eclampsia. *Lancet* II:1374, 1980.

20. Bodzenta, A., Thomson J.M., Poller L.: Prostacyclin activity in amniotic fluid in pre-eclampsia. *Lancet* II:650, 1980.

21. Bussolino F., Benedetto C., Massobrio M., Camussi G.: Maternal vascular prostacyclin activity in pre-eclampsia. *Lancet* II:702, 1980.

22. Lewis P.J., Shepherd G.L., Ritter J., Chan S.M.T., Bolton P.J., Jogee M., Myatt L., Elder M.G.: Prostacyclin and pre-eclampsia. *Lancet* I:559, 1981.

23. Remuzzi G., Zoja C., Marchesi D., Schieppati A., Mecca G., Misiani R., Donati M.B., de Gaetano G.: Plasmatic regulation of vascular prostacyclin in pregnancy. *Br. Med. J.* 282:512–514, 1981.

24. Redman C.W.G., Brennecke S.P., Mitchell M.D.: Prostaglandins and pre-eclampsia. *Lancet* I:731, 1981.
25. Remuzzi G., Cavenaghi A.E., Mecca G., Donati M.B., de Gaetano G.: Prostacyclin-like activity and bleeding in renal failure. *Lancet* II:1195–1197, 1977.
26. Saeed S.A., McDonald-Gibson W.J., Cuthbert J., Copas J.L., Schneider C., Gardiner P.J., Butt N.M., Collier H.O.J.: Endogenous inhibitor of prostaglandin synthetase. *Nature* 270:32–36, 1977.
27. Kant K.S., Pollak V.E., Weiss M.A., Glueck H.I., Miller M.A., Hess E.V.: Glomerular thrombosis in systemic lupus erythematosus: Prevalence and significance. *Medicine* (Baltimore) 60:71–86, 1981.
28. Mueh J.R., Herbst K.D., Rapaport S.I.: Thrombosis in patients with the lupus anticoagulant. *Am. Intern. Med.* 92(Part 1):156–159, 1980.
29. Thiagarajan P., Shapiro S.S., De Marco L.: Monoclonal immunoglobulin Mλ coagulation inhibitor with phospholipid specificity. *J. Clin. Invest.* 66:397–405, 1980.
30. Carreras L.O., Defreyn G., Machin S.J., Vermylen J., Deman R., Spitz B., Van Assche A.: Arterial thrombosis, intrauterine death and "lupus" anticoagulant detection of immunoglobulin interfering with prostacyclin formation. *Lancet* I:244–246, 1981.
31. Carreras L.O., Vermylen J.: "Lupus" anticoagulant and prostacyclin. *Lancet* I:665, 1981.
32. Marchesi D., Parbtani A., Frampton G., Livio M., Remuzzi G., Cameron J.S.: Thrombotic tendency in systemic lupus erythematosus. *Lancet* I:719, 1981.
33. Dormandy T.L.: Plasma antioxidant potential, in Remuzzi G., Mecca G., de Gaetano G. (eds.): *Hemostasis, Prostaglandins and Renal Disease.* New York, Raven Press, 1980, pp. 251–253.
34. Prostacyclin in Therapeutics. *Lancet* I:643–644, 1981. (Editorial)
35. Lewis P.J., Boylan P., Friedman L.A., Hensby C.N., Downing I.: Prostacyclin in pregnancy. *Br. Med. J.* 280:1581–1582, 1980.
36. Remuzzi G., Marchesi D., Mecca G., Misiani R., Rossi E., Donati M.B., de Gaetano G.: Reduction of fetal vascular prostacyclin activity in preeclampsia. *Lancet* II:310, 1980.
37. Hensby C.N., Lewis P.J., Hilgard P., Mufti G.J., Hows J., Webster J.: Prostacyclin deficiency in thrombotic thrombocytopenic purpura. *Lancet* II:748, 1979.
38. Budd G.T., Bukowski R.M., Lucas F.V., Cato A.E., Cocchetto D.M.: Prostacyclin therapy of thrombotic thrombocytopenic purpura. *Lancet* II:915, 1980.

Toxemia of Pregnancy and Prostaglandins

THOMAS F. FERRIS

Department of Medicine
University of Minnesota Hospitals
Minneapolis, Minnesota

Introduction

Striking changes occur in the cardiovascular system during pregnancy. Cardiac output increases in the first trimester of pregnancy and reaches a maximum of 30% to 40% above the nonpregnant level by the twenty-fourth week of gestation.[1] The rise in cardiac output during pregnancy is accompanied by an expanded extracellular volume and is associated with a striking fall in peripheral vascular resistance. The fall in peripheral resistance is frequently noted in the development of palmar erythema and spider telangiectases during pregnancy. Renal blood flow and glomerular filtration rate also increase early in pregnancy, with the increase occurring within four weeks of the last menstrual period.[2] In spite of the expanded extracellular fluid volume and increased renal blood flow, plasma renin rises early in pregnancy.[3] The cause of the increase in renin secretion in pregnancy has not been understood. The studies to be presented were designed to examine the possible role of prostaglandin synthesis in these cardiovascular changes and to propose a hypothesis for the pathophysiology of toxemia of pregnancy.

Methods

The animal studies were done in anesthetized pregnant New Zealand rabbits at about the twenty-sixth day of gestation. Uterine blood flow was measured by the injection into the left ventricle of approximately 200,000 radioactive microspheres either 19 ± 2 or 26 ± 2 μm in diameter labeled with either strontium-85 or cesium-141. Uterine and renal blood flows were determined by acid digestion of the organs at the completion of the experiment with calculation of the radioactivity in the digested organ. Cardiac output was measured by the timed blood withdrawal from the right femoral artery after injection of the microsphere. Plasma renin activity and urinary and plasma PGE were measured by radioimmunoassay using previously described methods.[4]

Results

Pregnancy is associated with striking increase in renin secretion, with an increase in plasma renin demonstrated in the first trimester. To examine whether the increase in renin and aldosterone secretion is necessary to compensate for the increased glomerular filtration rate and elevated progesterone secretion occurring in pregnancy, both of which might cause a propensity for urinary salt wasting, seven third trimester pregnant women were placed on 10 mEq sodium diets for seven days. There was no difference in the ability of the pregnant woman to conserve sodium. Urinary sodium fell to 10 mEq or below as quickly as in nonpregnant women, and weight loss was similar

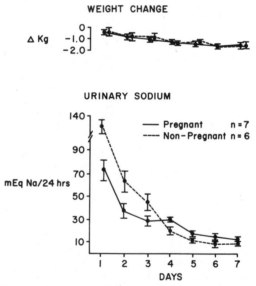

Fig 29–1.—Weight and urinary sodium excretion in pregnant women in their third trimester and in controls when on a 10 mEq sodium intake.

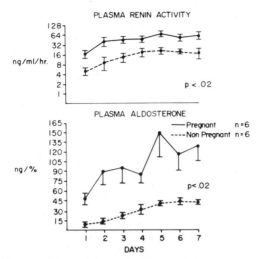

PLASMA RENIN ACTIVITY

ng/ml/hr.

p < .02

PLASMA ALDOSTERONE

——Pregnant   n=6
----Non Pregnant   n=6

ng / ‰

p< .02

DAYS

Fig 29-2.—Plasma renin activity and aldosterone in pregnant and nonpregnant women on a 10 mEq sodium intake.

(Fig 29-1). With the decrease in sodium intake, PRA and plasma aldosterone rose higher in pregnant than in nonpregnant women (Fig 29-2). Since the higher aldosterone might be necessary to prevent salt wasting, we examined the response to a 300 mEq sodium diet in pregnant and nonpregnant women. Although pregnant and nonpregnant women were excreting 300 mEq sodium in the urine by day 4, plasma renin and aldosterone did not suppress in pregnant women as in nonpregnant controls (Fig 29-3).

We believed that these findings indicated that factors other than sodium balance were causing the increase in renin secretion during pregnancy. Since renal prostaglandin synthesis plays a role in renin release, studies were carried out to determine urinary PGE excretion in pregnant women in their third trimester (Fig 29-4). Urinary PGE excretion was significantly higher in the pregnant women. Figure 29-5 demonstrates that peripheral venous PGE was also significantly elevated in pregnant women in their third trimester.

Studies have been conducted in pregnant rabbits in which uterine vein PGE concentration was found to be extraordinarily high, 172 ng/ml compared to 2.2 ng/ml in peripheral blood (Fig 29-6). Following the administration of indomethacin, uterine vein PGE concentration decreased from 172 ± 48 ng/ml to 23 ± 10 ng/ml and uterine blood flow fell from 17 ± 3.5 to 7.8 ± 1.3 ml/min (p .01) (Fig 29-7).

The pregnant uterus, like the kidney, is an organ with a high syn-

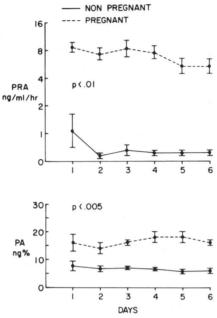

Fig 29–3.—Plasma renin activity (PRA) and plasma aldosterone in pregnant and nonpregnant women on a 300 mEq sodium intake.

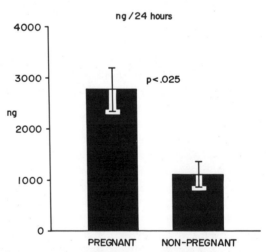

Fig 29–4.—Urinary PGE excretion in pregnant women in their third trimester and in nonpregnant women on an unrestricted diet.

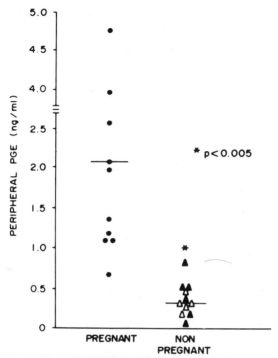

Fig 29-5.—Peripheral vein PGE concentration in pregnant and nonpregnant women on unrestricted diets.

thesis rate of both renin[5] and prostaglandin E. Since angiotensin is known to increase uterine blood flow and uterine vein PGE concentration in the pregnant rabbit,[6] dog,[7] and monkey,[8] we examined the question whether uterine synthesis of PGE was dependent upon angiotensin II. The angiotensin I converting enzyme inhibitor, Captopril, was administered to pregnant rabbits and its effect on uterine blood flow and uterine vein PGE concentration determined. Following Captopril, 5 mg/kg, administered intravenously, there was a significant reduction in mean arterial pressure from 102 ± 3 to 85 ± 4 mm Hg ($p < .01$) with no change in cardiac output, 492 ± 37 versus 480 ± 40 ml/min, uterine blood flow 15.5 ± 3 vs. 14.4 ± 3 ml/min, or renal blood flow 72 ± 5 vs. $81 \pm$ ml/min. A striking reduction in uterine vein PGE concentration, i.e., from 102 ± 17 to 29 ± 9 ng/ml, occurred, suggesting that PGE synthesis in the uterus of the pregnant rabbit is dependent upon angiotensin II (Fig 29-8). Uterine vein plasma renin activity rose from 11 ± 3 to 90 ± 19 ng/ml/hr and from 6 ± 1.6 to 62 ± 15 ng/ml/hr in the peripheral vein following Capto-

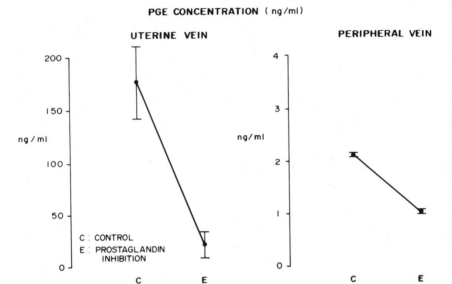

Fig 29–6.—Uterine vein and peripheral vein PGE in pregnant rabbits before (C) and after (E) indomethacin.

pril. Higher concentration of PRA was found in uterine vein than in peripheral vein before and after Captopril.

To determine whether these effects of angiotensin I blockade on uterine PGE synthesis had an effect on gestation, oral Captopril, either 2.5 or 5 mg/kg/day, was given to pregnant rabbits beginning on

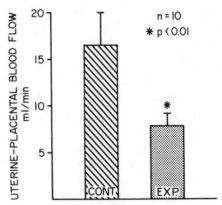

Fig 29–7.—Effect of prostaglandin inhibition on uterine-placental blood flow. The hatch bar denotes uterine blood flow before (CONT.) and the dotted bar after (EXP.) indomethacin in pregnant nephrectomized rabbits.

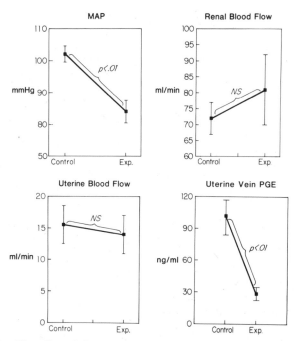

Fig 29–8.—The effect of Captopril on mean arterial pressure (MAP), renal blood flow, uterine blood flow, and uterine vein PGE concentration in pregnant rabbits.

the fifteenth day of gestation. In 12 control animals, 80 or 81 fetuses survived, whereas in 10 pregnant does receiving 2.5 mg/kg/day of Captopril, only 18 of 89 fetuses survived, and in 11 pregnant does receiving 5 mg/kg/day, only 6 of 8 fetuses survived (Fig 29–9). There was no change in arterial blood pressure during chronic administration of Captopril.

Discussion

The finding of increased PGE synthesis in both pregnant women and rabbits points to a potential role of prostaglandin synthesis in

Group	No.	Dose (mg/kg/d)	Fetal Survival	
Control	12	0	80/81	(99%)
Treated	10	2.5	18/89	(20%)
	11	5.0	6/80	(7.5%)

Fig 29–9.—The effect of chronic administration of Captopril to pregnant rabbits on fetal survival.

control of blood pressure and renin secretion during pregnancy. Gant et al. demonstrated a striking decrease in angiotensin sensitivity in normal pregnancy occurring as early as the tenth week of gestation.[9] Although clinical manifestations of toxemia did not develop until after the thirty-second week, there was a gradual increase in sensitivity demonstrated in women who developed toxemia from the eighteenth week of gestation (Fig 29–10). One might speculate that if the decrease in sensitivity to angiotensin in pregnancy is caused by prostaglandin synthesis, the increase in sensitivity in women with toxemia may be caused by decreased synthesis of vasodilating prostaglandins. Lewis et al. have recently reported elevated plasma and urinary 6-keto-PGF$_{1\alpha}$ in pregnant women in their third trimester.[10]

In addition to potentially playing a role in the development of hypertension, altered prostaglandin synthesis conceivably could be playing a role in many of the systemic manifestations of the disease (Fig 29–11). The increase in angiotensin sensitivity, reduction in uterine and renal blood flow, and fall in glomerular filtration rate all could be secondary to diminished prostaglandin synthesis. The reduction in renin and aldosterone secretion with toxemia might also reflect diminished renal PGI$_2$ synthesis.

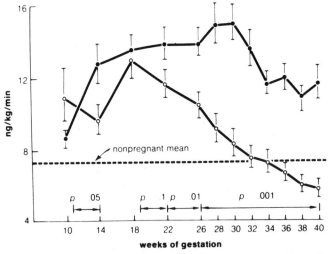

Fig 29–10.—Variations in angiotensin sensitivity during pregnancy. Comparison of mean angiotensin dose required to cause a 20-mm rise in diastolic blood pressure in 120 primigravidas who remained normotensive *(black circles)* and 72 primigravidas *(open circles)* in whom toxemia occurred. Nonpregnant mean dose is shown as a broken line.[9]

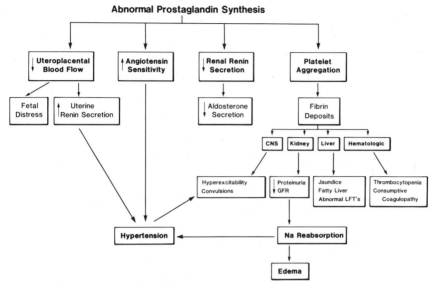

Fig 29–11.—A hypothesis for the pathophysiology of toxemia of pregnancy.

Several of the other features of the disease, i.e., fibrin deposits in kidney and liver, the thrombocytopenia, and consumptive coagulopathy in severe toxemia, point to activation of intravascular coagulation. One might speculate that a decrease in PGI_2 synthesis could set the stage for platelet aggregation, endothelial cell damage, and activation of clotting in small blood vessels throughout the body. If a balance normally exists between the aggregatory influence of thromboxane production in platelets and the antiaggregatory production of PGI_2 in vascular endothelium, an imbalance might occur in toxemia. Although PGI_2 synthesis may be elevated in pregnancy, pregnancy represents a shift toward enhanced clotting, with most clotting factors increased in pregnancy. Platelets have recently been reported to be more aggregable in late pregnancy and to contain higher thromboxane concentration.[11]

Obviously, a great deal more clinical and laboratory investigation will be needed to determine whether prostaglandin synthesis plays a role in toxemia. Of even greater importance would be an understanding of the factors that increase prostaglandin synthesis during pregnancy, since such a finding might lead to newer concepts in the treatment of human hypertension.

ACKNOWLEDGMENTS

This work was supported by National Institutes of Health Grant HL-17871.

REFERENCES

1. Ueland K., Navy M.J., Peterson E.N., Metcalf J.: Maternal cardiovascular dynamics. *Am. J. Obstet. Gynecol.* 104:856, 1969.
2. Davison J.M., Dunlop W.: Renal hemodynamics and tubular function in normal human pregnancy. *Kid. Int.* 18:152, 1980.
3. Weinberger M.H., Kramer N.J., Grim C.E., Petersen L.P.: The effect of posture and saline loading on plasma renin activity and aldosterone concentration in pregnant, non-pregnant, and estrogen-treated women. *J. Clin. Endocrinol. Metab.* 44:69, 1977.
4. Venuto R., O'Dorisio T., Stein J.H., Ferris T.F.: The effect of prostaglandin inhibition on uterine blood flow. *J. Clin. Invest.* 55:193, 1975.
5. Ferris T.F., Gorden P., Mulrow P.J. Rabbit uterus as a source of renin. *Am. J. Physiol.* 212:698, 1967.
6. Ferris T.F., Stein J.H., Kauffman J.: Uterine blood flow and uterine renin secretion. *J. Clin. Invest.* 51:2828, 1972.
7. Terragno N.A., Terragno D.A., Pacholczyk D., McGiff J.C.: Prostaglandins and the regulations of uterine blood flow in pregnancy. *Nature* 249:57, 1974.
8. Franklin G.O., Dowd A.J., Caldwell B.V., Speroff L.: The effect of angiotensin II on plasma renin activity and prostaglandins A, E, F levels in the uterine vein of the pregnant monkey. *Prostaglandins* 6:271, 1974.
9. Gant N.F., Daley G.L., Chand S., Walley P.J., MacDonald P.C.: A study of angiotensin II pressor response throughout primigravid pregnancy. *J. Clin. Invest.* 52:2682, 1973.
10. Lewis P.J., Boylan P., Friedman L.A., Hensby C.N., Dowing I.: Prostacyclin in pregnancy. *Br. Med. J.* 280:1581, 1980.
11. Ylikorkala O., Viinikka L.: Thromboxane A_2 in pregnancy and puerperium. *Br. Med. J.* 281:1601, 1980.

PGI_2, Indomethacin, and Heparin Promote Postischemic Neuronal Recovery in Dogs When Administered Therapeutically

J. M. HALLENBECK, D. R. LEITCH, A. J. DUTKA,
L. J. GREENBAUM, JR.
Naval Medical Research Institute
Bethesda, Maryland

Introduction

We have been interested in the factors that impair microvascular perfusion after ischemia. The fundamental hypothesis guiding our studies has been that acute ischemic tissue damage may initiate a sequential interaction between constituents in blood and elements in damaged tissue that can progressively increase resistance to microcirculatory flow.[1] This process has been viewed as causing a focal shutdown of slow flows in the injury zone. Previous studies have suggested that products of the "arachidonic acid cascade" may participate in the process of blood-damaged tissue interaction.[2] In these earlier studies, reversible central nervous system ischemia was produced in dogs by hydrostatically raising cerebrospinal fluid pressure to the level of mean aortic blood pressure for 35 minutes. Autoradiographic blood flow studies performed 30 minutes after this form of global neuraxis ischemia demonstrated zones of greatly impaired reperfusion in dogs receiving only heparin 300 units/kg. Therapeutic administration of PGI_2 and indomethacin, *beginning five minutes after* ischemia in heparinized animals, was shown to eliminate the zones of greatly reduced flow. Thus, PGI_2, and indomethacin appeared capable of counteracting the process leading to impairment of microvascular perfusion when given therapeutically to heparinized animals.

335

In these studies, blood flow was the primary variable of concern and no index of neuronal function was measured, so that conclusions could not be drawn regarding the potential capacity of this drug combination to promote neuronal recovery after ischemia. We therefore developed a model of reversible *focal* ischemia, in which the cortical sensory evoked response served as a quantifiable index of neuronal function. The influence of heparin, PGI_2, and indomethacin on postischemic nerve cell recovery was then investigated in this model.

Materials and Methods

Thirty-nine dogs were anesthetized with alpha chloralose 80 mg/kg, intubated, and mechanically ventilated. The right internal carotid artery was carefully catheterized and the femoral vessels were catheterized bilaterally. Each animal was placed in a stereotaxic apparatus, and steel screws were inserted into the skull for recording the cortical sensory evoked response. The recording electrode was positioned over the right sensorimotor cortex, and the reference electrode was embedded in the nasal bones at their distal extreme. The stimulating needle electrodes were inserted percutaneously next to the median nerve in the left upper foreleg. Four dogs served as controls and were not subjected to air embolism. Cortical sensory evoked potentials were measured and ^{14}C-iodoantipyrine autoradiographic blood flow studies[3] were performed in these animals. The remaining 35 dogs were handled as follows.

After preparation, several cortical sensory evoked responses were recorded and 50 µl of room air were gently flushed into the right internal carotid artery catheter and washed in with 500 µl of saline. After two minutes, another evoked response was recorded. If the response was suppressed, no more air was infused. If it was only partially suppressed, another 20 to 50 µl of air was delivered. By infusing 20 to 50 µl increments of air as necessary, the neuronal pool generating the cortical sensory evoked response was maintained in a state of suspended electrophysiologic function for one hour. After this period of ischemic suppression of the cortical sensory evoked response, a step was carried out which separated the animals into various groups. Animals received no therapy or one of several drug regimens, depending on the group to which they were assigned. For the next 15, 60, or 120 minutes, the cortical sensory evoked response was periodically measured to assess the degree of neuronal recovery. At the conclusion of this recovery period, a ^{14}C-iodoantipyrine autoradiographic blood flow study of cerebral blood flow was performed.

TABLE 30–1.—DESCRIPTION OF THE EXPERIMENTAL GROUPS

GROUP; NUMBER OF ANIMALS	DURATION OF ISCHEMIA (min)	DURATION OF RECOVERY (min)	PGI ng/kg/min	TREATMENT Indomethacin 4 mg/kg	Heparin 300 μ/kg
A. 4	None	–	0	0	0
B. 13	60	60	TRIS-HCL	–	–
C. 13	60	60	90–260	+	+
D. 2	60	15	TRIS-HCL	–	–
E. 3	60	15	90–150	+	+
F. 2	60	120	TRIS-HCL	–	–
G. 2	60	120	70–240	+	+

Table 30–1 defines the various groups. Four animals in group A were not exposed to ischemia. All other groups were subjected to 60 minutes of ischemia. Thirteen animals in group B, two animals in group D, and two animals in group F received no therapy. These groups differed with regard to duration of postischemic recovery: 60 minutes in group B, 15 minutes in group D, and 120 minutes in group F. Thirteen animals in group C, three animals in group E, and two animals in group G received the combination of PGI_2, indomethacin, and heparin. Again, the groups differed with regard to duration of postischemic recovery: 60 minutes in group C, 15 minutes in group E, and 120 minutes in group G.

Results and Discussion

The cortical sensory evoked response is a reproducible oscillation of cortical potential that is timelocked to a stimulus and can be extracted from concurrent, random EEG activity by serial recording and signal averaging techniques. This oscillation of cortical potential represents the composite shifts of membrane potential from a pool of nerve cells within the right lateral cortex in response to stimulation of the left median nerve.[4] When all of the cells depolarize at the right time, there is a normal response. The first positive fluctuation in potential can be designated P_1 and the first negative fluctuation accordingly designated N_1. The next positive peak would be P_2 and so on. By virtue of its relative reproducibility and stability, the peak-to-trough amplitude between waves P_1 and N_1 served as the quantifiable index of neuronal function in this study. The progression of cortical sensory evoked response changes formed a distinct pattern in the embolized animals. The normal evoked responses seen during the control period were morphologically similar in all groups, but there was interanimal variability with regard to P_1—N_1 amplitude. When the pool of responding nerve cells was deprived of oxygen and glucose by ischemia, the cortical neurons stopped firing and evoked response flattened. The number of nerve cells in the pool that regained the capacity to respond normally to the median nerve stimulation determined how much amplitude of the oscillation of cortical potential was recovered. Furthermore, the number of these nerve cells restored to normal depended on the degree and distribution of blood flow return.

Table 30–2 summarizes the evoked response recoveries observed in the various groups. The ratio of the peak-to-trough amplitude between P_1 and N_1 measured at the end of the recovery period, and the same amplitude measured in the control period was multiplied by 100 to yield the percent recovery. The major comparison is between the two groups followed for a 60-minute period of postischemic recovery. Each group is comprised of 13 animals, and the corresponding mean ± SD percent CSER recoveries are displayed for each group. The difference between these group means is significant at p much less than 0.01 by Wilcoxon Rank Sum test. CSER recoveries are also compared for untreated animals and animals receiving PGI_2, indomethacin, and heparin after 15 minutes and 120 minutes of postischemic recovery, respectively. The cumulative total volumes in microliters of embolic air from the two major groups followed for 60 minutes were 184 ± 79 μl (mean ± SD) for group B (TRIS-HCL) and 191 ± 49 μl for group C (PGI_2, indomethacin, heparin). None of the mean cumulative air doses deviated significantly among any of the groups. Further, there was no correlation between an animal's total air dose and its subsequent recovery as analyzed across all animals in this study.

Average brain blood flow rates by the ^{14}C iodoantipyrine technique were similar in the various groups. No correlation was found between these mean values and percent amplitude recovery of the evoked re-

TABLE 30–2.—MEAN ± SD OF THE PERCENT
RECOVERY OF CSERs IN THE VARIOUS
EMBOLIZED GROUPS

$$\frac{\text{PREFLOW AMPLITUDE}}{\text{CONTROL AMPLITUDE}} \times 100$$

TRIS-HCL	21 ± 9	(mean ± SD)
PGI_2, indomethacin, heparin	53 ± 19*	
	15 min	120 min
TRIS-HCL	11 ± 7	17 ± 3
PGI_2, indomethacin, heparin	47 ± 18	82 ± 49

*Significance of difference $p \ll 0.01$ by Wilcoxon Rank Sum.

sponse across the sample of embolized animals. Brain gray and white matter blood flows in ml/100 gm/min (mean ± SD) are tabulated for the right and left sides in Table 30–3. Blood flow from brain gray matter designates an unweighted average from the following structures: auditory cortex, sensorimotor cortex, visual cortex, anterior association cortex, anterior cerebral-middle cerebral watershed cortex, posterior cerebral-middle cerebral watershed cortex, caudate nucleus, thalamus, and hippocampus. Blood flow from brain white matter designates an unweighted average from the following structures: anterior centrum ovale, middle centrum ovale, corpus callosum, internal capsule, and optic radiations.

The spectrum of blood flows that cause suppression of electrophysiologic function have been demarcated by a number of studies.[5, 6] Neuronal excitability is reduced or eliminated by brain flows in the range of 12 to 20 ml/100 gm/minute. Analysis of the lower limits of gray and white matter blood flows occurring in animals from this study with a CSER recovery of 35% or better suggested threshold values of 15 ml/100 gm/minute for gray matter and 6 ml/100 gm/minute for white matter. Animals with flow rates below these thresholds and in what might be described as the "neuron-disabling" range posted CSER recoveries of 0 to 22%, with a mean ± SD of 14 ± 8%. In contrast, animals with flow rates above the neuron-disabling gray and white matter thresholds averaged 30 ± 19% CSER recovery. The difference between these means was significant at $p < 0.02$ by Wilcoxon Rank Sum.

Animals treated with PGI_2, indomethacin, and heparin were free of brain flows in the neuron-disabling range at all time points investigated. The focal adequacy of nutrient flow was in a state of flux in animals receiving TRIS-HCL buffer, as revealed by the 15-, 60-, and 120-minute sampling points. There was a definite tendency for the intragroup incidence of animals with low flow rates to decline be-

TABLE 30–3.—MEAN ± SD BRAIN BLOOD FLOWS FOR GRAY AND WHITE MATTER IN THE VARIOUS GROUPS

GROUP	RIGHT SIDE Gray Matter	White Matter	LEFT SIDE Gray Matter	White Matter
A. (Control)	65 ± 20	16 ± 2	76 ± 19	19 ± 4
B. (TRIS)	51 ± 23	14 ± 6	53 ± 21	15 ± 6
C. (P, I, H)	60 ± 58	15 ± 7	55 ± 56	15 ± 13
D. (TRIS)	50 ± 46	9 ± 6	49 ± 14	13 ± 4
E. (P, I, H)	64 ± 34	15 ± 4	48 ± 16	17 ± 4
F. (TRIS)	63 ± 30	16 ± 4	64 ± 20	14 ± 2
G. (P, I, H)	72 ± 40	15 ± 3	68 ± 29	18 ± 4

tween the 15-minute sampling point and the 120-minute sampling point in untreated animals.

The enhanced neuronal recovery in the group receiving PGI_2, indomethacin, and heparin group was reflected in blood flows performed 15 minutes into the recovery period. Autoradiograms from untreated animals revealed the persistence of low, neuron-damaging flow rates for 15 minutes into the recovery period. In contrast, brain blood flow in animals receiving PGI_2, indomethacin, and heparin had already returned to high levels by this time point.

The data indicate that therapeutic administration of heparin, PGI_2, and indomethacin, a drug combination that counteracts postischemic impairment of microvascular perfusion, can greatly enhance the recovery of nerve cells after ischemia. This raises the exciting prospect that this drug combination or related agents will provide a means of effectively preserving viable neurons in an ischemic injury zone and promoting their ultimate functional recovery.

ACKNOWLEDGMENTS

Naval Medical Research and Development Command, Research Task No. M0099PN001.1150. The opinions and assertions contained herein are the private ones of the writers and are not to be construed as official or reflecting the views of the Navy Department or the naval service at large. The experiments reported herein were conducted according to the principles set forth in the *Guide for the Care and Use of Laboratory Animals,* Institute of Laboratory Resources, National Research Council, DHEW, Pub. No. (NIH) 78-23.

We thank the Upjohn Company, Kalamazoo, Michigan, and Merck, Sharp & Dohme, West Point, Pennsylvania, for supplying drugs used in this study.

REFERENCES

1. Hallenbeck J.M.: Prevention of post-ischemic impairment of microvascular perfusion. *Neurology* 27:3–10, 1977.
2. Hallenbeck J.M., Furlow T.W. Jr.: Prostaglandin I_2 and indomethacin prevent impairment of post-ischemic brain reperfusion in the dog. *Stroke* 10:629–637, 1979.
3. Sakurada O., Kennedy C., Jehle J., et al.: Measurement of local cerebral blood flow in iodo [^{14}C] antipyrine. *Am. J. Physiol.* 234:H59–H66, 1978.
4. Iragui-Madoz V.J., Wiederholt W.C.: Far-field somatosensory evoked potentials in the cat. *Electroencephalogr. Clin. Neurophys.* 43:646–657, 1977.
5. Branston N.M., Symon L., Crockard H.A., et al.: Relationship between the cortical evoked potential and local cortical blood flow following acute mid-

dle cerebral artery occlusion in the baboon. *Exp. Neurol.* 45:195–208, 1974.

6. Heiss W.D., Hayakawa T., Waltz A.G.: Cortical neuronal function during ischemia. Effects of occlusion of one middle cerebral artery on single-unit activity in cats. *Arch. Neurol.* 33:813–820, 1976.

PART VII

PROSTAGLANDINS IN CARDIOPULMONARY BYPASS SURGERY

Interactions of Platelets with Artificial Surfaces

EDWIN W. SALZMAN

Beth Israel Hospital
Boston, Massachusetts

Increasing use of prosthetic devices has created a host of new syndromes produced by contact of the blood with artificial surfaces. The significance of these phenomena to a conference devoted to consideration of "Prostaglandins in Cardiovascular and Thrombotic Disorders" rests on the fact that platelets are the hemostatic elements most disturbed by blood-artificial surface interaction, and the complexities of their response intersect the paths of prostaglandin metabolism at many points. In patients bearing artificial heart valves, vascular grafts, or other prosthetic devices in contact with the blood or in those undergoing extracorporeal circulation for hemodialysis or cardiopulmonary bypass, activation of platelets by contact with foreign surfaces of the prosthesis leads to generation of prostaglandin endoperoxides and, subsequently, of thromboxane A_2. In the case of cardiopulmonary bypass, for example, the thromboxane concentration is sufficient to induce an important degree of platelet aggregation and coronary vasoconstriction, which may contribute to the morbidity of operations on the heart.[1] On the other hand, prostaglandins may also provide the possibility of new therapeutic interventions in syndromes of blood-surface interaction.

The consequences of contact of the blood with an artificial surface may sometimes be gross thrombosis in the device, perhaps with remote embolization, but are often more subtle.[2] There is apt to be accelerated consumption of platelets and labile clotting factors, which in some instances leads to thrombocytopenia, but in others may be manifest only by shortened platelet survival and measurably altered platelet function. Studies with labeled platelets have shown uptake of platelets by an arterial graft after implantation,[3] and there is per-

343

sistent shortening of platelet life span. Eventually platelet survival tends to become normal. On the basis of experiments in animals, this sequence was initially attributed to re-endothelialization of the prosthesis.[4] However, the explanation is probably more complicated, since there are major species differences in the rate and extent of endothelial coverage of a vascular graft, and in man, total re-endothelialization of a vascular graft is an unusual event. Clagett and associates have studied the rate of acquisition of the capacity to produce prostacyclin in vascular prostheses and have correlated this property in experimental animals with survival of labeled platelets and neointimal ("pseudo-intimal") coverage.[5] His group have also provided evidence for continued interactions of platelets with vascular grafts, reporting that platelets that circulate in the presence of an arterial prosthetic graft have, on the average, a subnormal content of serotonin, presumably because of continued low-grade secretion by the stimulated platelets.[6] The phenomenon is analogous to the partial release reaction observed in cardiopulmonary bypass,[7] in which an alleged acquired storage pool defect is alleged to make an important contribution to the bleeding tendency following open heart operations.

The earliest event observed upon contact of blood with an artificial surface is adsorption of plasma proteins and formation of an adsorbed film which precedes the adhesion of the platelets by some tens of seconds.[8] Because of the large size of platelets and their small number relative to plasma proteins, diffusion of protein molecules to the surface always antedates the arrival of platelets. Thus the platelet never sees a bare surface. The nature of the artificial surface is revealed to the potentially adherent platelet by the nature of the adsorbed film, i.e., by its composition and by the configuration of the adsorbed protein molecules. There is evidence that fibrinogen must be a constituent of the interfacial layer in order for platelets to adhere to artificial surfaces,[9] and it is claimed that the attractiveness of a surface for platelets can be correlated with the concentration of fibrinogen in the adsorbed surface coat.[10] This is almost certainly an oversimplification. Whether the ubiquitous adhesive protein fibronectin is also involved is unclear. Fibronectin appears to be present in platelet storage granules and to be secreted in the course of the release reaction,[11] but it is also a normal constituent of plasma, and it would be difficult to rule out its participation. The role of von Willebrand's factor in these interactions is also uncertain. There is evidence that this large molecule is involved as a binding protein in platelet adherence to collagen in connective tissue,[12] and it participates also in the adherence of platelets to glass beads.[13] Given time and a low blood shear rate, however, platelets are able to adhere to collagen or glass even in the absence of von Willebrand's factor, and so it is certain that the molecule is not essential for these reactions.

Once adherent to a surface, platelets spread on it, generate thromboxane A_2, secrete the contents of intracellular storage granules, and become attractive to other platelets, not necessarily in that order. The sequence is analogous to the events that lead to platelet aggregation in vitro when stimulated by "aggregating agents" such as ADP. The intimacies of the mechanism of stimulation of the platelet by adherence to a surface are not understood.

Platelet aggregation occurs to various degrees on different surfaces, under the influence of thromboxane A_2 generation and secreted ADP. Whether the process leads to accumulation of a gross platelet thrombus or is limited to transient collision of platelets with the artificial surface, followed by their return to the bloodstream to be removed from the circulation elsewhere in the body, depends to a large extent on the local dynamics of blood flow. In arteries and in connecting tubes of extracorporeal circuits, brisk flow prevents the local build-up of a platelet aggregate and sweeps the platelets altered by surface contact downstream to be removed by the liver and spleen before their appointed time, thus accounting for the shortened survival of labeled platelets, whereas in the headers and reservoirs of an artificial kidney, recirculating eddies may permit the accumulation of a substantial mass of platelets.

Controlling factors in the interaction of platelets with artificial surfaces are the nature of the surface, the fluid mechanics of the system, and the reactivity of the blood, to borrow from Virchow's triad.

Although from common experience one must conclude that the nature of an artificial surface influences its reactivity with the blood, there is evidence that platelets adhere to virtually all such surfaces. Platelets have been found to adhere in roughly the same number to materials of widely varying physical properties,[14] but the subsequent events of secretion and aggregation may differ to a large extent on various surfaces, and under most conditions platelet-platelet interactions apparently predominate over platelet-surface interactions in their influence on the macroscopic manifestation of thrombosis.

There is not complete agreement concerning the features of a surface that dictate its reactivity with platelets. Such aspects as net surface charge, roughness or smoothness, reversible work of adhesion as determined by microcalorimetry, water wettability, critical surface tension, and other parameters derived from measurements of contact angle have each proven inadequate by itself to describe a surface with sufficient sensitivity to predict its behavior in contact with the blood.[15]

We studied different aspects of surface chemistry in vitro in a system in which whole blood anticoagulated with citrate was pumped from below through a column of beads of the material to be tested.[16] Effluent blood was collected and tested for retention of platelets on the bead column and secretion of platelet constituents. It should be noted that such an experimental model, using citrated blood, ignores the possible effects of thrombin generated by activation of the intrinsic clotting system. Such information should be sought in collateral experiments, for it is likely that, if present, thrombin contributes in an important way to platelet-surface interaction. For example, clinical experience shows that thromboembolic complications of radiographic angiography can be largely prevented through the prophylactic administration of heparin, which blocks the platelet changes induced by thrombin, although it enhances platelet reactivity in response to other agonists.

We studied a series of acrylates and methacrylates varying in length of the alkyl side chain.[17] These polymers are of interest as artificial materials, since they can be readily fabricated in great variety in prosthetic devices demanding a range of physical properties. It can be seen that retention of platelets on the bead column and secretion of platelet constituents are direct correlates of the alkyl chain length, polymethyacrylate (side chain length = 1) being least reactive and polylauryl acrylate (chain length = 12) being most reactive. The methacrylates show a similar rank order of reactivities. The hydrocarbon-like surfaces of the higher alkane acrylates and methacrylates may lead to strong hydrophobic interactions with adsorbed protein molecules and to irreversibility of adsorption, as Brash has shown.[18]

In other experiments,[19] a copolymer of polymethyl acrylate and polystyrene was studied, varying the relative mole fractions of the acrylate and styrene. As the polymer composition varied from 100% methyacrylate to 100% styrene, platelet reactivity increased, reaching a maximum at about 40% styrene, beyond which the copolymers behaved like pure styrene. These experiments suggest that aromatic groups such as the styrene phenyl are highly reactive with platelets, of course, through the intermediary of adsorbed plasma protein.

That simply avoiding hydrophobic interactions is not sufficient to achieve passivity toward platelets is illustrated by our experience with polyvinyl alcohol and copolymers of aromatic diisocyanates, the so-called polyureas.[19] Both of these classes of polymers are hydrophilic and are capable of strong hydrogen bonding. These proved to be strongly reactive with platelets, behavior that may also have been influenced by their partial crystallinity.

The foregoing conclusions are reinforced by studies of a series of segmented polyurethanes, copolymers consisting of potentially reactive "hard segments" (by virtue of their intensely hydrogen-bonding urea or urethane moieties), which serve to cross link intervening "soft segments" of linear polyethers.[20] These polymers undergo phase separation during fabrication, and their reactivity turns out to be a direct function of the relative concentration of hard segments at the polymer-blood interface. Among the polyether soft segments, which are much less reactive than the hard segments and predominate at the interface when the surface that is ultimately to come into contact with the blood is formed against air or the hydrophobic surface of a mold, platelet reactivity varies with the chain length of the polyether: polytetramethylene oxide (PTMO) is more reactive than polypropylene oxide (PPO), which is more reactive than polyethylene oxide (PEO). The latter is very hydrophilic and, in fact, water-soluble unless cross-linked, but lacks hydrogen atoms capable of hydrogen bonding. We find that the platelet reactivity of the polymers decreases as their water content increases and that this attractiveness to platelets parallels their ability to adsorb thrombin, and perhaps other proteins.[21] Thus, as with the acrylate series, increasing hydrophobicity gives increasing platelet reactivity, and increasing hydrophilicity, increasing blandness, so long as the hydrophilic nature of the polymer does not result from a capacity for electrostatic interactions or from the presence of potentially hydrogen bonding hydrogens. Materials fabricated according to this prescription approach theoretical blandness with respect to platelets and show great promise in vivo in studies of their effects on the survival of labeled platelets,[22] a system in which so-called "medical grade" silicone rubber, polytetrafluorethylene (Teflon), and polyvinyl chloride, all materials widely used in clinical applications, prove much more reactive.

An alternative approach that has received widespread interest and sporadic clinical application has been the attachment to surfaces of biologically active antithrombotic molecules, of which the most widely studied has been heparin.[23] Heparin does not, of course, block the earliest steps in the intrinsic clotting system, nor does it inhibit platelet reactions except those induced by thrombin, and so there is no reason a priori why bound heparin should be expected to confer thromboresistance on a surface. Nonetheless, surfaces with heparin attached electrostatically, usually to a quaternary amine group, sometimes with cross-linking by gluteraldehyde, have shown encouraging clinical results in such acute applications as intraoperative artery-to-artery shunts, although their behavior in more chronic situations has been erratic at best.

When heparin is fixed to a surface primarily by ion pairing, it may exchange with charged plasma species and desorb. This may or may not be detrimental to thromboresistance of the surface, but it seriously complicates any attempt to understand the mechanism of action of the surface, since its nonthrombogenic character could be due either to an intrinsic property or to the anticoagulant effect of desorbed heparin in the layer of blood that bathes the surface. To avoid confusion by desorption of heparin bonded by electrostatic interactions, we studied various techniques for covalently linking heparin to surfaces.[23] We found that surfaces to which heparin was covalently bound, which did not leach measurable quantities of heparin, could in fact be thromboresistant, provided the heparin was bound in such a fashion that it retained its capacity to adsorb antithrombin III. Heparin-coated surfaces appeared not to be passive toward platelets by nature,[24] but rather to promote platelet activation, as has been shown to be the case for heparin in solution.[25] However, adsorption of antithrombin and formation of an antithrombin-heparin complex served to inactivate the heparinized surface. In some cases, the technique for preparation of a heparin-coated surface retained heparin's catalytic activity, i.e., its ability to enhance thrombin-antithrombin interaction, but this property was not critical for inactivation of a heparin-coated surface by antithrombin adsorption. Thus, surfaces such as heparin-Sepharose, which complexed antithrombin in high concentration, but had no heparin catalytic activity and did not enhance the rate of thrombin neutralization by antithrombin,[23] were made passive by adsorption of antithrombin, just as was a copolymer of heparin and polymethyacrylate, in which the chemistry of bonding preserved heparin's biologic activity. Development of new polymers that capitalize on these findings may more closely approach the ideal of a truly thromboresistant artificial material.

No totally nonthrombogenic artificial surface having yet been developed, however, designers of artificial organs have had to pay attention to other factors, such as optimization of hemodynamic design, avoiding areas of flow separation and recirculating eddies, which might prolong the residence time of activated platelets or clotting factors. Failing this, designers of devices such as prosthetic heart valves or auxiliary ventricles have accepted the inevitable formation of a thin layer of thrombus at the interface with blood and have relied on surface roughness to keep the thrombotic film in place and thus prevent the complicating embolization that might be a greater hazard. Such an approach is clearly unsuitable for extracorporeal circuits such as those employed in hemodialysis or cardiopulmonary bypass and has its limitations also in intravascular prostheses, where even a limited layer of thrombus may interfere with valve closure or impinge on the lumen of the arterial graft.

Given such shortcomings of reliance on fluid dynamics and the lack of totally thromboresistant artificial surfaces, the use of certain prosthetic devices in contact with the blood is at present necessarily dependent on inhibition of blood reactivity by antithrombotic drugs. Conventional anticoagulation with heparin or, in the longer term, vitamin K antagonists may reduce the contribution of the intrinsic clotting system to surface-induced thrombosis, but has limited efficacy toward platelet-surface interaction except that secondarily produced by the influence of thrombin. Drugs that alter platelet function are more attractive in this regard. For practical purposes the agents available include those that interfere directly with formation of a platelet-platelet or platelet-protein-platelet complex, such as probably is the case for dextran, or those that interfere with the more intimate aspects of platelet behavior by elevation of platelet cyclic AMP (e.g., adenosine, prostaglandins, dipyridamole) or by blocking the formation of thromboxane A_2 (e.g., aspirin and other nonsteroidal anti-inflammatory agents). Decalcifying agents, such as EDTA, and local anesthetics, antihistamines, and other "membrane stabilizers," which alter calcium homeostasis in the platelet, are effective in vitro but inapplicable in vivo because they lack selectivity and have intolerable effects on other organs. Their regional use during hemodialysis in experimental animals has been reported,[26] but there appears to be no similar experience in man.

In long-term applications, there is evidence that anti-inflammatory drugs that inhibit platelet cyclo-oxygenase may have a useful antithrombotic effect in prosthesis-induced platelet thrombosis. For example, sulfinpyrazone and aspirin have been shown to increase the longevity of arteriovenous shunts for hemodialysis[27, 28] and, in combination with oral anticoagulants, to reduce the rate of thromboembolic events in patients with prosthetic heart valves.[29] On the other hand, their use has been disappointing in patients with prosthetic arterial grafts,[30] in whom they have failed to yield any improvement in long-term graft patency.

In the short term, administration of aspirin reduces platelet consumption during hemodialysis, but at the cost of a significant increase in bleeding complications,[31] which are also frequent after cardiopulmonary bypass in patients who have received aspirin.[32] Aspirin and such drugs lack the property of prompt reversibility of action, a feature that would be essential to their successful use during cardiopulmonary bypass or hemodialysis. Otherwise their protective value against platelet consumption would be offset by a persistent paralysis of platelet function after conclusion of the period of extracorporeal circulation. Furthermore, cyclo-oxygenase inhibitors, while able to inhibit platelet aggregation, do not prevent the adhesion of platelets to artificial surfaces, which does not require thromboxane generation.[33] The adhesion of individual platelets without aggregation may be sufficient to produce significant thrombocytopenia when the surface area of the prosthetic device is large, as in hemodialysis or membrane oxygenation, and may also interfere with the function of a device designed for transfer of gases or solutes by intruding on the process of diffusion.

Drugs that increase platelet cyclic AMP, particularly the prostaglandins and related compounds, are more promising. In sufficient dosage, they block platelet adhesion to surfaces as well as platelet aggregation and secretion.[33] Furthermore their action is reversible and their duration of action limited: with PGE_1, by degradation during passage of the compound through the lung and, with PGI_2, by its short biological half-life at neutral pH, which permits its regional use, confining its effect to the extracorporeal circuit, e.g., in hemodialysis[34] or in partial bypass for extracorporeal membrane oxygenation.[35] More detailed consideration of the use of prostaglandins for preservation of platelet number and function during extracorporeal circulation will be found elsewhere in the proceedings of this conference.

Our own experience has shown that animals given prostacyclin in sufficient dosage may have complete preservation of platelet number and virtually normal platelet function during oxygenation with a membrane or bubble oxygenator,[36] but the concentration of infused prostacyclin required to preserve platelet function is sufficiently high to lead to significant vasodilatation and hypotension. The infusion dose sufficient to preserve a normal platelet count is lower and better tolerated, but unless prostacyclin paralyzes platelet function during bypass, subsidence of the effect of the drug after completion of extracorporeal circulation leaves a profound defect in platelet function, which is apt to reduce the benefit of normal platelet number. Contrary to early reports,[37] prostacyclin does not eliminate the need for heparin during cardiopulmonary bypass;[36] the use of PGI$_2$ with omission of heparin leads to the interesting syndrome of DIC without platelet consumption. On the other hand, the slower flows involved in hemodialysis apparently allow prostacyclin to be used as the sole antithrombotic agent during this procedure.[34] Development of a new generation of prostacyclin analogues or similar compounds with a larger therapeutic ratio, maximizing inhibition of platelet aggregation and minimizing vasodilation, would be a valuable step toward wider use of this fascinating family of compounds.

ACKNOWLEDGMENTS

Original work reported from the authors laboratory was supported by grants # HL25066 and HL20079 from the N.H.L.B.I.

REFERENCES

1. Davies G.C., Sobel M., Salzman E.W.: Elevated plasma fibrinopeptide A and thromboxane B$_2$ levels during cardiopulmonary bypass. *Circulation* 61:808, 1980.
2. Berger S., Salzman E.W.: Thromboembolic complications of prosthetic devices, in Spaet T. (ed.): *Progress in Hemostasis and Thrombosis, Vol. II.* New York, Grune and Stratton, 1974.
3. Dewanjee M.K., Fuster V., Kaye M.P., Josa M.: Imaging platelet deposition with ^{111}In-labeled platelets in coronary artery bypass grafts in dogs. *Mayo Clin. Proc.* 53:327–331, 1978.
4. Harker L.A., Slichter S.J., Sauvage L.R.: Platelet consumption by arterial prostheses: the effects of endothelialization and pharmacologic inhibition of platelet function. *Ann. Surg.* 186:594, 1977.
5. Clagett G.P., Hufnagel H., Carter R., Gregory W., Robinowitz M., Bedynek J.L., Maddox Y., Ramwell P.W., Collins G.J., Rich N.M.: Vascular prosthetic pseudo-intima produces PGI$_2$. *Circulation* 62(suppl III):272, 1980.
6. Clagett G.P., Russo M., Hufnagel H., Collins G.J., Rich N.M.: Platelet serotonin changes in dogs with prosthetic aortic grafts. *J. Surg. Res.* 28:223–229, 1980.
7. Beurling-Harbury C., Galvan C.A.: Acquired decrease in platelet secretory ADP associated with increased postoperative bleeding in post-cardiopulmonary bypass patients and in patients with severe valvular heart disease. *Blood* 52:13–23, 1978.
8. Scarborough D.E., Mason R.G., Dalldorf F.G., Brinkhous K.M.: Morphologic manifestations of blood-solid interfacial reactions: A scanning and transmission electron microscopic study. *Lab. Invest.* 20:164–169, 1969.
9. Zucker M.B., Vroman L.: Platelet adhesion induced by fibrinogen adsorbed onto glass. *Proc. Soc. Exp. Biol. Med.* 131:318, 1969.
10. Olsson P., Blomback B., Lagergren H., Larsson R., Tomikava M.: Interaction of platelets with surface-bound or conjugated fibrinogen. *Biblthca. Haemat.* 44:134–138, 1978.
11. Ginsberg M.H., Painter R.G., Birdwell C., Plow E.F.: The detection, im-

munofluorescent localization, and thrombin induced release of human platelet-associated fibronectin antigen. *J. Supramol. Struct.* 11:167–174, 1979.

12. Weiss H.J., Tschopp T.B., Baumgartner H.R.: Impaired interaction (adhesion-aggregation) of platelets with the subendothelium in storage-pool disease and after aspirin ingestion. *N. Engl. J. Med.* 293:619–623, 1975.

13. Salzman E.W.: The measurement of platelet adhesiveness: a simple *in vitro* technique demonstrating an abnormality in von Willebrand's disease. *J. Lab. Clin. Med.* 62:724, 1963.

14. Friedman L.I., Liem H., Grabowski E.F., Leonard E.F., McCord C.W.: Inconsequentiality of surface properties for initial platelet adhesion. *Trans. Am. Soc. Artif. Intern. Org.* 16:63–73, 1970.

15. Salzman E.W.: Nonthrombogenic surfaces: critical review. *Blood* 38:509, 1971.

16. Lindon J.N., Collins R.E.C., Coe N.P., Jagoda A., Brier-Russell D., Merrill E.W., Salzman E.W.: *In vivo* assessment of thromboresistant materials by determination of platelet survival. *Circ. Res.* 46:84, 1980.

17. Brier-Russell D., Salzman E.W., Lindon J., Handin R., Merrill E.W., Dincer A.K., Wu J.: *In vitro* assessment of interaction of blood with model surfaces: acrylates and methacrylates. *J. Colloid Interface Sci.* 81:311–318,1981.

18. Brash J.L., Uniyal S.: Dependence of albumin-fibrinogen simple and competitive adsorption on surface properties of biomaterials. *J. Polymer Sci.:Polymer Sympos.* 66:377–389, 1979.

19. Merrill E.W., Salzman E.W., Sa Da Costa V., Brier-Russell D., Wolfe L.C., Dincer A., Wu J.J., Pape P., Lindon J.N.: Molecular factors in blood polymer interactions: Hydrophobic, hydrophilic, hydrogen bonding and aromatic. *AIChE Sympos.* (In Press).

20. Sa Da Costa V., Brier-Russell D., Salzman E.W., Merrill E.W.: ESCA studies of polyurethanes: Blood platelet activation in relation to surface composition. *J. Colloid Interface Sci.* 80:445–452, 1981.

21. Sa Da Costa V., Brier-Russell D., Trudel G.E., Waugh D.F., Salzman E.W., Merrill E.W.: Polyether-polyurethane surfaces: Thrombin adsorption, platelet adsorption and ESCA scanning. *J. Colloid Interface Sci.* 76:594, 1980.

22. Lindon J.N., Rodvien R., Brier D., Greenberg R., Merrill E.W., Salzman E.W.: *In vitro* assessment of interaction of blood with model surfaces. *J. Lab. Clin. Med.* 92:904, 1978.

23. Salzman E.W., Silane M., Lindon J.N., Brier-Russell D., Dincer A., Rosenberg R., Labarre D., Merrill E.W.: Thromboresistance of heparin-coated surfaces, in Brown W.V., Mann K.G., Roberts H.R., Lundblad R.L. (eds.): *The Chemistry and Biology of Heparin.* New York, Elsevier North-Holland, 1981, pp. 435–448.

24. Lindon J.N., Rosenberg R., Merrill E., Salzman E.W.: Interaction of human platelets with heparinized agarose gel. *J. Lab. Clin. Med.* 91:47, 1978.

25. Salzman E.W., Rosenberg R.D., Smith M.H., Lindon J.N., Favreau L.: Effect of heparin and heparin fractions on platelet aggregation. *J. Clin. Invest.* 65:84, 1980.

26. Scharschmidt B.F., Martin J.F., Shapiro L.J., Plotz P.H., Berk P.D.: The

use of calcium chelating agents and prostaglandin E_1 to eliminate plate-let and white blood cell losses resulting from hemoperfusion through un-coated charcoal, albumin-agarose gel, and neutral and cation exchange resins. *J. Lab. Clin. Med.* 89:110–119, 1977.

27. Kaegi A., Pineo G.F., Shimizu A., Trivedi H., Hirsh H., Gent M.: The role of sulfinpyrazone in the prevention of arterio-venous shunt throm-bosis. *Circulation* 52:497–499, 1975.
28. Harter H.R., Burch J.W., Majerus P.W., Stanford N., Delmez J.A., An-derson C.B., Weerts C.A.: Prevention of thrombosis in patients on he-modialysis by low-dose aspirin. *New Engl. J. Med.* 301:577, 1979.
29. Dale J., Myhre E., Storstein O., Stormorken H., Efskind L.: Prevention of arterial thromboembolism with acetylsalicylic acid. *Am. Heart J.* 94:101–111, 1977.
30. Blakely J.A., Pogoriler G.: A prospective trial of sulfinpyrazone after pe-ripheral vascular surgery. *Thromb. Haemostas.* 38:238, 1977.
31. Lindsay R.M., Prentice C.R.M., Ferguson D., Burton J.A., McNicol G.P.: Reduction of thrombus formation on dialyser membrane by aspirin and RA233. *Lancet* I:1287–1290, 1972.
32. Torosian M., Michelson E.L., Morganroth J., MacVaugh H. III: Aspirin-and coumadin-related bleeding after coronary-artery bypass graft sur-gery. *Ann. Intern. Med.* 89:325–328, 1978.
33. Salzman E.W., Lindon J.N., Brier D., Merrill E.W.: Surface induced platelet adhesion, aggregation, and release. *Proc. N.Y. Acad. Sci.* 283:114–127, 1977.
34. Zusman R.M., Rubin R.H., Cato A.E., Cocchetto D.M., Crow J.W., Tol-koff-Rubin N.: Hemodialysis using prostacyclin instead of heparin as the sole antithrombotic agent. *New Engl. J. Med.* 304:934–939, 1981.
35. Coppe D., Wonder T., Snider M., Salzman E.W.: Preservation of platelet number and function during extracorporeal membrane oxygenation by regional infusion of prostacyclin, in Vane J., Bergstrom S. (eds.): *Pros-tacyclin.* New York, Raven Press, 1979, pp. 371–382.
36. Coppe D., Sobel M., Seamans L., Levine F., Salzman E.W.: Prostacyclin preserves platelet function and number during cardiopulmonary bypass. *J. Thorac. Cardiovasc. Surg.* 81:274, 1981.
37. Longmore D.B., Bennett G., Gueirrara D., Smith M., Buntin S., Moncada S., Reed P., Read N.G., Vane J.R.: Prostacyclin: a solution to some prob-lems of extracorporeal circulation. *Lancet* I:1002–1005, 1979.

Damaging Effects of Cardiopulmonary Bypass

EUGENE H. BLACKSTONE, JOHN W. KIRKLIN,
ROBERT W. STEWART, DENNIS E. CHENOWETH

Department of Surgery, University of Alabama in
Birmingham; Scripps Clinic and Research Foundation,
La Jolla, California

Cardiac surgery is performed today in hundreds of centers and in practically every country of the world. Development and expansion of cardiac surgery was made possible by the combined discovery of heparin and the introduction of clinically usable pump-oxygenator support systems for cardiopulmonary bypass.[1] Although bulky, complex, and nonphysiologic substitutes for the heart and lungs, these support systems are usually so well tolerated that in some situations (e.g., coronary artery bypass grafting) hospital mortality in good centers approaches zero.[2, 3] Since much of the cardiac surgery done today is in such situations, even relatively inexperienced centers have low (but not approaching zero) mortality. When work is limited to such situations, it is easy to gain the impression that cardiopulmonary bypass is an innocuous tool.

We believe, however, that damaging effects of cardiopulmonary bypass occur in every patient. But, like all other incremental risk factors, they become apparent as a source of important morbidity and mortality only under special circumstances, such as when very complex kinds of heart disease are repaired, particularly in the very young, the very old, or the very ill.[4]

For example, in the 13¹/₂-year period from January 1967 to July 1980, 355 infants, less than three months old, underwent cardiac surgery at the University of Alabama in Birmingham.[5] In half (174), cardiopulmonary bypass was required for repair of their cardiac lesion. Their hospital mortality rate, though decreasing substantially over the years, has remained consistently higher than for patients

355

with complex heart disease whose surgery did not require use of cardiopulmonary bypass. A dozen (7%) of these 174 babies experienced hemorrhagic pulmonary edema without a hemodynamic basis, one kind of result of the damaging effects of cardiopulmonary bypass. In contrast, this phenomenon occurs in only about one in 2000 patients undergoing coronary artery bypass grafting. The same kinds of contrasts between good-risk adult patients and these infants are obtained after comparison of the incidences of important postoperative oliguria, intense vasoconstriction, perfusion deficits, and bleeding diatheses.[6]

In this paper we will discuss the nature of the damaging effects of cardiopulmonary bypass, then present our current working hypothesis concerning the mechanism of the damage. Finally, we will indicate some directions for future research and development which may lead to preventing or neutralizing the damaging effects of cardiopulmonary bypass in the future.

Nature of the Damaging Effects of Cardiopulmonary Bypass

The manifestations of the damaging effects of cardiopulmonary bypass are highly variable, ranging from subtle and inconsequential to fulminant and lethal. They include hemorrhagic pulmonary edema despite low left atrial pressure, bleeding tendencies, increased susceptibility to infection, increased interstitial water, fever, intense vasoconstriction (resulting in hemodynamic and metabolic problems), and breakdown of red blood cells (resulting in hemoglobinemia, hemoglobinurea, and anemia). These result in variable organ dysfunction, referred to by some as a "postperfusion" syndrome. The dysfunction is transient and inconsequential in most good-risk patients. But even in them it may occasionally necessitate prolonged and expensive respiratory or renal support or transfusions and re-entry for diffuse bleeding. No doubt the characteristics of the patient, his lesion, the conduct of his perfusion and operation, and the management of his postoperative care all interact to increase or decrease the probability that the abnormal state of cardiopulmonary bypass will produce manifest damage in that particular patient. That cardiopulmonary bypass is generally well tolerated may only attest to the remarkable resilience of the human organism.

Over the past 25 years, considerable progress has been made to increase the overall safety of cardiopulmonary bypass. One of the most important was the abandonment of a whole blood prime in favor of hemodilution. It has resulted in better perfusion of the microcirculation, less hemolysis due to lower viscosity and shear rates, less renal dysfunction, fewer transfusion reactions, a lower incidence of hepatitis, and decreased costs. The introduction of hypothermia, made practical by the introduction of an efficient heat exchanger,[7] has greatly increased the flexibility of cardiopulmonary bypass as a surgical tool and has provided an extra margin of safety against failures of the support systems. A number of other improvements can be cited, including improved gas exchange capacity, so that adequate flow rates can be achieved, and the introduction of cardiotomy filters. On the other hand, improved cardiopulmonary bypass safety has been disappointingly difficult to demonstrate for such theoretically advantageous advances as membrane oxygenation[8, 9] and pulsatile flow.[10-16] This has led us to conclude that there is something fundamental about blood's circulating outside its normal endothelial channels, which masks the potential benefits of such innovations.

Hypothesis

A great deal of information has accumulated concerning measurable abnormalities occurring during cardiopulmonary bypass. Hemostatic mechanisms are abnormal in disproportion to the amount of heparin administered;[17] blood cell constituents are changed in number and function; plasma proteins are denatured; gaseous and particulate emboli are identifiable; and a wide variety of vasoactive and otherwise biologically active substances are detectable (usually by indirect assay only). Yet, the prevention or neutralization of the untoward effects of cardiopulmonary bypass has drawn little attention. In part, this is due to the low incidence of clinical problems under normal circumstances. Even so, progress has been slow, perhaps because there has been no unifying concept inter-relating the various cellular and humoral abnormalities found.

We have recently developed just such a unifying concept. Although a great oversimplification, the concept is that the patient on cardiopulmonary bypass experiences a *whole body inflammatory reaction* from the sudden switching into action of multiple inter-related cellular and humoral cascades by the *exposure of blood to abnormal events*. The biologic activity of these reactions was never intended for systemic circulation, its being developed over eons to act as defense against *local* injury (such as a simple cut or splinter or burn). We have developed this concept over the past 2¹/₂ years from our analysis and synthesis of our own data, those of others working in the area of cardiopulmonary bypass, and those coming from recent advances in immunology, hematology, cell biology, biochemistry, physiology, and pharmacology. As we reviewed this information, we have been encouraged to think that eventually the damaging effects of cardiopulmonary bypass will be prevented or neutralized, and that this will result in a decreased mortality and morbidity associated with cardiac surgery, an extended scope of cardiac surgery, and a reduced cost and complexity of postoperative care.

Exposure of Blood to Abnormal Events

The exposure of blood to abnormal events has separate, well-known effects on formed and unformed blood elements. The abnormal events include *exposure to unphysiologic surfaces, exposure to shear stresses,* and *incorporation of abnormal substances.* The separate effects on the formed and unformed blood elements are highly inter-related and, we believe, are best understood as a *generalized* manifestation of the body's integrated inflammatory response to *local* injury.

EXPOSURE TO UNPHYSIOLOGIC SURFACES.—Damage initiated by contact of blood with a nonendothelial surface is, other things being equal, greater the larger the proportion of blood in the boundary layer where surface effects occur. Thus, the oxygenating area is the most critical surface. The surface may be gas (generally 100% oxygen) accompanied by "defoaming" surfaces, or it may be a membrane. Unphysiologic surfaces have direct and indirect effects on *platelets,* which result in platelet clumps that may embolize,[18] a reduction in platelet number,[19, 20] and a reduction in platelet adhesive and aggregating properties.[21-23] This initial clumping of platelets on foreign surfaces affects the platelet surface characteristics, allows calcium influx into the cells, and, in the presence of phospholipase and available membrane phospholipids, leads to the formation of arachidonic acid.[24] This fatty acid becomes oxidized via the cyclo-oxygenase pathway to thromboxane A_2, a potent stimulator of platelet aggregation and of vasoconstriction.[25] Thromboxane A_2, ADP, and vasoactive polypeptides are released from the platelets, propagating the clumping and eventually leading to liberation of α-granule proteins, some of which promote vascular permeability.[26] These same platelet-released substances can trigger leukocyte aggregation as well. Thus, thromboxane B_2, the degradation product of thromboxane A_2, has been shown in experimented animals to rise early during cardiopulmonary bypass, although it subsequently falls as prostacyclin is synthesized (as documented by a rise in its degradation product 6-keto-PGF$_{1\alpha}$).[27] Platelets so stimulated are temporarily or permanently refractory to further participation in hemostasis. These effects are probably the most important cause of postcardiopulmonary bypass bleeding diatheses.

Exposure of blood to nonphysiologic surfaces also affects *leukocytes* and *erythrocytes,*[28] although shear stresses (q.v.) probably have more important direct effects.

Carrier proteins are significantly damaged by blood's exposure to nonbiologic surfaces.[29] Denatured proteins increase plasma viscosity and the clumping of red cells, making them vulnerable to shear forces. Denaturation of gamma globulins (increased at a blood-gas interface and decreased by the presence of albumin on artificial membranes[30, 31]) may contribute to the humoral and cellular immune defects present after cardiopulmonary bypass.[32, 33]

Damage to the proteins constituting the *humoral amplification systems* has more complex and widespread effects. These are systems that respond to small stimuli with a self-propagating reaction. They include coagulation, fibrinolysis, complement, and kallikrein cascades. In intact man these are modulated in the blood stream by potent inhibitors of proteolytic enzymes (α_2-macroglobulin, α_1-antitrypsin, antithrombin III, C1-inactivator),[34–36] but are active at localized areas of injury. Cardiopulmonary bypass is perhaps the only situation in which the whole body is exposed directly to the results of activation of these substances.

No doubt *Hageman factor* (factor XII) is activated (denatured or uncoiled) almost immediately after the start of cardiopulmonary bypass by the massive contact of blood with nonbiologic surfaces.[37] The evidence for this is indirect; it includes demonstrating fibrinopeptide A from fibrinogen activation,[38] bradykinin, and plasmin during cardiopulmonary bypass, all by-products of Hageman factor activation. Activated Hageman factor initiates the *coagulation cascade.* Thus, despite "adequate" heparinization, microcoagulation continues, generating fibrin and consuming coagulation factors.[19]

The *fibrinolytic cascade* is probably activated,[39] plasminogen being transformed into the fibrinolytic agent plasmin, which has been demonstrated in patients shortly after initiation of cardiopulmonary bypass.[40] This transformation is facilitated by kallikrein, which results from Hageman factor activation; thus, the fibrinolytic cascade may be initiated indirectly by the activation of factor XII. Plasmin also activates complement, prekallikrein, and possibly Hageman factor, so that activation of plasminogen can trigger all the humoral amplification systems.

A third humoral amplification system involves *complement,* a group of circulating glycoproteins that act in concert to form a self-assembling biologic system, which functions as the primary humoral mediator of antigen-antibody (classic pathway) and foreign surface (alternative pathway) reactions to injury.[41] Complement, once activated, produces anaphylatoxins[42] (C3a, C5a) which lead to increased vascular permeability, smooth muscle contraction, histamine release from mast cells, and promotion of leukocyte chemotaxis, aggregation, free radical production, and lysosomal enzyme release.[43, 44] The usefulness of this in response to localized injury is obvious, but the problems of a whole body response to cardiopulmonary bypass are also obvious.

Complement activation occurs when blood contacts nonbiologic surfaces[45] and perhaps, by way of Hageman factor, thrombin, and plasmin. The adverse effects of complement activation are: (1) depletion of components necessary for normal immune responses, and (2) intravascular production of anaphylatoxins. As regards (1), post-bypass serum has a decreased ability to inhibit the growth of certain bacteria.[32] As regards (2), in response to C5a production, pulmonary sequestration of neutrophils and neutropenia develop during cardiopulmonary bypass[46, 47] (as they do during hemodialysis[48] and nylon fiber leukapheresis[49]). C5a-activated neutrophils can ultimately produce toxic free-radicals and release lysosomal enzymes,[50] which may cause endothelial injury and lead to increased pulmonary capillary permeability and diffusion abnormalities.[51] Using highly sensitive radioimmunoassay techniques, we have recently demonstrated a marked rise in C3a during the course of cardiopulmonary bypass, accompanied by pulmonary leukosequestration.[52] In vitro testing has demonstrated that among the factors that may be responsible for the production of anaphylatoxins are the materials used in constructing the oxygenating portions of the heart-lung apparatus.

The mechanistic sequence by which anaphylatoxins and neutrophils interact to produce a final biologic effect is still under intense study. At least one sequence is becoming clear. C5a binds to neutrophil receptors, alters the fluidity of the phospholipid membrane, and (again, with calcium) elicits oxidation of arachidonic acid to form leukotrienes via the lipoxygenase pathway. Leukotrienes are those formerly elusive substances which were termed "slow reactive substance of anaphylaxis." When released from leukocytes, they cause potent vasoconstriction, decreased pulmonary compliance, and elevated vascular resistance.[53] They provide a powerful chemotactic stimulus, augmenting that of C5a.[54, 55] Inhibition of leukotriene synthesis leads to inhibition of C5a activity.[56] Other effects of complement-derived anaphylatoxins are thought to be mediated by products of the arachidonic acid cascade as well, for they are inhibited by prostacyclin and nonsteroidal anti-inflammatory agents which are believed to exert their primary effects upon prostaglandin synthesis. For example, these substances prevent C5a-induced adhesion of neutrophils to foreign surfaces[57, 58] and the release of histamine from basophils.[57] Other mediators for anaphylatoxin activity include platelet activating factor,[60] which in the presence of C5a, leads to increased vascular permeability.

A fourth amplification system involves *kallikrein*. Contact activation of Hageman factor initiates the kallikrein cascade-producing kinins. The biologic activity of kinins is to increase vascular permeability, dilate arterioles, initiate smooth muscle contraction, and elicit pain.[61] In turn, kallikrein activates Hageman factor and plasminogen, demonstrating again the complex interactions among the various reactions of blood to a nonphysiologic experience. Important amounts of bradykinin can be demonstrated during cardiopulmonary bypass.[62] Hypothermia itself apparently results in bradykinin production, and immaturity (for example, infants) results in less effective bradykinin elimination.[63] Exclusion during cardiopulmonary bypass of the pulmonary circulation, the main site of bradykinin elimination, reduces the organism's ability to cope with circulating kinins.

Like the biologic activity of complement anaphylatoxins, the activity of the kinins is probably mediated and amplified via cofactors. For example, bradykinin may act via alteration of membrane phospholipids to ultimately produce prostaglandins such as PGE_2[64] and leukotrienes,[65] which act with bradykinin *in concert* to elicit such "kinin-like" biologic activities as enhanced vascular permeability and edema, hallmarks of the damaging effects of cardiopulmonary bypass.[66–68]

Thus, events initiated at an unphysiologic surface can directly or indirectly activate a host of the body's normal primary and secondary defense mechanisms. Rather than remaining localized, the effects of these humoral and cellular mediators of inflammation are amplified and disseminated throughout the body during cardiopulmonary bypass.

SHEAR STRESSES.—Shear stresses, generated by blood pumps, suction systems, acceleration of blood, and cavitation at the end of the arterial cannula, are probably the most important direct abnormal events as regards *leukocytes*. During cardiopulmonary bypass, an initial leukopenia develops, returning to (or above) baseline values after about two hours.[69] Similar changes occur without an oxygenator in the system.[70] The changes seem, in part, the result of movement of leukocytes out of the vascular spaces. Leukocytes injured by shear stresses release their cytotoxic granular components. This release may not be a passive phenomenon, however, but may be a programmed response to injury. For example, degranulation may be facilitated by products of arachidonic acid oxidation, since PGE_1 or phosphodiesterase inhibitors greatly decrease the shear-related release of leukocyte β-glucuronidase and alkaline phosphatase.[71]

Erythrocytes are also damaged during cardiopulmonary bypass by shear stresses. This damage results in either immediate lysis of erythrocytes with release of free hemoglobin, or subhemolytic damage resulting in a shortened life span and in delayed hemolysis. The amount of hemolysis and liberated free hemoglobin increases linearly with increased shear rate.[28] Hemolysis is much less without the oxygenator in the system,[72] and bubble oxygenators produce more hemolysis than membrane oxygenators.[8, 9]

INCORPORATION OF ABNORMAL SUBSTANCES.—During cardiopulmonary bypass, blood inadvertently has incorporated into it micro and macro air bubbles, bits of fibrin, tissue debris, defoaming agents, and so forth. Shed blood which has contacted injured tissues contains thromboplastinogen, a coagulation activator, and its aspiration into the extracorporeal system must contribute to activation of the coagulation cascade (and thereby all the other cascades).

Preventing or Neutralizing the Damaging Effects of Cardiopulmonary Bypass

In what ways might this new conceptual approach to the damaging effects of cardiopulmonary bypass help us in developing a rational program of research and development aimed at ultimate prevention or neutralization? Certainly, if the mechanism is, indeed, exposure of blood to abnormal events leading to a whole body inflammatory response, it is unlikely that the solution will be a simple one. Nature has provided us with a complex, highly integrated, robust, cellular and humoral defense mechanism, which will be difficult to "fool." What may be very compatible with one of its components is recognized as foreign to another, and the entire system is soon activated. It is, thus, not surprising that the search for a perfectly biocompatible synthetic surface has met with considerable frustration, research in this area revealing, for example, that interfacial free energy and the polar characteristics of artificial surfaces have completely opposite effects on humoral versus cellular components of the coagulation system. Artificial surfaces might be somewhat "inactivated" by being coated with plasma albumin.[73, 74] More promising might be surfaces that are locally pharmacologically active,[72] although *many* cascades must be modulated by such a scheme.

Another approach is via systemic pharmacologic intervention. Heparin is the familiar example of this approach. Other interventions include massive corticosteroid administration moments before expected complement activation.[75] Aprotinin, given to neutralize the effects of bradykinin and plasmin, has been tried,[76] and some advocate infusing prostacyclin or phosphodiesterase inhibitors to moderate the cellular response.[77–80] It is unlikely that a single pharmacologic agent will suffice to control all aspects of the inflammatory reaction, however.

For the time being, we are directing our efforts to documenting and clarifying the roles of mediators of inflammation in the damaging effects of cardiopulmonary bypass. As yet, the state of the art is too dependent upon indirect bioassays that may yield misleading results in the setting of blood's having been exposed massively to abnormal events. With increasingly more direct assays available to us from others, those we have developed with our colleagues, and others we are attempting to develop, we are seeking to discover clear associations, even if not cause-effect ones, between the measured mediators of inflammation and the clinical manifestations of the damaging effects of cardiopulmonary bypass. We are also developing experimental models of cardiopulmonary bypass that will yield clinically translatable results about the mechanisms of the damage and its amelioration.

Although such research and development will take some years, we are encouraged to believe that some day cardiac surgeons may be able to manage patients following low-risk coronary bypass operations with even greater simplicity than at present. An even more germaine possibility is that safe and definitive operations with rapid, simple, and inexpensive postoperative convalescence might be performed in situations that at present are limited by the damaging effects of cardiopulmonary bypass.

ACKNOWLEDGMENTS

Dr. Chenoweth acknowledges that portions of this work were done during the tenure of an Established Investigatorship from the American Heart Association. Drs. Stewart and Blackstone were supported in part by Program Project Grant HL-11310 from the National Heart, Lung, and Blood Institute.

REFERENCES

1. Kirklin J.W.: Open-heart surgery at the Mayo Clinic. *Mayo Clin. Proc.* 55:339–341, 1980.
2. Barnhorst D.A., Oxman H.A., Connolly D.C., Pluth J.R., Danielson G.K., Wallace R.B., McGoon D.C.: Isolated replacement of the aortic valve with the Starr-Edwards prosthesis: A 9 year review. *J. Thorac. Cardiovasc. Surg.* 70:113–118, 1975.
3. Rizzoli G., Blackstone E.H., Kirklin J.W., Pacifico A.D., Bargeron L.M. Jr.: Incremental risk factors in hospital mortality rate after repair of ventricular septal defect. *J. Thorac. Cardiovasc. Surg.* 80:494–505, 1980.
4. Kirklin J.W.: A letter to Helen. *J. Thorac. Cardiovasc. Surg.* 78:643–654, 1979.
5. Kirklin J.K., Blackstone E.H., Kirklin J.W., McKay R., Pacifico A.D., Bargeron L.M. Jr.: Intracardiac surgery under 3 months of age: Incremental risk factors for hospital mortality. *Am. J. Cardiol.* 48:500–506, 1981.
6. Kirklin J.K., Blackstone E.H., Kirklin J.W., McKay R., Pacifico A.D., Bargeron L.M. Jr.: Intracardiac surgery under 3 months of age: Postoperative predictors of hospital death in acute cardiac failure. Am. J. Cardiol. 48:507–515, 1981.
7. Brown I.W., Smith W.W., Emmons W.O.: An efficient blood heat exchanger for use with extracorporeal circulation. *Surgery* 44:372–377, 1958.
8. Alon L., Turina M., Gattiker R.: Membrane and bubble oxygenator: A clinical comparison in patients undergoing aortocoronary bypass procedures. *Herz* 4:56–62, 1979.
9. Clark R.E., Beauchamp R.A., Magrath R.A., Brooks J.D., Ferguson T.B., Weldon C.S.: Comparison of bubble and membrane oxygenators in short and long perfusions. *J. Thorac. Cardiovasc. Surg.* 78:655–666, 1979.
10. Jacobs L.A., Klopp E.H., Seamone W., Topaz S.R., Gott V.L.: Improved organ function during cardiac bypass with a roller pump modified to deliver pulsatile flow. *J. Thorac. Cardiovasc. Surg.* 58:703–712, 1969.
11. Trinkle J.K., Helton N.E., Bryant L.R., Griffen W.O.: Pulsatile cardiopulmonary bypass. Clinical evaluation. *Surgery* 68:1074–1078, 1970.
12. Taylor K.M., Bain W.H., Maxted K.J., Hutton M.M., McNab W.Y., Caves P.K.: Comparative studies of pulsatile and nonpulsatile flow during cardiopulmonary bypass. I. Pulsatile system employed and its hematologic effects. *J. Thorac. Cardiovasc. Surg.* 75:569–573, 1978.
13. Taylor K.M., Bain W.H., Maxted K.J., Hutton M.M., McNab W.H., Caves P.K.: Comparative studies of pulsatile and nonpulsatile flow during cardiopulmonary bypass. II. The effects on adrenal secretion of cortisol. *J. Thorac. Cardiovasc. Surg.* 75:574–578, 1978.
14. Taylor K.M., Wright G.S., Bain W.H., Caves P.K., Beastall G.S.: Comparative studies of pulsatile and nonpulsatile flow during cardiopulmonary bypass. III. Response of anterior pituitary gland to thyrotropin-releasing hormone. *J. Thorac. Cardiovasc. Surg.* 75:579–584, 1978.
15. Mavroudi C.: To pulse or not to pulse. *Ann. Thorac. Surg.* 25:259–271, 1978.
16. Singh R.K.K., Barratt-Boyes B.G., Harris E.A.: Does pulsatile flow im-

prove perfusion during hypothermic cardiopulmonary bypass? *J. Thorac. Cardiovasc. Surg.* 79:827–832, 1980.

17. Harker L.A., Malpass T.W., Branson H.E., Hessel E.A. II, Slichter S.J.: Mechanism of abnormal bleeding in patients undergoing cardiopulmonary bypass: Acquired transient platelet dysfunction associated with selective α-granule release. *Blood* 56:824–834, 1980.

18. Edmunds L.H. Jr., Saxena N.C., Hillyer P., Wilson T.J.: Relationship between platelet count and cardiotomy suction return. *Ann. Thorac. Surg.* 25:306–310, 1978.

19. Kalter R.D., Saul C.M., Wetstein L., Soriano C., Reiss R.F.: Cardiopulmonary bypass. Associated hemostatic abnormalities. *J. Thorac. Cardiovasc. Surg.* 77:427–435, 1979.

20. Han P., Turpie A.G.G., Butt R., LeBlanc P., Genton E., Gunstensen S.: The use of B-thromboglobulin release to assess platelet damage during cardiopulmonary bypass. Presented at the Combined Meeting of the Royal Australasian College of Surgeons and Royal Australasian College of Physicians, Sydney, Australia, February 24–29, 1980.

21. Addonizio V.P. Jr., Strauss J.F. III, Colman R.W., Edmunds L.H. Jr.: Effects of prostaglandin E_1 on platelet loss during in vivo and in vitro extracorporeal circulation with a bubble oxygenator. *J. Thorac. Cardiovasc. Surg.* 77:119–126, 1979.

22. Friedenberg W.R., Myers W.O., Plotka E.D., Beathard J.N., Kummer D.J., Gatlin P.F., Stoiber D.L., Ray J.F. III, Sautter R.D.: Platelet dysfunction associated with cardiopulmonary bypass. *Ann. Thorac. Surg.* 25:298–305, 1978.

23. Bharadwaj B.B., Chong G.: Effects of extracorporeal circulation on structure, function, and population distribution of canine blood platelets. Presented at the Combined Meeting of the Royal Australasian College of Surgeons and Royal Australasian College of Physicians, Sydney, Australia, February 24–29, 1980.

24. Gerrard J.M., White J.G.: Prostaglandins and thromboxanes: "Middlemen" modulating platelet function in hemostasis and thrombosis, in Spaet T.H. (ed.): *Progress in Hemostasis and Thrombosis, Vol. 4.* New York, Grune and Stratton, 1978, pp. 87–125.

25. Cohen I.: Platelet structure and function role of prostaglandins. *Ann. Clin. Lab. Sci.* 10:187–194, 1980.

26. Holmsen H.: Prostaglandin endoperoxide—thromboxane synthesis and dense granule secretion as positive feedback loops in the propagation of platelet responses during "the basic platelet reaction." *Thromb. Haemostas.* (Stuttg.) 38:1030–1041, 1977.

27. Zapol W.M., Peterson M.B., Wonders T.R., Kong D., Watkins W.D.: Plasma thromboxane and prostacyclin metabolites in sheep partial cardiopulmonary bypass. *Trans. Am. Soc. Artif. Intern. Organs* 26:556–560, 1980.

28. Solen K.A., Whiffen J.D., Lightfoot E.N.: The effect of shear, specific surface, and air interface on the development of blood emboli and hemolysis. *J. Biomed. Materials Res.* 12:381–399, 1978.

29. Lee W.H. Jr., Krumbhoar D., Fonkalsrud E.W., Schjeide O.A., Maloney J.V. Jr.: Denaturation of plasma proteins as a cause of morbidity and death after intracardiac operations. *Surgery* 50:29–39, 1961.

30. Pruitt K.M., Stroud R.M., Scott J.W.: Blood damage in the heart-lung machine (35651). *Proc. Soc. Exp. Biol. Med.* 137:714–718, 1971.
31. Scott J: Mechanism of gamma globulin denaturation. Doctoral Dissertation, University of Alabama in Birmingham, 1970.
32. Hairston P., Manos J.P., Graber C.D., Lee W.H. Jr.: Depression of immunologic surveillance by pump-oxygenator perfusion. *J. Surg. Res.* 9:587–593, 1969.
33. Fong I.W., Baker C.B., McKee D.C.: The value of prophylactic antibiotics in aorta-coronary bypass operations. A double-blind randomized trial. *J. Thorac. Cardiovasc. Surg.* 78:908–913, 1979.
34. Harpel P.C., Rosenberg R.D.: α_2-macroglobulin and antithrombin-heparin cofactor: Modulators of hemostatic and inflammatory reactions, in Spaet T.H. (ed.): *Progress in Hemostasis and Thrombosis, Vol. 3.* New York, Grune and Stratton, 1976, pp. 145–189.
35. Heimburger N., Haupt H., Schwick H.G.: Proteinase inhibitors of human plasma, in Fritz H., Tschesche H. (eds.): *Proceedings of the International Research Conference on Proteinase Inhibitors.* New York, Walter de Gruyter, 1971, pp. 1.
36. Heimburger N.: Biochemistry of proteinase inhibitors from human plasma: A review of recent developments, in Fritz H., Tschesche H., Greene L.J. (eds.): *Bayer Symposium on Proteinase Inhibitors.* Berlin, Springer-Verlag, 1974, p. 14.
37. Feijen J.: Thrombogenesis caused by blood–foreign surface interaction, in Kenedi R.M., Courtney J.M., Gaylor J.D.S., Gilchrist T. (eds.): *Artificial Organs.* Baltimore, University Park Press, 1977, pp. 235–247.
38. Davies G.C., Sobel M., Salzman E.W.: Elevated plasma fibrinopeptide A and thromboxane B_2 levels during cardiopulmonary bypass. *Circulation* 61:808–814, 1980.
39. Lambert C.J., Marengo-Rowe A.J., Leveson J.E., Green R.H., Theile J.P., Geisler G.F., Adam M., Mitchel B.F.: The treatment of postperfusion bleeding using epsilon-aminocaproic acid, cryoprecipitate, fresh-frozen plasma, and protamine sulfate. *Ann. Thorac. Surg.* 28:440–444, 1979.
40. Backmann F., McKenna R., Cole E.R., Najafi H.: The hemostatic mechanism after open-heart surgery. I. Studies on plasma coagulation factors and fibrinolysis in 512 patients after extracorporeal circulation. *J. Thorac. Cardiovasc. Surg.* 70:76–85, 1975.
41. Muller-Eberhard H.J.: Complement. *Ann. Rev. Biochem.* 44:697–724, 1975.
42. Holobut W., Modrzejewski E., Stazka W.: Irrigation sanguine et consommation d'oxygene de divers organes en temperature normale et en hypothermie. *J. Physiol. (Paris)* 61:507–517, 1969.
43. Grant J.A., Durpee E., Goldman A.S., Schultz D.R., Jackson A.L.: Complement-mediated release of histamine from human leukocytes. *J. Immunol.* 114:1101–1106, 1975.
44. Goldstein I.M., Brai M., Osler A.G., Weissmann G.: Lysosomal enzyme release from human leukocytes: Mediation by the alternate pathway of complement activation. *J. Immunol.* 111:33–37, 1973.
45. Birek A., Duffin J., Glynn M.F.X., Cooper J.D.: The effect of sulfinpyrazone on platelet and pulmonary responses to onset of membrane oxygen-

ator perfusion. *Trans. Am. Soc. Artif. Int. Organs* 22:94–100, 1976.

46. Hammerschmidt D.E., Stroncek D.F., Bowers T.K., Lammi-Keefe C.J., Kurth D.M., Ozalins A., Nicoloff D.M., Lillehei R.C., Craddock P.R., Jacob H.S.: Complement activation and neutropenia occurring during cardiopulmonary bypass. *J. Thorac. Cardiovasc. Surg.* 81:370–377, 1981.

47. Wilson J.W.: Pulmonary morphologic changes due to extracorporeal circulation: A model for 'the shock lung' at cellular level in humans, in Forscher B.K., Lillehei R.C., Stubbs S.S. (eds.): *Shock in Low- and High-Flow States.* Proceedings of a Symposium at Brook Lodge, Augusta, Michigan. Amsterdam, Excerpta Medica, 1972, pp. 160–171.

48. Craddock P.R., Fehr J., Dalmasso A.P., Brigham K.L., Jacob J.S.: Pulmonary vascular leukostasis resulting from complement activation by dialyzer cellophane membranes. *J. Clin. Invest.* 59:879–888, 1977.

49. Hammerschmidt D.E., Craddock P.R., McCullough F., Kronenberg R.S., Dalmasso A.P., Jacob H.S.: Complement activation and pulmonary leukostasis during nylon fiber filtration leukapheresis. *Blood* 51:721–730, 1978.

50. Sacks T., Moldow C.F., Craddock P.R., Bowers T.K., Jacob H.S.: Oxygen radicals mediate endothelial cell damage by complement-stimulated granulocytes. *J. Clin. Invest.* 61:1161–1167, 1978.

51. Craddock P.R., Fehr J., Brigham K.L., Kronenberg R.S., Jacob H.S.: Complement and leukocyte-mediated pulmonary dysfunction in hemodialysis. *N. Engl. J. Med.* 296:769–774, 1977.

52. Chenoweth D.E., Cooper S.W., Hugli T.E., Stewart R.W., Blackstone E.H., Kirklin J.W.: Complement activation during cardiopulmonary bypass. *N. Engl. J. Med.* 304:497–503, 1981.

53. Sirois P., Borgeat P., Jeanson A., Roy S., Girard G.: The action of leukotriene B$_4$ (LTB$_4$) on the lung. *Prostaglandins Med.* 5:429–444, 1980.

54. Goetzl E.J., Woods J.M., Gorman R.R.: Stimulation of human eosinophil and neutrophil polymorphonuclear leukocyte chemotaxis and random migration by 12-L-hydroxy-5,8,10,14-eicosatetraenoic acid. *J. Clin. Invest.* 59:179–183, 1977.

55. Palmer R.M.J., Stepney R.J., Higgs G.A., Eakins K.E.: Chemokinetic activity of arachidonic acid lipoxygenase products on leukocytes of different species. *Prostaglandins* 20:411–418, 1980.

56. Regal J.F., Pickering R.J.: C5a-induced tracheal contraction: Effect of an SRS-A antagonist and inhibitors of arachidonate metabolism. *J. Immunol.* 126:313–316, 1981.

57. McGillen J., Patterson R., Phair J.P.: Adherence of polymorphonuclear leukocytes to nylon: Modulation by prostacyclin (PGI$_2$), corticosteroids, and complement activation. *J. Infect. Dis.* 141:382–388, 1980.

58. Boxer L.A., Allen J.M., Schmidt M., Yoder M., Baehner R.L.: Inhibition of polymorphonuclear leukocyte adherence by prostacyclin. *J. Lab. Clin. Med.* 95:672–678, 1980.

59. Marone G., Hammarstrom S., Lichtenstein L.M.: An inhibitor of lipoxygenase inhibits histamine release from human basophils. *Clin. Immunol. Immunopathol.* 17:117–122, 1980.

60. Lotner G.Z., Lynch J.M., Betz S.J., Henson P.M.: Human neutrophil-derived platelet activating factor. *J. Immunol.* 124:676–684, 1980.

61. Ellison N., Behar M., MacVaugh H. III, Marshall B.E.: Bradykinin, plasma protein fraction and hypotension. *Ann. Thorac. Surg.* 29:15–19, 1980.

62. Pang L.M., Stalcup S.A., Lipset J.S., Hayes C.J., Bowman F.O. Jr., Mellins R.B.: Increased circulating bradykinin during hypothermia and cardiopulmonary bypass in children. *Circulation* 60:1503–1507, 1979.

63. Friedli B., Kent G., Olley P.M.: Inactivation of bradykinin in the pulmonary vascular bed of newborn and fetal lambs. *Circ. Res.* 33:421–427, 1973.

64. Bell R.L. Baenziger N.L., Majerus P.W.: Bradykinin-stimulated release of arachidonate from phosphatidyl inositol in mouse fibrosarcoma cells. *Prostaglandins* 20:269–274, 1980.

65. Bray M.A., Cunningham F.M., Ford-Hutchinson A.W., Smith M.J.H.: Leukotriene B_4: A mediator of vascular permeability. *Br. J. Pharmacol.* 72:483–486, 1981.

66. Breckenridge I.M., Digerness S.B., Kirklin J.W.: Increased extracellular fluid after open intracardiac operation. *Surg. Gynec. Obstet.* 131:53–56, 1970.

67. Pacifico A.D., Digerness S., Kirklin J.W.: Regression of body compositional abnormalities of heart failure after intracardiac operations. *Circulation* 42:999–1008, 1970.

68. Parker D.J., Karp R.B., Kirklin J.W., Bedard P.: Lung water and alveolar and capillary volumes after intracardiac surgery. *Circulation* 45(suppl I):139–146, 1972.

69. Kusserow B., Larrow R., Nichols J.: Perfusion- and surface-induced injury in leukocytes. *Fed. Proc.* 30:1516–1520, 1971.

70. Kusserow B.K., Machanic B., Collins F.M. Jr., Clapp J.F. III.: Changes observed in blood corpuscles after prolonged perfusions with two types of blood pumps. *Trans. Am. Soc. Artif. Int. Organs* 11:122–126, 1965.

71. McIntire L.V., Stockwell D.J., Martin R.R., Sybers H.D.: Leukocyte response to mechanical trauma—antiplatelet drug effects. *Trans. Am. Soc. Artif. Intern. Organs* 26:289–293, 1980.

72. Lindsay R.M., Mason R.G., Kim S.W., Andrade J.D., Hakim R.M.: Blood surface interactions. *Trans. Am. Soc. Artif. Intern. Organs* 26:603–610, 1980.

73. Packham M.A., Evans G., Glynn M.F., Mustard J.F.: The effect of plasma proteins on the interaction of platelets with glass surfaces. *J. Lab. Clin. Med.* 73:686–697, 1969.

74. Addonizio V.P. Jr., Macarak E.J., Nicolaou K.C., Edmunds L.H., Colman R.W.: Effects of prostacyclin and albumin on platelet loss during in vitro simulation of extracorporeal circulation. *Blood* 53:1033–1042, 1979.

75. Hammerschmidt D.E., White J.G., Craddock P.R., Jacob H.S.: Corticosteroids inhibit complement-induced granulocyte aggregation. *J. Clin. Invest.* 63:798–803, 1979.

76. Nagaoka H., Katori M.: Inhibition of kinin formation by a kallikrein inhibitor during extracorporeal circulation in open-heart surgery. *Circulation* 52:325–332, 1975.

77. Addonizio V.P. Jr., Macarak E.J., Niewiarowski S., Colman R.W., Edmunds L.H. Jr.: Preservation of human platelets with prostaglandin E_1

during in vitro simulation of cardiopulmonary bypass. *Circ. Res.* 44:350–357, 1979.

78. Addonizio V.P. Jr., Strauss J.F. III, Macarak E.J., Colman R.W., Edmunds L.H. Jr.: Preservation of platelet number and function with prostaglandin E_1 during total cardiopulmonary bypass in rhesus monkeys. *Surgery* 83:619–625, 1978.

79. Plachetka J.R., Salomon N.W., Larson D.F., Copeland J.G.: Platelet loss during experimental cardiopulmonary bypass and its prevention with prostacyclin. *Ann. Thorac. Surg.* 30:58–63, 1980.

80. Longmore D.B., Gueirrara D., Bennett G., Smith M.: Prostacyclin: A solution to some problems of extracorporeal circulation. *Lancet* I:1002–1005, 1979.

Hemodynamic and Platelet-Preserving Effects of Prostacyclin During Cardiopulmonary Bypass

MICHAEL P. KAYE, KEVIN A. PETERSON,
CARL R. NOBACK, MRINAL K. DEWANJEE

Mayo Clinic and Foundation
Rochester, Minnesota

It has been suggested that prostacyclin (PGI_2), a known inhibitor of platelet aggregation, might be useful as a "platelet preservative" during cardiopulmonary bypass. Accordingly, animal studies were conducted to determine the platelet preservation effect of prostacyclin, and initial clinical studies were conducted on patients undergoing cardiopulmonary bypass to determine the hemodynamic effects of a constant infusion of prostacyclin.

Materials and Methods

ANIMAL STUDIES

Thirteen mongrel dogs weighing between 15 and 20 kg were studied. Seven dogs (group 1) served as controls and were given an anticoagulant (3 mg/kg heparin) prior to cardiopulmonary bypass. Six dogs (group 2) were given 1 mg/kg of heparin and a continuous infusion of 25 ng/kg/min of prostacyclin in a buffered solution, administered by a Harvard pump through a jugular venous line, from 15 minutes prior to bypass to 15 minutes after bypass (total $1^{1}/_{2}$ hours.). In addition, 50 ng/ml of prostacyclin was added to the oxygenator priming solution. In all other ways the two study groups were treated identically.

Sixteen to 20 hours prior to instituting cardiopulmonary bypass, platelets from the experimental animals were labeled with indium-111. Immediately preceding the operation the dogs were given 25 μCi of iodine-125 human serum albumin and then anesthetized with pentobarbital and placed on a respirator. After suitable preparation and following a left thoracotomy, systemic heparinization was induced with 3 mg/kg of heparin given intravenously, and the femoral artery and right atrium were cannulated for cardiopulmonary bypass. Bypass was established using a BOS 5 Bentley oxygenator with silicone rubber tubing and a nonocclusive Mayo-Gibbons pump. All oxygenators were primed with 1000 cc of Plasma-lyte solution. All dogs were subjected to cardiopulmonary bypass for one hour, including the period of systemic hypothermia at 25°C for 30 minutes. At the completion of bypass, all blood was returned to the animal, the oxygenator gently flushed with one liter of Plasma-lyte, the polyurethane core removed from the oxygenator and measured for indium-111 in a modified ionization chamber. Five-milliliter samples of blood were removed prior to institution of bypass and at 5, 10, 20, 30, 60, 120, 180, and 240 minutes after initiation of bypass. From each sample a 1.2-ml aliquot was centrifuged at 25,000 g for 10 minutes. Plasma supernatant was removed and the samples measured for indium-111 and iodine-125 with a gamma well counter. The gamma ray spectrometers were adjusted to incorporate the 28 to 35 keV peaks of iodine-125 and the 174, 247, and 421 keV peaks of indium-111, and a cross-over correction for indium-111 was made. Indium-111 deposition on the oxygenator was expressed as indium-111 in the oxygenator (cpm) divided by total indium-111 injected corrected for decay. Significance was determined by nonparametric Wilkoxon-Mann-Whitney rank sum tests. Platelet destruction was measured by determining the amount of the plasma-bound indium-111 and expressed as indium-111 in plasma divided by indium-111 in whole blood at the time the sample was taken. Platelet concentration was measured by determining platelet-bound indium concentration and was expressed as percentage of platelet-bound indium in prebypass blood. Iodine-125-labeled human serum albumin levels measured in six animals were expressed by blood iodine-125 level at time t divided by blood iodine-125 level prebypass. Mean plasma-bound indium-111, platelet-bound indium-111, and iodine-125 serum human albumin levels were calculated with standard deviations and graphed vs. time on bypass.

CLINICAL STUDIES

Six adult patients undergoing coronary artery bypass graft procedures were studied after giving informed written consent. After induction of anesthesia, a 7F Swan-Ganz thermodilution catheter was placed via the right internal jugular vein. Radial artery cannulation had previously taken place. Enflurane served as the primary anesthetic agent. After sternotomy and prior to bypass, an anesthetic steady-state was reached, at which point cardiac output was determined with an Edwards cardiac output computer. Heart rate, systolic pressure, diastolic pressure, pulmonary artery pressure, pulmonary capillary wedge pressure, and right atrial pressures were recorded. Infusion of prostacyclin at a rate of 10 ng/kg/min, via Harvard pump, was begun. The foregoing variables were then recorded each minute for 10 minutes, allowing calculation of cardiac index, stroke volume, stroke volume index, systemic vascular resistance, pulmonary vascular resistance, and rate pressure product.

Results

ANIMAL STUDIES

Platelet destruction as indicated by increases in the ratio of plasma indium-111 to whole blood indium-111 was notably different in the heparin (group 1) as opposed to the heparin-prostacyclin (group 2) treated animals (Fig 33–1). In the group 1 animals, plasma to whole blood ratios of indium-111 increased from a prebypass control value of $6 \pm 1\%$ to $34 \pm 7\%$ one hour following the initiation of bypass and then declined slowly to a level of $18 \pm 7\%$ three hours following bypass. In marked contrast, plasma to whole blood ratios from the animals in group 2 increased from a prebypass control of $5 \pm 2\%$ to only $15 \pm 5\%$ after one hour of bypass. The 28% increase in platelet lysis

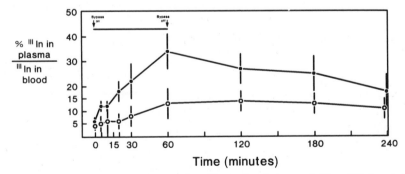

Fig 33–1.—Platelet lysis expressed as the ratio of plasma indium-111 to whole blood indium-111 plotted against time prior to, during, and following 1 hour of cardiopulmonary bypass in dogs. Mean ± S.D. of group 1 (7 dogs—heparin only ●——●) and group 2 (6 dogs—heparin and prostacyclin ○——○) ($p < 0.01$ at 60 min).

in group 1 is significantly greater than the 10% in group 2 (P <0.01). Likewise, in group 2, the ratio of plasma indium-111 to whole blood indium-111 (11.4%) was lower three hours following termination of bypass.

In group 1, platelet-bound indium-111 declined in the first 5 minutes following initiation of bypass to 40 ± 7% of control values (Fig 33–2). Platelet-bound indium-111 continued to decline for 20 minutes and remained low, being 25 ± 6% after one hour. Platelet-bound indium-111 levels rose to 37 ± 7% at three hours following termination of bypass. In group 2, platelet-bound indium-111 declined in the first 5 minutes to 38 ± 8% of control value and remained steady, being 35 ± 5% after the completion of one hour of bypass. Following bypass, platelet-bound indium-111 levels in group 2 increased, and at three hours postbypass they were 54 ± 7%. Hemodilution, which accounts for a portion of the decrease in platelet-bound indium-111, was quantitated by using iodine-125-albumin concentration, and these data points are superimposed upon Figure 33–2 to give an estimation of the drop in platelet concentration due to dilution by oxygenator prime. Although some iodine-125-albumin is absorbed onto the extracorporeal circuit,[1] total absorbed albumin fraction is small, and thus accurately reflects dilution. Iodine-125-radioactivity declined to 66 ± 7% after 5 minutes of bypass, remained at that level, and after one hour of bypass was 68 ± 8%. Following bypass, iodine-125-albumin slowly increased to 73 ± 8% at four hours. This correlates well with expected dilution due to the 1000 cc of clear prime and a total blood volume calculated as 8% of body weight.

Following the completion of bypass, and when all of the contents of

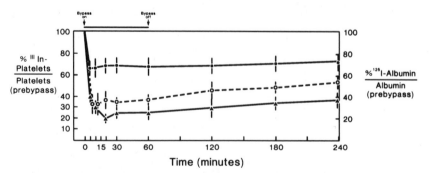

Fig 33–2.—Platelet concentrations expressed as the ratio of indium-111-labeled platelets during and following bypass to prebypass control levels. Iodine-125 albumin levels plotted as an index of hemodilution occurring during and following bypass. ▲——▲ = control animals; ○——○ = prostacyclin-treated animals; ●——● = ^{125}I-albumin reference for dilution.

the oxygenator and arterial line had been returned to the animal, the oxygenators, which had been flushed with normal saline, were disassembled and the polyurethane core counted in a modified scintillation counter. This polyurethane mesh of the oxygenators used in group 1 experiments was found to contain 20 ± 5% of the total injected indium-111 (corrected for decay). In the oxygenators from the group 2 animals, the core contained only 11 ± 3% of the injected indium-111, a value significantly (P <0.01) less than that of the group 1 oxygenators.

CLINICAL STUDIES

Vasodilation occurred in each patient, with four of six patients requiring methoxamine after prostacyclin infusion to attain pre-infusion blood pressure. Hemodynamic data are presented in Table 33–1. Significant findings include a 39% increase in cardiac index, after 10 minutes of prostacyclin infusion, from an average of 2.14 ± 0.22 to 3.48 ± 0.27 L/min/m² (P <0.02). Concurrently, systemic vascular resistance decreased by 49% at 10 minutes, from 1720 ± 191 to 872 ± 91 dynes·cm·sec^{-5}, (P <0.02). Heart rate and rate pressure product remained unchanged, whereas mean arterial pressure decreased 14% and stroke volume index increased 46%.

Discussion

Cardiopulmonary bypass has been demonstrated to result in a decrease in circulating platelet count, presumably following platelet deposition and platelet destruction in the extracorporeal circuit.[2, 3] Resulting deficits of platelet number and function impair hemostasis and may result in significant postoperative complications.[4, 5] Because of the dynamics of platelet sequestration, mobilization, activation, and deposition during cardiopulmonary bypass, data concerning platelet dynamics during bypass have been difficult to achieve. With the introduction of indium-111-labeling techniques, a new tool has been made available for the study of such platelet kinetics and platelet deposition.[6] Platelets labeled with indium-111 release very little radioactive label during activation or degranulation,[7] and significant loss of the indium-111 label occurs only upon platelet destruction. Since indium-111 lost into blood remains bound to protein, possibly transferrin,[6] the ratio of serial plasma-indium-111 concentrations to those of whole blood indium-111 make an excellent in vivo indicator of continuing platelet destruction. This characteristic, in addition to

TABLE 33–1.—Hemodynamic Effects of Prostacyclin*

GROUP	CARDIAC INDEX (L/MIN/M²)	SYSTEMIC VASCULAR RESISTANCE (DYNES/CM/SEC⁻⁵)	STROKE VOLUME INDEX (ML BEAT/M²)	MEAN ARTERIAL PRESSURE (MM HG)	HEART RATE (BEATS/MIN)	RATE PRESSURE PRODUCT (BEATS MM HG/MIN)
Control	$2.14 \pm .2$†	1720 ± 191	35 ± 5	94 ± 3.4	63 ± 3.6	8545 ± 720
10 min after infusion begun	$3.48 \pm .3$	872 ± 91	51 ± 5	81 ± 3.7	72 ± 4.8	8581 ± 298
p <	.02	.02	.02	.05	NS	NS
% △	+39	−49	+46	−14	—	—

*Infusion constant at 10 ng/kg/min.
†Mean ± SE.

the excellent recovery and high yield of gamma emissions of indium-111-labeled platelets, allows for a sensitive examination of platelet response to cardiopulmonary bypass.

Twenty percent of injected radioactive platelets in our heparinized control group were sequestered by the bubble oxygenator during one hour of cardiopulmonary bypass. Significantly less (P <0.01) platelet sequestration occurred in the oxygenators in the presence of prostacyclin. Plasma-indium-111 levels in controls increased serially from 6% of total whole blood indium-111 prior to bypass to 33% one hour after initiation of bypass. This significant increase in plasma indium-111 indicates that large numbers of platelets were destroyed during the bypass procedure. In the presence of prostacyclin, platelet destruction was significantly reduced (P <0.01) with plasma-indium-111 levels rising to only 15% of whole blood indium-111 levels. Finally, in animals treated with prostacyclin, total indium-111-labeled platelet levels remained at higher values during the operation and increased more rapidly postoperatively, achieving 56% of prebypass levels at three hours postbypass compared to only 36% in the control groups. The mechanism by which prostacyclin preserves platelets during bypass is not well understood. Possible mechanisms of platelet destruction include platelet membrane damage by shearing forces either by contact with foreign material with partial release of platelet content, or by contact with the blood-gas interface in the bubble oxygenator.[5] Presumably, by increasing platelet adenylate cyclase and, consequently, the inhibition of platelet activation, the trauma of surface contact is reduced. Nonspecific platelet damage induced by high flow rates might be expected to remain unchanged.

Notably, in both experimental bypass groups a large drop in platelet concentration occurs within five minutes of initiation of bypass, which cannot be accounted for by hemodilution alone. This drop in circulating platelet levels probably represents a large initial absorption of platelets onto the extracorporeal surface or sequestration within the experimental animal. Such an initial absorption might be expected, since prostacyclin in this dose does not appear to totally prevent surface adhesion.[8-10] Our data demonstrating deposition of platelets on the polyurethane base of oxygenator tend to confirm this hypothesis.

In summary, we have developed a sensitive technique for determining platelet dynamics and destruction during cardiopulmonary bypass. Using this technique, we have demonstrated that the reversible inhibition of platelet activity by prostacyclin results in higher intraoperative and postoperative platelet counts during cardiopulmonary bypass. This effect is associated with a significant decrease in platelet destruction and a reduction of platelet uptake by the oxygenator.

Preliminary human studies indicate that prostacyclin is a potent vasodilator in anesthetized man. From these preliminary data we may surmise that if prostacyclin is to be used as an intrabypass platelet preservative, it may also be useful in controlling intrabypass hypertension.

REFERENCES

1. Addonizio V.P. Jr., Macarak E.J., Nicolaou K.C., Edmunds L.H. Jr., Colman R.W.: Effects of prostacyclin and albumin on platelet loss during in vitro simulation of extracorporeal circulation. *Blood* 53:1033–1042, 1979.
2. Hennessy V.L. Jr., Hicks R.E., Niewiarowski S., Edmunds L.H. Jr., Colman R.W.: Function of human platelets during extracorporeal circulation. *Am. J. Physiol.* 232:H622–628, 1977.
3. McKenna R., Bachmann F., Whittaker B., Gilson J.R., Weinberg M. Jr.: The hemostatic mechanism after open heart surgery. *J. Thorac. Cardiovasc. Surg.* 70:298–308, 1975.
4. Andersen M.N., Hambraeus G.: Physiologic and biochemical responses to prolonged extracorporeal circulation. Experimental studies during four-hour perfusion. *Ann. Surg.* 153:592–598, 1961.
5. Bick R.L.: Alterations of hemostasis associated with cardiopulmonary bypass: pathophysiology, prevention, diagnosis, and management, in Mammen E.F. (ed.): *Seminars in Thrombosis and Hemostasis.* New York, Stratton Intercontinental, 1976, pp. 59–82.
6. Thakur M.L., Welch M.J., Joist J.H., Coleman R.E.: Indium-111-labeled platelets: Studies on preparation and evaluation of in vitro and in vivo functions. *Thromb. Res.* 9:345–357, 1976.
7. Joist J.H., Baker R.K., Thakur M.L., Welch M.J.: Indium-111-labeled human platelets: uptake and loss of label and in vitro function of labeled platelets. *J. Lab. Clin. Med.* 92:829–836, 1978.
8. Cazenave J.P., Dejana E., Kinlough-Rathbone R., Packham M.A., Mustard J.F.: Platelet interactions with endothelium and the subendothelium: the role of thrombin and prostacyclin. *Haemostasis* 8:183–192, 1979.
9. Fry G.L., Czervionke R.L., Hoak J.C., Smith J.B., Haycraft D.L.: Platelet adherence to cultured vascular cells: Influence of prostacyclin (PGI_2). *Blood* 55:271–275, 1980.
10. Curwen K.D., Gimbrone M.A. Jr., Handin R.I.: In vitro studies of thromboresistance: The role of prostacyclin (PGI_2) in platelet adhesion to cultured normal and virally transformed human vascular endothelial cells. *Lab. Invest.* 42:366–374, 1980.

Experiences with Use of Prostacyclin in Open Heart Surgery

K. RÅDEGRAN, C. ARÉN, N. EGBERG,
C. PAPACONSTANTINOU, A.-C. TEGER-NILSSON

*Departments of Thoracic Surgery and Clinical
Chemistry, Sahlgrenska sjukhuset, Göteborg;
Department of Thoracic Surgery and Laboratory of Blood
Coagulation Disorders, Karolinska Sjukhuset,
Stockholm, Sweden*

Introduction

It has been shown under conditions of in vitro simulated cardiopulmonary bypass (CPB)[1], in experiments on dogs[2,3] as well as in patients undergoing open heart surgery,[4,5,6] that prostacyclin improves the preservation of platelets and their function. As our earliest studies in man indicated that a prostacyclin dosage of 20 ng/kg/min or less during CPB was insufficient,[4] we subsequently turned to dosages of 50 to 100 ng/kg/min. In the present report we will attempt to sum up some of our experiences with these higher dosages in patients randomly assigned to prostacyclin treatment or control groups.[5,6] We have not attempted to perform a blind study because of the pronounced arterial hypotension that accompanies high-dosage prostacyclin treatment, alerting surgeons and anesthetists to the nature of the infusion. The studies were approved by the Ethics Committees of the Karolinska sjukhuset and the Sahlgrenska sjukhuset.

Material and Methods

Adult patients scheduled for surgery of acquired heart disease were randomly assigned to prostacyclin treatment or control groups. The first 45 patients (groups 1 and 2) were operated upon at the Karolinska sjukhuset in Stockholm by a group of 10 surgeons. Valvular and coronary surgery were approximately equally represented. The last 20 patients (group 3) were all operated upon at the Sahlgrenska sjukhuset, Göteborg, and underwent aortocoronary saphenous vein bypass performed by only two surgeons (K.R. and C.A.). CPB was by roller pump and bubble oxygenator primed with a crystalloid solution. General hypothermia to a rectal temperature of 25 to 28°C and cold hyperkalemic cardioplegia were employed. The perfusion rate was generally 2.2 L/m^2 body surface area with a reduction to 1.5 L/m^2 (Stockholm) or 40 ml/kg (Göteborg) during hypothermia. Cardiotomy reservoir filters but no arterial line filters were used, and free use of cardiotomy suction was allowed. Unless otherwise stated, patients were given heparin, 3 mg/kg, before cannulation, and 50 to 75 mg were added to the pump prime. Anticoagulation was checked intraoperatively by the activated clotting time (Hemochron). Prostacyclin was dissolved in a pH 10.5 glycine buffer (Upjohn) and infused into the venous line of the extracorporeal circuit. Blood samples were drawn into appropriate anticoagulants from wide-bore cannulae in the superior vena cava, by needle puncture of the right atrial appendage (group 3) and during bypass from the extracorporeal circuit. Platelet counts in whole blood were determined by particle counters (Clay-Adams Ultra-Flo 100 or Linson 401 A) and are reported with correction for changes in hematocrit. Heparin and antithrombin III concentrations in plasma were measured with chromogenic substrate methods.[7, 8] Fibrinopeptide A was determined by radioimmunoassay.[9] Platelet aggregation induced by ADP and collagen was studied in a Payton dual channel aggregometer on platelet-rich plasma prepared by centrifugation immediately after collection.

GROUP 1.—Ten patients received prostacyclin 50 ng/kg/min for the first 30 minutes of CPB, with another 12 patients serving as controls (Table 34–1).

GROUP 2.—Fourteen patients received prostacyclin 100 ng/kg/min throughout CPB except for the last 5 to 20 minutes. Nine patients served as controls.

GROUP 3.—Eleven patients received prostacyclin 50 ng/kg/min except for the last 10 minutes of CPB. Nine patients did not receive prostacyclin. In this group, the patients receiving prostacyclin were given heparin, 2 mg/kg, before aortic cannulation, and control patients were given heparin, 3 mg/kg. More detailed descriptions of methodology and results are presented elsewhere.[5, 6]

STATISTICS.—All data are reported as $\bar{x} \pm$ S.D. Significance testing was by Student's t test.

TABLE 34–1.—PATIENT DATA AND PROSTACYCLIN DOSAGE
DURING CPB

GROUP	NO. PATIENTS	NO. FEMALES	AGE (YR)	CPB TIME (MIN)	PROSTACYCLIN (NG/KG/MIN)
1	12	6	60 ± 7	103 ± 45	No
	10	3	57 ± 8	119 ± 40	50, 30
2	9	0	54 ± 10	104 ± 33	No
	14	2	61 ± 6	111 ± 34	100
3	9	1	53 ± 9	130 ± 36	No
	11	1	60 ± 8	134 ± 20	50

Results

COMPLICATIONS AND DEATHS

There were three deaths among the 30 control patients and one death among the 35 patients who received prostacyclin (Table 34–2). Two control and two prostacyclin patients had to undergo a second operation because of bleeding. In one of the latter cases, the cause of bleeding was clearly a puncture hole in the brachiocephalic vein after premature removal of a Swan-Ganz catheter introduced at this site. The other bleeding incident was in a man with triple valve disease, functional group IV, and compromised liver function. He bled diffusely postoperatively and subsequently died in myocardial failure. Severe cerebral damage occurred in two control patients in whom CPB was prolonged by several hours because of poor cardiac function. Neither of these two patients regained consciousness and they subsequently died. One patient receiving prostacyclin was operated on for calcific aortic stenosis and coronary bypass and suffered right hemiparesis postoperatively; partial recovery was achieved. Another patient was mildly confused for three days, but recovered completely. Several years previously, he had had a similar episode in conjunction with a febrile illness.

INTRAOPERATIVE AND POSTOPERATIVE BLEEDING

Intraoperative bleeding was measured in groups 1 and 2. Prostacyclin infusion did not affect intraoperative bleeding, which was 971 ± 536 ml in control patients and 810 ± 243 ml in patients who received prostacyclin. Postoperatively (until 7.00 a.m. the day after surgery), bleeding was respectively 665 ± 238 and 572 ± 263 ml. These patients were operated upon by a group of 10 surgeons for a variety of acquired cardiac disorders. In group 3 (which was com-

TABLE 34–2.—Complications and Deaths in 35 Prostacyclin and 30 Control Patients

PATIENT	AGE/SEX	GROUP	OPERATION	PROSTACYCLIN (NG/KG/MIN)	COMMENTS
M.M.	58/F	1	Coronary bypass	No	Prolonged CPB. Cerebral damage. Died in sepsis 30 days postop.
L.H.	71/F	1	AVR + MVR	No	Prolonged CPB. Died 6 hours postop.
T.F.	66/M	2	Coronary bypass	No	Prolonged CPB. Cerebral damage. Died 3 days postop.
S.L.	53/M	2	Coronary bypass	No	Reoperated on for bleeding, IMA bed.
S.H.	42/M	3	Coronary bypass	No	Reoperated on for bleeding.
S.G.	70/M	2	AVR + ACB	100	Reoperated on for bleeding, puncture hole, brachiocephalic vein. Right hemiparesis, partial recovery.
E.R.	61/M	2	AVR + MVR + TAP	100	Reoperated on for diffuse bleeding. Died after 3 days in myocardial failure.
L.W.	70/M	3	Coronary bypass	50	Confusion for 3 days. Complete recovery.

prised of 20 patients who underwent aortocoronary vein bypass performed by only two surgeons), control patients bled postoperatively 550 ± 338 ml (one patient reoperated for bleeding not included); and prostacyclin-treated patients bled 352 ± 61 ml. This difference is not statistically significant, but the number of patients studied is as yet small. Combined data from all three groups reveal a probably significant difference (p <0.053, Mann-Whitney test) in blood loss between control (630 ± 271 ml) and prostacyclin-treated patients (499 ± 240 ml).

EFFECTS ON PLATELET COUNT AND PLATELET AGGREGABILITY

Infusion of prostacyclin 50 or 100 ng/kg/min significantly improved the preservation of the platelet count during and after CPB (combined data from all groups presented in Fig 34–1). Even when prostacyclin was infused for only the first 30 minutes of bypass, this resulted in preservation of the platelet counts during CPB. It does not reach statistical significance in this group, however, probably because of the small number of experiments. Platelet aggregation induced by ADP or collagen was abolished during CPB by infusion of prostacyclin 100 ng/kg/min. Following termination of the infusion,

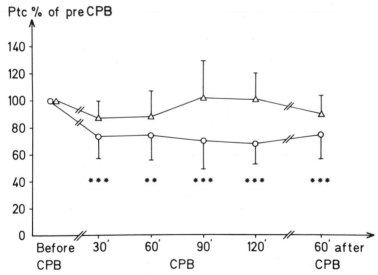

Fig 34–1.—Platelet count in percent of pre-CPB value with corrections for hemo-dilution in all prostacyclin (△) and control patients (○) from groups 1–3. (**, p<0.01; ***, p<0.001.)

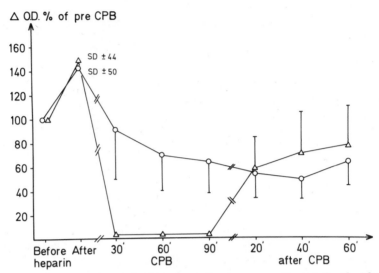

Fig 34–2.—ADP-induced platelet aggregation in seven patients infused with prostacyclin 100 ng/kg/min (△) and in nine control patients from group 2. The maximal extent of aggregation (change in light transmission or optical density) in the sample taken before heparinization was denoted 100%.

aggregability returned, although not to prebypass level. There was a tendency to better ADP-induced aggregation in prostacyclin patients than in control patients following CPB (Fig 34–2).

Effects on Arterial Blood Pressure and Systemic Vascular Resistance

Infusion of prostacyclin 50 or 100 ng/kg/min lowered the aortic mean blood pressure during CPB to sometimes as low as 10 mm Hg, but generally to around 30 mm Hg for the 50-ng dosage and to 20 mm Hg for the 100-ng dosage. When prostacyclin infusion was stopped in group 1 patients (after 30 minutes of bypass), the aortic blood pressure gradually increased to the same level as in the control patients (Fig 34–3A). Interestingly, a similar increase, albeit a little delayed and slightly less pronounced, was observed also in group 3 patients in spite of continued infusion of prostacyclin. The decrease, as well as the subsequent increase, in aortic blood pressure observed in group 1 prostacyclin patients was caused mainly by changes in systemic vascular resistance (SVR calculated as aortic mean pressure in mm Hg divided by pump flow in liters/minute). In group 2 patients

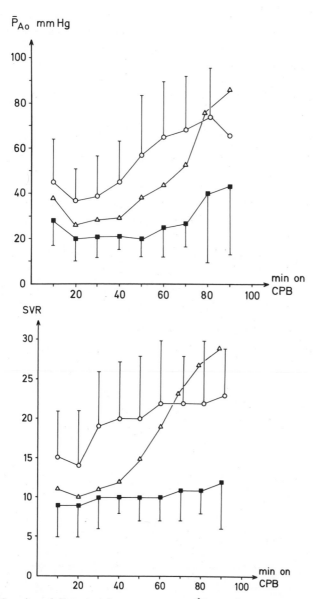

Fig 34–3.—**A** and **B**, arterial mean pressure ($\bar{P}$Ao) and systemic vascular resistance (SVR) in control patients (combined from groups 1 and 2–○), patients infused with prostacyclin 50 ng/kg/min for the first 30 minutes of bypass (group 1–△) or 100 ng/kg/min throughout almost the entire CPB (group 2–■). Data presented as mean and standard deviation. For improved picture clarity, S.D. has been omitted for group 1 prostacyclin patients.

infused with prostacyclin 100 ng/kg/min, the SVR remained low throughout the infusion period (Fig 34–3*B*). The hematocrit was stable at 28% to 30% during CPB. Vasopressors or increased pump flows were not used to counteract the effects of prostacyclin on aortic blood pressure.

EFFECTS ON THE COAGULATION SYSTEM

In group 3 the activated clotting time (Hemochron) after 10 minutes of CPB was over 800 seconds in the prostacyclin patients and 508 ± 117 seconds in the control patients. There was then a gradual decline of the ACT in the prostacyclin patients, so that after two hours of bypass no difference remained. One prostacyclin-treated and five control patients received supplemental heparin injections during CPB. The heparin concentrations remained stable during CPB at an average of 1.8 units/ml in prostacyclin-treated patients, but decreased in control patients from about 3 units/ml to 2.4 units/ml by the end of bypass. No significant change in antithrombin III concentration was observed during CPB. The fibrinopeptide A concentration in plasma was also assessed in these patients and was low (less than 1 ng/ml) throughout bypass. After CPB there was a moderate increase in fibrinopeptide A concentration in both prostacyclin and control patients.

Discussion

It is often proposed that hemostatic disturbances during CPB may result in bleeding or cerebral damage caused by microembolization of platelet aggregates and fibrin. In our opinion, by far the greatest danger is that of embolization. Faulty surgical technique and poor management of the cardiopulmonary bypass could result in embolism of air or of formed particles from, for example, calcified valves. However, even in the best of hands there are instances of postoperative bleeding or cerebral damage that defy simple explanation. These instances are the ones that conceivably could be prevented by the use of reversible platelet inhibition in addition to standard anticoagulant treatment, i.e., heparin, during CPB. Prostacyclin has many of the desirable characteristics of such an inhibitor, since it is potent, rapidly degraded in vivo, and has a shortlived effect on platelets. Our earliest investigations were undertaken to gain experience in the clinical use of prostacyclin during CPB and to provide a baseline for further more controlled and directed investigations, such as have been commenced in our group 3 patients.

It is now quite clear that the use of prostacyclin in adequate dosage results in a significant protection of the platelet count during and after CPB. It is important to note, however, that the relatively high average platelet counts late during bypass in prostacyclin-treated patients may reflect, to a degree, an actual increase in platelet count caused by disaggregation of platelet aggregates or recruitment of new circulating platelets. For this reason it may be preferable to start prostacyclin infusion before CPB is begun. Others have demonstrated in animal experiments[3] and in vitro[1] that prostacyclin may also prevent the platelet release reaction and possibly protect platelet function. Whether or not these beneficial effects will be reflected in a reduced incidence of excessive postoperative bleeding and neurologic damage remains to be proven. The combined data from our investigations now begin to support the assumption that postoperative bleeding is actually reduced by prostacyclin infusion during CPB. However, because of the low frequency of serious bleeding when surgery is properly performed, definitive proof will require the study of a larger number of patients.

The possible prevention of cerebral damage during CPB is perhaps the most important aspect of the use of prostacyclin. Improved reperfusion of the brain following ischemia[10] or prevention of the build-up of thrombi on stenosed vessel segments[11] may be of particular significance. Prevention of the formation of platelet and fibrin microemboli in the bypass circuit may be of importance, particularly when CPB is of long duration. Of potential value in the prevention of brain damage is that prostacyclin permits the safe use of arterial line filters,[2] removing air and formed particles from the bypass circuit.

As used by us, prostacyclin infusion was accompanied by a pronounced arterial hypotension during CPB. Hypotension of such severity is usually avoided because of the potential danger of brain damage. It is surprising and gratifying that in the 35 patients who were exposed to such hypotension in our study, there was only one incident of overt neurologic damage, i.e., hemiparesis in a man operated upon for calcific aortic stenosis.

Prostacyclin was found to have effects apart from those observed on the platelet count and the arterial blood pressure. It also prolonged the activated clotting time early during bypass. The reason for its decreasing effect late during bypass is not known but may involve release into the blood stream during CPB of substances such as biogenic amines. It is possible, however, that a dosage of 50 ng/kg/min is insufficient, since the effect on the systemic vascular resistance also decreased during the late phase of CPB. This phenomenon did not occur with the 100-ng dose.

Prostacyclin made it possible to safely reduce the heparin dose from 3 to 2 mg/kg, as shown by ACT, fibrinopeptide A, and fibrinogen measurements. Also, the heparin level remained constant during CPB in prostacyclin-treated patients, whereas there was a gradual decline in control patients. We do not know whether this is the result of a difference in breakdown and excretion or due to inhibited release of the antiheparin platelet factor 4. It is not our belief that prostacyclin should be used as the only anticoagulant[2, 3] during CPB for cardiac surgery. It is possible, however, that for prolonged extracorporeal circulation, particularly as used in some patients with acute pulmonary insufficiency, a reduced heparin dosage in combination with prostacyclin may be of real advantage.

ACKNOWLEDGMENTS

Prostacyclin for this study was supplied by Upjohn Ltd., Crawley, England.

REFERENCES

1. Addonizio V.P. Jr., Macarak E.J., Nicolau K.G., Edmunds L.H. Jr., Colman R.W.: Effects of prostacyclin and albumin on platelet loss during in vitro simulation of extracorporeal circulation. *Blood* 53:1033, 1979.
2. Longmore D.B., Bennet G., Gueirrara D., Smith M., Bunting S., Moncada S., Reed P., Read N.G., Vane J.E.: Prostacyclin: A solution to some problems of extracorporeal circulation. Experiments in greyhounds. *Lancet* I:1002, 1979.
3. Coppe D., Sobel M., Seamans L., Levine F., Salzman E.: Preservation of platelet function and number by prostacyclin during cardiopulmonary bypass. *J. Thorac. Cardiovasc. Surg.* 81:274, 1981.
4. Rådegran K., Papaconstantinou C.: Prostacyclin infusion during cardiopulmonary bypass in man. *Thromb. Res.* 19:267, 1980.
5. Rådegran K., Egberg N., Papaconstantinou C.: Effects of prostacyclin during cardiopulmonary bypass in man. *Scand. J. Thorac. Cardiovasc. Surg.* Submitted for publication, 1981.
6. Rådegran K., Arén C., Teger-Nilsson A.-C.: Prostacyclin infusion during extracorporeal circulation for coronary bypass surgery. Read at the 61st Annual Meeting of the American Association for Thoracic Surgery (1981) and submitted for publication in *J. Thorac. Cardiovasc. Surg.*
7. Teien A.N., Lie M., Abildgaard U.: Assay of heparin in plasma using a chromogenic substrate. *Thromb. Res.* 8:413, 1976.
8. Ödegård O.R., Lie M., Abildgaard U.: Heparin co-factor activity measured with an amidolytic method. *Thromb. Res.* 6:287, 1975.

9. Nossel H.L., Younger L.R., Willner G.D., Procopez T., Canfield R.E., Butler V.P.: Radioimmunoassay of human fibrinopeptide A. *Proc. Nat. Acad. Sci.* 68:2350, 1971.
10. Hallenbeck J.M., Turlow T.W. Jr.: Prostaglandins influence nutrient perfusion in brain during the postischemic period, in Vane J.R., Bergström S. (eds.): *Prostacyclin.* New York, Raven Press, 1979, pp. 229–310.
11. Aiken J.W., Gorman R.R., Shebuski R.J.: Prostacyclin prevents blockage of partially obstructed coronary arteries, in Vane J.R., Bergström S. (eds.): *Prostacyclin.* New York, Raven Press, 1979, pp. 311–321.

The Use of Prostacyclin in Cardiopulmonary Bypass: Roundtable Discussion*

MODERATOR: O.I. LINET

DR. LINET: During the past two days, several speakers have stressed the need for controlled studies evaluating the effects of prostacyclin and prostaglandin E_1 in various clinical disorders. Controlled studies have been performed with prostacyclin in cardiopulmonary bypass (CPB). The available data concerning the effects of prostacyclin upon CPB in animals are summarized in Table 35–1.

Prostacyclin was infused into the venous line during bypass. In all studies prostacyclin maintained or increased the platelet count during and, where measured, after CPB. Maintenance or improvement of platelet function was observed in all studies where this parameter was analyzed.

No effect on perfusion pressure was observed in lambs,[1] whereas in dogs variable hypotension and low perfusion pressure were observed during prostacyclin infusion.[4, 6]

The results achieved with prostacyclin in human studies are summarized in Table 35–2.

Prostacyclin was usually infused into the venous line both before and during CPB. The dosages used varied greatly, especially in the open-label studies.[7, 8, 10] As in animal experiments, prostacyclin preserved the platelet count and function during and sometimes after the CPB. However, a complete normalization of platelet count and function was not achieved. The clinical significance of these observations is not clear. However, the potential endpoint of reduction in blood loss is clearly important and was observed in one patient[7] and

---

*This chapter is a partial transcript of the discussion, held May 9, 1981, in Chicago, Illinois.

TABLE 35–1.—Effects of Prostaglandin on Cardiopulmonary Bypass in Animals

REFERENCE	COPPE ET AL.[1]	LONGMORE ET AL.[2]	PLACHETKA ET AL.[3]	VAN DEN DUNGEN ET AL.[4]	KOSHAL ET AL.[5]	COPPE ET AL.[6]
Species	Lamb	Dog	Dog	Dog	Dog	Dog
Dose (ng/kg/min)	80	50 and 100	~12	50–100	500	20–80
Maintenance or ↑ platelet count	Yes	Yes	Yes	Yes	Yes	Yes
Maintenance or improvement of platelet function	Yes	Yes	Not reported	Yes	Yes	Yes
Perfusion pressure	No effect	Not reported	Not reported	Variable hypotension	Not reported	Low
Other effects	Not reported	Normal fibrinogen levels, ↓ filter deposits	Not reported	Normal fibrinogen levels, bleeding times	↓ heparin dose; no protamine	Shorter bleeding times

TABLE 35–2.—PROSTACYCLIN IN CARDIOPULMONARY BYPASS IN MAN

STUDY	FABIANI ET AL.[7] (Open)	BUNTING ET AL.[8] Open	BUNTING ET AL.[8] Double-Blind	WALKER ET AL.[9] (Double-Blind)	RÅDEGRAN ET AL.[10] (Open)	LONGMORE ET AL.[11] (Double-Blind)
No. of Pts. (D=Drug, C=Control)	1 D	10 D 10 C	12 D 15 C	21 D 22 C	22 D 7 C	12 D 11 C
Dose (ng/kg/min)	25 and 64	4–64; 8–120	12.5 and 25	10 and 20	2–50	10 and 20
Platelet count preservation	Yes	Yes	Yes	Yes	Yes	Yes
Platelet function preservation	Not reported	Yes	Yes	Yes	Not reported	Yes
Blood loss reduction	Yes	Not reported	NS	NS	Not reported	Yes
Perfusion pressure	→	→	→	Not reported	→	Unchanged
Additional observation in D	Not reported	Not reported	↓ Urine output; ACT prolonged	↓ Filter weight; fibrinogen unchanged	ACT prolonged	ACT prolonged; heparin dose ↓; PT, PTT, fibrinogen unchanged

NS = not significant. ACT = activated clotting time.

in two controlled studies (Longmore et al.[11] and Rådegran, see p. 379). By contrast, reduction in blood loss was not observed in the studies of Bunting et al.[8] or Walker et al.[9] Obviously, more controlled studies with large numbers of patients are needed to verify this important clinical endpoint.

Other changes observed during prostacyclin infusion included decreased urine output in one study,[8] prolongation of activated clotting time (ACT),[8, 10, 11] and decrease in heparin requirement for effective anticoagulation.[11] The possibility of decreasing the required heparin dose was also documented in dogs.[5]

DR. L. KAIJSER (Karolinska Institute, Stockholm, Sweden): We studied the production of prostacyclin in 15 patients undergoing aortic valve replacement who were on CPB and cardioplegia. Patients had no detectable atherosclerotic changes in their coronary arteries and had only moderately increased heart size. Blood was sampled from arterial catheters and the coronary sinus before, during, and for the first 60 minutes after cardioplegia when the patient was taken off CPB. Cardioplegia was induced by the infusion of 1,000 ml of cooled Ringer's solution into the left coronary artery followed by a slow constant infusion of 25 ml/min of diluted blood.

Before cardioplegia the arterial concentration of prostacyclin measured by radioimmunoassay was about 200 ng/L, which is about 10 times the basal level. This was probably due to the release of prostacyclin from the pulmonary circulation by the artificial ventilation. Before cardioplegia no significant arterial-coronary sinus difference was found. Cardioplegia produced progressively increasing release of prostacyclin. At the end of cardioplegia, the arterial coronary sinus difference was minus 100 ng/L.

A pronounced increase in arterial prostacyclin concentration occurred (up to 300 ng/L) when, after the cardioplegic period, the pulmonary circulation of the patient was reperfused and the patient was taken off CPB. Levels returned to precardioplegic concentrations within 30 minutes.

Thus, cardioplegia leads to the production of prostacyclin in the coronary vascular bed. The arterial concentrations of prostacyclin during cardioplegia were of the same magnitude as when we infused prostacyclin intravenously into healthy volunteers in doses of about 12 ng/min/kg of body weight. On the other hand, in Dr. Rådegran's studies about a 4-fold higher infusion rate was needed to induce the beneficial effect of prostacyclin in CPB. Therefore, it could be presumed that addition of prostacyclin into the cardioplegic solution might be beneficial.

DR. RÅDEGRAN: I would like to ask a question of Dr. Salzman. After prostacyclin infusion, we get quite a remarkable prolongation of activated clotting time (ACT). But as time goes on, the ACT decreases to the same values as in control patients, despite the fact that the heparin concentration remains constant.

DR. SALZMAN: This phenomenon might be related to variations in platelet factor 4 (PF4) released by platelets. The prostacyclin effect may begin to wear off during the infusion. This could be followed by an elevation of PF4, which could offset the heparin effect.

DR. LINET: Bunting and Moncada[12] showed that addition of prostacyclin to blood or platelet-rich plasma, both containing heparin, prolonged the kaolin ACT. As I showed previously, the ACT was prolonged after prostacyclin in several studies.[8, 10, 11] In one animal[5] and one clinical study[11] it was possible to decrease the heparin dose during CPB. Since you, Dr. Rådegran, did investigate the possibility of lowering heparin dosage during prostacyclin infusion, would you comment on this?

DR. RÅDEGRAN: I agree with Dr. Salzman that it is not possible to eliminate heparin entirely from CPB, even when prostacyclin is administered concomitantly. However, we were able to decrease the heparin dosage to 2 mg/kg body weight. Even with blood heparin concentration of 1.8 units/ml there was no fibrinogen consumption and no fibrinopeptide A production. So, as far as I can tell from our limited experience, it is safe to use the lowered heparin dose during CPB along with prostacyclin infusion.

DR. LINET: We have in the audience Dr. J. Crow, who is one of the authors of a paper that appeared recently in the *New England Journal of Medicine.*[13] This work showed that it was possible to perform renal hemodialysis completely without heparin when prostacyclin was administered. Since we are dealing here with a type of extracorporeal circulation other than CPB, I think it would be of interest to hear Dr. Crow's comments.

DR. CROW (Burroughs-Wellcome Research Laboratories, Durham, NC): The Wellcome Laboratories sponsored two studies with the objective of substituting heparin for prostacyclin in dialyzing patients with chronic renal failure. The studies were conducted by Drs. Rubin and Zusman (Massachusetts General Hospital) and by Drs. Dunn and Smith (University Hospitals, Cleveland). Each of about 25 patients received two dialyses using a bicarbonate dialysant. Prostacyclin, 4 ng/kg/min, was infused for 10 minutes just prior to the first dialysis, followed by an infusion of 4 ng/kg/min into the arterial line of the dialyzer at the start of dialysis. The dose of prostacyclin during dialysis was adjusted according to the cardiovascular response. During the second dialysis, each patient received standard low-dose heparin as the sole anticoagulant, but no prostacyclin. Patients receiving prostacyclin during dialysis had decrements in BUN and creatinine similar to those on standard heparin dialysis. There were no other effects of prostacyclin on hematologic measurements or blood chemistries. Data from the Cleveland Center suggested that the dialysis with prostacyclin was more efficient in clearing BUN and creatinine than the standard heparin dialysis. Studies are ongoing in patients with acute renal failure with a high risk of bleeding. The objective is to demonstrate a decrease in blood loss when prostacyclin is substituted for heparin in dialyses. Preliminary data are encouraging.

DR. LINET: Dr. Blackstone, can we hear your opinion whether prostacyclin could be of clinical importance in CPB?

DR. BLACKSTONE: I really don't know at present, and that's why we are doing the study. The amount of blood spared, as shown today, i.e., about 150 cc, is perhaps statistically significant, but does not seem to be clinically significant. On the other hand, the studies were being conducted in patients in whom you might say bleeding is not the problem. If PGI_2 were conspicuously effective in sparing blood loss, then, theoretically, upon cessation of cardiopulmonary bypass the wound should be as dry as if a normal operation had been done. I have not yet heard that this has happened: mediastinal tubes are still being used. If one could show that PGI_2 absolutely eliminated postoperative bleeding, even for low-risk operations, that would significantly simplify postoperative management in these patients.

DR. LINET: Dr. Kaye, as you mentioned in your talk, prostacyclin, by virtue of its vasodilatory properties, could possibly be used to prevent the hypertension that occurs in about 14% to 40% of the patients during and after bypass. Would you comment please?

DR. KAYE: Any comments that I might make would be speculative. Prostacyclin is effective and you can control the hypertension very nicely. One consideration here is the fact that in the past we ascribed this hypertension to the increase of the catecholamines associated with bypass. It could well be that this is related more to thromboxane A_2 release, with resultant vasoconstriction. Maybe we are neutralizing this effect with the prostacyclin infusion.

A further word of caution in using prostacyclin as the sole agent during cardiopulmonary bypass: The other panelists have mentioned some of the systemic problems. I think one peculiar to cardiopulmonary bypass is associated with cross-clamping of the aorta. We attempted this on a few occasions, utilizing short cross-clamping times.

Following the arteriotomy we have found clots in one of the coronary vessels. This potential event should rule against the use of prostacyclin without heparin during bypass.

I think it is very difficult to evaluate the possibility of decreasing bleeding because we are dealing with a mixed group of patients. Individuals who have had no previous surgery and are undergoing bypass of a single coronary artery will not experience much bleeding. Therefore it is almost impossible to show any statistical difference in blood loss. In patients who undergo double- or triple-valve corrections or multiple coronary artery operations, we may be able to see a significant difference in blood loss. We have done some studies in this regard and our subjective feeling in complex operations is that the operative field is considerably drier when PGI_2 is used. However, we have been unable to document this with clarity.

REFERENCES

1. Coppe D., Wonders T., Snider M., Salzman E.W.: Preservation of platelet number and function during extracorporeal membrane oxygenation by regional infusion of prostacyclin, in Vane J.R., Bergstrom S. (eds.): *Prostacyclin*. New York, Raven Press, 1979, pp. 371–383.
2. Longmore D.B., Gueirrara D., Bennett G., Smith M.: Prostacyclin: A solution to some problems of extracorporeal circulation: Experiments in greyhounds. *Lancet* I:1002–1005, 1981.
3. Plachetka J.R., Salomon N.W., Larson D.F., Copeland J.G.: Platelet loss during experimental cardiopulmonary bypass and its prevention with prostacyclin. *Ann. Thorac. Surg.* 30(1):58–63, 1980.
4. van den Dungen J.J.A.M., Velders A.J., Karliczek G.F., Homan van der Heide J.N., Wildevuur Ch.R.H.: Platelet preservation during cardiopulmonary bypass (CPB) with prostaglandin (PGE_1) and prostacyclin (PGI_2). *Trans. Am. Soc. Artif. Intern. Organs* XXVI:481–486, 1980.
5. Koshal A., Krausz M., Hechtman H., Collins J., Cohn L.: Prostacyclin (PGI_2) preserves platelet number and function during and after cardiopulmonary bypass (CPB). Abstracts of the 53rd Scientific Sessions, 1980, pp. III-323.
6. Coppe D., Sobel M., Seamans L., Levine F., Salzman E.: Preservation of platelet function and number by prostacyclin during cardiopulmonary bypass. *J. Thorac. Cardiovasc. Surg.* 81:274–278, 1981.
7. Fabiani J.N., Deloche A., Dubost C.: Extracorporeal circulation of autotransfusion: the use of prostacyclin. *La Nouvelle Presse Med.* 9:1961–1962, 1980.
8. Bunting S., O'Grady J., Fabiani J.N., Terrier E., Moncada S., Vane J.R., Dubost Ch.: Cardiopulmonary bypass in man: effects of prostacyclin. Presented during Symposium, Clinical Pharmacology of Prostacyclin. London, UK, August 11, 1980.
9. Walker I.D., Davidson J.F., Faichney A., Wheatley D., Davidson K.: Prostacyclin in cardiopulmonary bypass surgery. Presented during Sympo-

sium, Clinical Pharmacology of Prostacyclin. London, UK, August 11, 1980.
10. Rådegran K., Papaconstantinou C.: Prostacyclin infusion during cardiopulmonary bypass in man. *Thromb. Res.* 19:267–270, 1980.
11. Longmore D.B., Hoyle P.M., Gregory A., Bennett J.G., Smith M.A., Osivand T., Jones W.A.: Prostacyclin administration during cardiopulmonary bypass in man. *Lancet* I:800–803, 1981.
12. Bunting S., Moncada S.: Prostacyclin, by preventing platelet activation, prolongs activated clotting time in blood and platelet rich plasma and potentiates the anticoagulant effect of heparin. *Br. J. Pharmacol.* 69(2):268P–269P, 1980.
13. Zusman R.M., Rubin R.H., Cato A.E., Cocchetto D.M., Crow J.W., Tolkoff-Rubin N.: Hemodialysis using prostacyclin instead of heparin as the sole antithrombotic agent. *N. Engl. J. Med.* 304:934–939, 1981.

Index

A

Acetylcholine, 185
Acetylsalicylic acid (*see* Aspirin)
Acrocyanosis, 191
Acrylates, 346
Actomyosin, 26
Adenosine
    diphosphate, 4, 57
        threshold aggregating
            concentrations of, 62
    monophosphate, cyclic, 4, 21, 57
        levels, platelet, and TMB, 26
Adenylate cyclase, 21, 64, 177
ADP, 4, 57
    threshold aggregating concentrations
        of, 62
Agglutinins: cold, 192
Airway response (in monkey), 246
    to *Ascaris serum* antigen, 246
    to BW755C, 249
    to ETYA, 249
    to ionophore, 248–249
    to prostaglandin
        E_1, 246
        F_{2a}, 246
    to slow reacting substance, 248
Albumin: effect on prostacyclin stability,
    43–45
Aldosterone, plasma
    during pregnancy, 327, 328
    prostacyclin effects on, 145, 236
Almitrine, 186
Amaurosis fugax, 169
AMP (*see* Adenosine, monophosphate)
Amputation: for peripheral vascular
    disease, 175
Anaphylatoxins, 360
Anaphylaxis, slow reacting substance of,
    360
    airway response to (in monkey), 248
Ancrod: in Raynaud's syndrome, 194
Angina pectoris, 18, 145
    prostacyclin in, 146
    stable, 273
        (*See also* Coronary, prostacyclin and
        thromboxane levels)
    supply and demand forms of, 296

Angina pectoris, unstable, 295–309
    (*See also* Coronary, prostacyclin and
        thromboxane levels)
    pharmacologic approaches, 299–301
    prostaglandin in, 297–299
    prostaglandin E_1 in, 301–305
        angiographic effects of (in dog), 301,
            302
        clinical efficacy of, 304
        hemodynamic effects of, 301, 303
Angiography
    effects of prostaglandin E_1 in angina
        on (in dog), 301, 302
    thromboembolic complications of, 346
Angiotensin
    I, 184–185
    II, 135
        effects of prostacyclin on, 145, 236
        prostanoid release and,
            antiaggregatory, 184–185
    sensitivity, during pregnancy, 332
Anticoagulant: lupus, 321
Antigen: *Ascaris serum,* airway
    responses to (in monkey), 246
Anti-inflammatory drugs: nonsteroidal,
    16, 50–51
Antimycin, 4–5
Antiplatelet effects: of prostacyclin
    infusion, 143–144
Anti-thrombin III, 311
Antithrombotic activity: vascular
    endothelium in, 316
α_1-Antitrypsin, 359
Aortocoronary vein bypass, 383
Aortoiliac disease, 164, 165–166
    symptoms of, 171
Aprostadil (*see* Prostaglandin, E_1)
Aprotinin: during cardiopulmonary
    bypass, 363
Apyrase, 4, 5–6
    effect on clot retraction, 61
Arachidonate, 1, 2, 3
Arachidonic acid, 3, 6, 15, 50
    in angina, 298–299
    15-hydroxyperoxy, 7
    metabolism, 85

399